Walter Hofmann, Johannes Aufenanger, Georg Hoffmann (Eds.)
Laboratory Diagnostic Pathways

Walter Hofmann, Johannes Aufenanger,
Georg Hoffmann (Eds.)

Laboratory Diagnostic Pathways

Clinical Manual of Screening Methods
and Stepwise Diagnosis

Translated by Matthew Schlecht

2nd updated and expanded edition

DE GRUYTER

Editors

Prof. Dr. med. Dipl. Chem. Walter Hofmann
Department für Klinische Chemie
Medizet des Städt. Klinikums München GmbH
Kölner Platz 1, 80804 München
walter.hofmann@klinikum-muenchen.de

Prof. Dr. med. Georg Hoffmann
Verlag Trillium GmbH
Hauptstr. 12b
82284 Grafrath
ghoffmann@trillium.de

Prof. Dr. med. Johannes Aufenanger
Klinikum Ingolstadt GmbH
Institut für Laboratoriumsmedizin
Krumenauerstr. 25
85049 Ingolstadt
johannes.aufenanger@klinikum-ingolstadt.de

Translated by
Matthew Schlecht, PhD
Word Alchemy
Newark, DE, USA

This book contains 87 Figures and 50 Tables.

ISBN 978-3-11-045367-6
e-ISBN (PDF) 978-3-11-045508-3
e-ISBN (ePUB) 978-3-11-045389-8

Library of Congress Cataloging in Publication data
A CIP catalog record for this book is available from the
Library of Congress.

German National Library Bibliographic Information
The German National Library has registered this publication in the German National Bibliography; detailed
bibliographic information can be accessed via the
internet at: http://dnb.dnb.de

The publisher has taken great pains with authors and
editors to ensure that the reproduction of all the information contained in this book (programs, methods,
quantities, dosages, applications, etc.) is reprinted
exactly to reflect the state of knowledge at the time this
work was completed.
Despite careful manuscript preparation and sentence
correction, errors cannot be completely ruled out. The
authors, editors and publisher consequently assume
no responsibility and no consequential or other liability
arising in any way from use of the information contained in the work or portions thereof.

The reproduction of common names, trade names,
trademarks and the like in this book does not warrant the assumption that such names can be used by
anyone without restriction. Rather, these are frequently
legally protected, registered trademarks, even if they
are not specifically identified as such.

© 2016 by Walter de Gruyter GmbH, Berlin/Boston
Cover art: dina2001/iStock/thinkstock
Image editing: Andreas Hoffmann, Berlin
Satz: LVD GmbH, Berlin
Printing and binding: CPI books GmbH, Leck
♾ Printed on acid-free paper
Printed in Germany

www.degruyter.com

Preface to the 2nd Edition

The "Handbook of Clinical Laboratory Diagnostic Pathways" appeared in July 2012 after several years of preparation under the auspices of the German Society for Clinical Chemistry and Laboratory Medicine (DGKL), and was sold out four months later. A second printing in early 2013 was also soon sold out. An e-book version with unlimited availability has already made the work accessible to a broader group of users on hospital intranets.

Such remarkable success is unusual for a textbook of laboratory diagnostics, and surprised both the publisher and the editors. The book appears to have arrived at exactly the right time, and obviously satisfies the rapidly growing demand for practical instructions in the creation of diagnostic pathways within the German Diagnosis Related Groups (DRG) fee-per-case system (see Preface to the first edition on page vi). Shortly before this second edition went to press, the German Association of Statutory Health Insurance Doctors (KBV) Center of Excellence Laboratory introduced a compendium containing information on the ordering and billing of laboratory services, in which a chapter was devoted to the role of the medical laboratory in stepwise diagnostics. This was unmistakably inspired by ideas from the present book, and has our full support: "In the course of a medically and scientifically meaningful stepwise diagnosis, a first step employs sensitive exploratory or screening procedures as the basis for the diagnosis. The findings from these procedures can then inform the selection of suitable (i.e., more specific; author's note) examination methods for subsequent use in the diagnostic process."

The Handbook was also well received in Germany's neighboring countries; in the meantime, a working group has been established under the auspices of the editors with representatives of professional associations from Austria, Switzerland and Liechtenstein, and we hope for representation from additional nations in the future. Some colleagues from this working group, however, have also pointed to the risk of misuse of diagnostic paths for purely economic purposes – for example, by medical cost controllers or utilization analysts. It is emphasized throughout this book that the decision trees presented are in no way binding; in particular, no inference regarding reimbursement should be drawn from the absence of a laboratory parameter in a path diagram.

Prof. Karl Lackner, longtime President of DGKL, concluded his review of the first edition with these words: "In our fast-paced times, it would behoove the authors to update this book on a regular basis so that its relevance will be preserved in the future." We heeded this call sooner than expected, and have gladly accepted the challenge; within only a few months' time, we contacted the nearly 30 authors to organize the updating of their chapters.

The main focus was on reviewing and updating the cited guidelines as well as elimination of the errors and inconsistencies that are inevitable in a first edition. The new material added includes subchapters on screening and stepwise diagnosis in the "Diagnostic Strategies" section, as well as a chapter on ejaculate testing with the current German Medical Association Quality Assurance Directive (RiliBÄK 2011). Also noteworthy is the updated chapters on diseases of the thyroid, liver and pancreas.

We thank everyone involved for their tremendous dedication, and also the readers and reviewers of the first edition who offered their suggestions for improvement.

Munich, Ingolstadt,
Grafrath, August 2013

Walter Hofmann
Johannes Aufenanger
Georg Hoffmann

Preface to the 1st Edition

With a timely recognition of the impending pressures of economic change, some German hospitals began to increase their competitiveness starting in the year 2000 by adopting management practices from the private sector. These models and methods originally arose in the anglophone countries, where they had been in use since the 1990s and were known as "clinical pathways" for optimizing and managing business processes in clinical practice. The considerable delay in the introduction of the clinical pathway concept in Germany was mainly due to the relatively late introduction of the fee-per-case system (diagnosis-related groups, DRGs) in 2003 and 2004 – some twenty years later than in the US and Canada, and more than ten years after the United Kingdom.

Amidst the turbulent and growing needs for practical guidance in creating and implementing such pathways, the present book sought to address this demand. The timing couldn't be better, in our opinion, because after a time lag of a few years now in Germany, recognition of the requirement for standardized remuneration according to standardized processes has come quite rapidly into focus, as has been the case everywhere else the DRGs have been introduced. When clinical treatment courses are reinvented day to day, or are left to the gut feelings of individuals, costs quickly run out of control.

This handbook focuses on a hitherto neglected aspect of clinical pathways: optimization of the diagnostic processes. Although this idea seems obvious, the "treatment pathways" concept stands in the foreground in most of the previously published textbooks because the treatments cost significantly more than the diagnoses, at least at first glance. On closer inspection, however, the optimization of the diagnostic processes warrants at least as high a medical and economic priority, because the correct diagnosis must precede every course of treatment. Beginning with an incorrect or ineffective diagnosis invariably increases the required time and costs of all the subsequent clinical processes. IT-based diagnostic pathways furnish correct diagnoses at the earliest possible juncture, do not overlook any important tests, and avoid unnecessary requirements.

The clinical laboratory assumes a key role at this early stage because it provides large quantities of information quickly and inexpensively without burdening the patients and staff too much. In addition, the ordering of laboratory tests via modern hospital and laboratory information systems (HIS and LIS) is increasingly paperless and rule-based, which considerably facilitates daily work in the wards. After reading this book, readers should be able to develop and implement diagnostic pathways themselves, without having to reinvent the wheel. Nevertheless, it should be recalled in prospect that the exemplified pathways featured here represent only a small part of the larger spectrum of laboratory diagnostics, and a limit will be reached when confronted with a complex problem. Thus, there will likely to be no shortage of material for a next edition. Contributions in other interesting specialist areas, such as hematology, immunology or neurology, are already in preparation.

The authors of this book are members of the DGKL* interdisciplinary working group, which has been concerned with diagnostic pathways since 2005. We take this opportunity to thank this specialist organization, all of the authors, and the publisher, Walter de Gruyter, for their helpful cooperation.

Munich, Ingolstadt,   *Walter Hofmann*
Grafrath, October 2011   *Johannes Aufenanger*
                                Georg Hoffmann

* German Society for Clinical Chemistry and Laboratory Medicine, www.dgkl.de

Contents

List of Authors IX

I General Information

1	Introduction	3
1.1	**Definitions**	3
1.1.1	Legal Rulings	5
1.2	**Historical Development**	5
1.3	**Diagnostic Strategies**	7
1.3.1	Stepwise Diagnosis or Profile Diagnosis	10
1.3.2	Diagnostic Quality Criteria	12
1.3.3	Stepwise Diagnosis during Screening of Clinically Unremarkable Persons...	14
1.4	**Outlook**	15

2	Implementation...............................	17
2.1	**Organizational Requirements in the Hospital**	17
2.2	**Economic Impacts**	19
2.3	**Implementation of Information Technology**	21

II Specialist Section

3	Practical Examples for Screening Examinations	27
3.1	**Internist Admissions Screening**	27
3.2	**Acute Poisoning**	38
3.2.1	Acute Drug Intoxication....................	39
3.2.1.1	Forms and Origins of Acute Drug Intoxication.....................................	39
3.2.2	Toxidromes	41
3.2.2.1	Anticholinergic Toxidrome...............	41
3.2.2.2	Cholinergic Toxidrome	41
3.2.2.3	Hallucinogenic Toxidrome	44
3.2.2.4	Opiate/Opioid Toxidrome.................	44
3.2.2.5	Sedative/Hypnotic Toxidrome	44
3.2.2.6	Sympathomimetic Toxidrome	47
3.2.3	Acute Poisoning of Unknown Origin ..	47
3.2.3.1	Forms and Origins of Acute Poisoning of Unknown Origin	47
3.2.3.2	Decision Tree for Acute Poisoning of Unknown Origin	47
3.3	**Extravascular Fluids**	52
3.3.1	Cerebrospinal Fluid Fistula Diagnostics	52

3.3.2	Peritoneal Dialysis Diagnostics	53
3.3.3	Chyle Diagnostics	55
3.3.4	Urine Leakage Diagnostics	55
3.3.5	Effusion Diagnostics	56
3.3.5.1	Ascites...	56
3.3.5.2	Pleural Effusion	57
3.3.5.3	Pericardial Effusion..........................	58

4	Practical Examples of Targeted Stepwise Diagnosis	61
4.1	**Endocrinology**	61
4.1.1	Thyroid Gland..................................	61
4.1.1.1	Hyperthyroidism...............................	61
4.1.1.2	Hypothyroidism................................	62
4.1.1.3	Pre- and Post-analytical Principles....	62
4.1.1.4	Laboratory Analysis	62
4.1.2	Adrenal Glands................................	67
4.1.2.1	Cushing Syndrome	67
4.1.2.2	Clarification of Cushing Syndrome	74
4.1.2.3	Hypocortisolism...............................	75
4.2	**Diabetes and Metabolism**	83
4.2.1	Diabetes Mellitus	83
4.2.1.1	Diagnosis and Risk Assessment	83
4.2.1.2	Gestational Diabetes Mellitus (GDM)	86
4.2.1.3	Monitoring Diabetes Mellitus	90
4.2.2	Lipid and Lipoprotein Metabolism	93
4.2.2.1	Assessment of Cardiovascular Risk...	93
4.2.2.2	Differential Diagnosis of Lipid Metabolism Disorders......................	97
4.2.3	Porphyrias	99
4.2.3.1	Neurovisceral Attacks	99
4.2.3.2	Photodermatoses	104
4.3	**Liver and Pancreatic Disorders**	107
4.3.1	Hepatobiliary Disorders	107
4.3.1.1	Non-Alcoholic Fatty Liver Disease (NAFLD)..	111
4.3.1.2	Acute Viral Hepatitis	111
4.3.1.3	Jaundice...	115
4.3.2	Pancreatic Diseases.........................	119
4.3.2.1	Acute Pancreatitis............................	119
4.3.2.2	Chronic Pancreatitis	123
4.4	**Kidneys and Efferent Urinary Tract** ...	128
4.4.1	Ruling Out Disorders of the Kidneys and Efferent Urinary Tract................	129
4.4.1.1	Medical History and Clinical Picture..	129
4.4.1.2	Pre- and Post-analytical Principles of Laboratory Diagnost ics	129
4.4.1.3	Basic Diagnostics	130
4.4.1.4	Analysis...	131

4.4.2 Stepwise Diagnostics of the
Glomerular Filtration Rate 132
4.4.2.1 Stages of Chronic Renal failure 132
4.4.2.2 Analysis and Calculation of the
Glomerular Filtration Rate 132
4.4.3 Stepwise Diagnostics of Proteinuria .. 135
4.4.3.1 Forms of Proteinuria 135
4.4.3.2 Decision Tree for Proteinuria 135
4.4.3.3 Quantification of Proteinuria 135
4.4.3.4 Further Diagnostics.......................... 137
4.4.3.5 Biomarkers and Proteomics.............. 139
4.4.4 Stepwise Diagnostics of Hematuria ... 139
4.4.4.1 Decision Tree for Hematuria 139
4.4.5 Stepwise Diagnostics of Leukocyturia 141
4.4.5.1 Decision Tree for Leukocyturia.......... 141
4.4.5.2 Further Diagnostics.......................... 143
4.4.5.3 Tubulointerstitial Kidney Disorders ... 144
4.4.6 Implementation of the Diagnostic
Pathways in a Hospital and
Laboratory Information System
(HIS, LIS)....................................... 144

4.5 **Hematology – Introduction and
Overview** 148
4.5.1 General Hematology 148
4.5.1.1 Erythropoiesis 148
4.5.1.2 Megakariopoiesis – Thrombopoiesis 148
4.5.1.3 Leukopoiesis – Generation of
Myeloid Cell Lines........................... 149
4.5.1.4 Lymphopoiesis 149
4.5.1.5 Hematopoiesis Disorders 149
4.5.2 Specialized Hematology –
Pathologies, Disorders, Diagnosis,
Differentiation 150
4.5.2.1 Anemia 150
4.5.2.2 Eosinophilia................................... 150
4.5.2.3 Hemolysis 151
4.5.2.4 Monoclonal Gammopathy 158
4.5.2.5 Leukocytosis 158
4.5.2.6 Lymphocytosis 161
4.5.2.7 Neutropenia 162
4.5.2.8 Pancytopenia 163
4.5.2.9 Polycythemia 163

4.6 **Coagulation disorders** 168
4.6.1 Diagnostic Pathways for Coagulation
disorders 168
4.6.1.1 Isolated aPTT Prolongation.............. 168
4.6.1.2 Isolated Quick Time Reduction 168
4.6.1.3 Bleeding Diathesis 171
4.6.1.4 Acute Venous Thromboembolism...... 172
4.6.1.5 Heparin-induced Thrombocytopenia
(Type 2 HIT) 173
4.6.1.6 Thrombophilia................................ 173

4.7 **Neurological Disorders** 186
4.7.1 Neurological Laboratory Diagnostics . 186

4.7.1.1 Characteristics of Neurological
Laboratory Diagnostics 186
4.7.1.2 Cerebrospinal Fluid Diagnostic
Parameters 186
4.7.1.3 Pre-analytics in Cerebrospinal Fluid
Diagnostics.................................... 186
4.7.2 Diagnostic Pathways and Procedures 187
4.7.2.1 Clinical Spectrum and Underlying
Guidelines from Clinical Professional
Associations 187
4.7.2.2 Acute Meningitis 187
4.7.2.3 Opportunistic CNS Infections 189
4.7.2.4 Suspected SAH/Bloody Cerebrospinal Fluid 190
4.7.2.5 Radicular Syndromes....................... 190
4.7.2.6 Meningeal carcinomatosis 192
4.7.2.7 Chronic Inflammatory CNS Disorders 194
4.7.2.8 Inflammatory Cerebrospinal Fluid
Syndrome of Unknown Origin........... 199
4.7.2.9 Dementia Syndromes....................... 199
4.7.2.10 Wilson's disease 200
4.7.3 Authors and Working Group 201
4.7.3.1 Spokesperson for the Working Group 201
4.7.3.2 Members of the Working Group 201
4.7.3.3 Objective of the Neurology Working
Group 201

4.8 **Autoimmune disorders** 201
4.8.1 Rheumatoid Arthritis Diagnostics 201
4.8.1.1 Diagnostic Scheme 202
4.8.1.2 Additional Reflections on Differential
Diagnosis....................................... 202
4.8.2 Systemic Lupus Erythematosus 203
4.8.2.1 Laboratory Diagnostics 204
4.8.2.2 Reflections on Differential Diagnosis 204

4.9 **Allergy Diagnostics – Diagnostic
Pathways** 204
4.9.1 Food Allergy Diagnostics.................. 204
4.9.2 Inhalation Allergy Diagnostics 208
4.9.3 Insect Venom Allergy Diagnostics 208
4.9.4 Drug Allergy Diagnostics 208

4.10 **Ejaculate Analysis and Quality
Assurance in Male Fertility
Laboratories** 210
4.10.1 Introduction 210
4.10.2 Pre-analytics and Macroscopic
Physical Examination of Ejaculate..... 210
4.10.3 Microscopic Examination of Ejaculate 212
4.10.4 Further Biochemical Testing of
Ejaculate....................................... 215
4.10.5 Quality Assurance in Ejaculate
Analysis.. 215

Index 221

List of authors

Prof. Dr. med. Dipl.-Biol. Johannes Aufenanger
Klinikum Ingolstadt GmbH
Institut für Laboratoriumsmedizin
Krumenauerstr. 25, 85049 Ingolstadt
E-Mail:
johannes.aufenanger@klinikum-ingolstadt.de

(Chapters 1.3, 2.2, 3.1)

Prof. Dr. med. Dr. troph. Dr. h.c. Max G. Bachem †

(Chapter 4.3)

Dipl. Chem. Dörte Brödje
Philipps-Universität Marburg
Klinische Chemie und Molekuläre Diagnostik
Baldingerstraße, 35043 Marburg
E-Mail: broedje@med.uni-marburg.de

(Chapter 4.8)

Dr. rer. nat. Fritz Degel
Klinikum Nürnberg
Institut für Klinische Chemie
Prof.-Ernst-Nathan-Straße 1, 90419 Nürnberg
E-Mail: degel@Klinikum-nuernberg.de
(Chapter 3.2)

Dr. med. Dr. rer. nat. Herbert Desel
GIZ Giftinformationszentrale Nord
Universitätsmedizin Göttingen
Robert-Koch-Str. 40, 37075 Göttingen
E-Mail: hdesel@med.uni-goettingen.de

(Chapter 3.2)

Prof. emeritus Dr. med. Jochen H.H. Ehrich
Pädiatrische Nieren-, Leber- und Stoffwechseler-
krankungen,
Medizinische Hochschule, Hannover
Carl-Neuberg-Straße 1, 30625 Hannover
E-Mail: ehrich.jochen@mh-hannover.de

(Chapter 4.4)

Dr. med. Norbert Felgenhauer
Klinikum rechts der Isar
TU München
Ismaninger Straße 22, 81675 München
E-Mail: n.felgenhauer@lrz.tu-muenchen.de

(Chapter 3.2)

Prof. Dr. med. Walter G. Guder
Marianne-Plehn-Str. 4
81825 München
E-Mail: walter.guder@extern.lrz-muenchen.de

(Chapters 1.2, 1.3, 4.4)

Dr. rer. nat. Jürgen Hallbach
Städtisches Klinikum München GmbH
Department Klinische Chemie
Kölner Platz 1, 80804 München
E-Mail: juergen.hallbach@klinikum-muenchen.de

(Chapter 3.2)

Prof. Dr. med. Georg Hoffmann
Verlag Trillium GmbH
Hauptstr. 12b, 82284 Grafrath
E-Mail: ghoffmann@trillium.de

(Chapters 1, 1.3, 2.1, 2.2, 2.3)

Oliver Hofmann
L.L.M., Rechtsanwalt
Jägerstr. 7a, 82008 Unterhaching
E-Mail: oliverhofmann86@googlemail.com

(Chapter 1.1)

Prof. Dr. med. Dipl. Chem. Walter Hofmann
Department für Klinische Chemie
Medizet des Städt. Klinikums München GmbH
Kölner Platz 1, 80804 München
E-Mail: walter.hofmann@klinikum-muenchen.de

(Chapters 1.1, 2.1, 4.4)

Priv.-Doz. Dr. med. Matthias Imöhl
Labordiagnostisches Zentrum (LDZ)
Universitätsklinikum Aachen
Pauwelsstraße 30, 52074 Aachen
E-Mail: mimoehl@ukaachen.de

(Chapter 4.1)

Prof. i.R. Dr. med. Frieder Keller
Nephrologie, Innere Medizin 1,
Universitätsklinikum Ulm
Albert-Einstein-Allee 23, 89070 Ulm
E-Mail: frieder.keller@uniklinik-ulm.de

(Chapter 4.4)

Prof. Dr. med. Elisabeth Minder
Zentrallabor
Stadtspital Triemli
Birmensdorferstraße 497, 8063 Zürich
Schweiz
E-Mail: Elisabeth.Minder@triemli.zuerich.ch

(Chapter 4.2)

Dr. med. Julia Poland
KABEG Klinikum Klagenfurt am Wörthersee
Institut für Labordiagnostik und Mikrobiologie
Feschnigstraße 11, 9020 Klagenfurt
Österreich
E-Mail: julia.poland@kabeg.at

(Chapter 4.5)

Prof. Dr. med. Harald Renz
Universitätsklinikum Giessen/Marburg
Klinische Chemie und Molekuläre Diagnostik
Baldingerstr. 1, 35043 Marburg
E-Mail: renzh@med.uni-marburg.de

(Chapters 4.8 and 4.9)

Priv.-Doz. Dr. med. Christian Martin Schambeck
Hämostasikum München
Haderunstr. 10 , 81375 München
E-Mail: christian.schambeck@haemostasikum.de

(Chapter 4.6)

Prof. Dr. med. Jürgen Scherberich
Internistische Praxis KfN
Seybothstr. 65
81545 München
E-Mail: j.scherberich@web.de

(Chapter 4.4)

Prof. Dr. med. Thomas Seufferlein
Zentrum für Innere Medizin
Klinik für Innere Medizin I
Universitätsklinikum Ulm
Albert-Einstein-Allee 23D-89070 Ulm
E-Mail: thomas.seufferlein@uniklinik-ulm.de

(Chapter 4.3)

Prof. Dr. med. Marco Siech
Chirurgische Klinik I
Ostalb-Klinikum Aalen
Im Kälblesrain 1, 73430 Aalen
E-Mail: chirurgie1.sekretariat@ostalb-klinikum.de

(Chapter 4.3)

Prof. Dr. med. Dr. rer. nat. Pranav Sinha †

(Chapter 4.5)

Prof. Dr. med. Axel Stachon
Westpfalz-Klinikum GmbH
Institut für Laboratoriumsmedizin
Hellmut-Hartert-Str. 1, 67655 Kaiserslautern
E-Mail: astachon@westpfalz-klinikum.de

(Chapter 4.1)

Prof. Dr. med. Arnold von Eckardstein
Universitätsspital Zürich
Institut für Klinische Chemie
Raemistraße 100, 8091 Zürich
Schweiz
E-Mail: arnold.voneckardstein@usz.ch

(Chapter 4.2)

Dr. med. Manfred Wolfgang Wick
LMU-Klinikum der Universität München
Institut für Klinische Chemie
Marchioninistr. 15, 81377 München
E-Mail: Manfred.Wick@med.uni-muenchen.de

(Chapter 4.7)

Priv.-Doz. Dr. med. Eray Yagmur
Labordiagnostisches Zentrum (LDZ)
Universitätsklinikum RWTH-Aachen
Pauwelsstr. 30, 52074 Aachen
MVZ Dr. Stein+Kollegen
Wallstr. 10, 41061 Mönchengladbach
E-Mail: eyagmur@ukaachen.de,
eyagmur@labor-stein.de

(Chapters 3.3, 4.9, 4.10)

Interdisciplinary Neurology Working Group

(see Chapter 4.7)

- Dr. med. Manfred Wolfgang Wick, Klinische Chemie, LMU München
- Dr. Hans Jürgen Kühn, Klinische Chemie, Uni Ulm
- Prof. Dr. Markus Otto, Klinische Chemie, Uni Ulm
- Dr. Dr. Manfred Uhr, MPI für Psychiatrie, München
- PD Dr. Hela-Felicitas Petereit, Neurologie, Heilig-Geist-Krankenhaus, Köln
- Prof. Brigitte Wildemann, Neurologie, Uni Heidelberg
- Prof. Dr. Hayrettin Tumani, Neurologie, Uni Ulm

(Chapter 4.7)

I: General Information

1 Introduction

Georg Hoffmann

Diagnosis and therapy are the two cornerstones of all the medical activity in a hospital. By definition, these two concepts are clearly distinguished as the "identification" and "treatment" of diseases. Certainly, if one considers the underlying clinical processes, they cannot always be strictly separated from each other: diagnostic procedures can be quite therapeutic in character – for example, the excision of a tumor during a colonoscopy – and conversely, diagnoses can sometimes only be confirmed once a therapeutic approach has either succeeded or failed. By and large, it has always been considered axiomatic in the field of medicine that, "it is ordained that diagnosis comes before therapy". Diagnosis provides the framework for a targeted selection among treatment options; expressed differently, efficient treatment is impossible without a targeted diagnosis.

Accordingly, on both didactic and organizational grounds, it makes sense to divide the overall concept of clinical pathways into diagnostic and therapeutic pathways. On the other hand, one should not speak of "clinical treatment pathways" to mean clinical pathways, especially in the clinical setting, since this would suggest that diagnosis is a subset of treatment. The concept of "clinical pathways" originated in the anglophone countries, where the more appropriate term "Clinical Care Pathway" is known, but uncommon.

In recent years, the term "diagnostic pathway" has received considerable public attention as an independent management concept; Google gave approximately 30,000 entries for "diagnostische Pfade" on German websites in early 2013, in which the top rankings were devoted to the activities of

Clinical Pathways	
Diagnostic Pathways (diagnosis pathways)	Therapeutic Pathways (treatment pathways)

Figure 1.1 Clinical pathways are divided into diagnostic pathways and therapeutic pathways. The terms "diagnosis pathway" or "treatment pathway" can be used interchangeably.

the DGKL society, which gave rise to this book. In 2009, the first decision trees were published by one of the present authors in a laboratory diagnostic textbook (Renz, 2009), in the form shown in the cover art. The response to this compact representation was so positive that the publisher approached the editors with a request to create a monograph on laboratory diagnostics based on decision trees. In such a work, the graphics would be systematized so as to serve as a rapid guide for doctors in clinical practice, and so their software implementation should be as simple as possible.

The book is divided into two parts, general and specialized. The first part includes theoretical foundations and practical implementation proposals, while the second contains typical examples of screening tests in the case of an unknown diagnosis, and of the targeted stepwise diagnosis to be employed when a particular disease is suspected.

Walter Hofmann, Oliver Hofmann

1.1 Definitions

Diagnostic pathways – as a subset of clinical pathways – first appeared in the medical literature only in the 1990s. Thus, at present, there is still some overlap with established terms such as diagnostic recommendations, guidelines, or directives. This can lead to significant misunderstandings; while the terms appear to have the same meaning, they actually do not.

Figuratively speaking, the diagnostic pathways in treatment procedures are analogous to using a navigator device while driving a car: They are based on guidelines and directives (corresponding to a road map) – without which they would not lead to the destination (i.e., the diagnosis). It isn't absolutely necessary to follow the guidance from the navigator device, but it behooves one to do so. When justified, however, departure from the guidance can be necessary or could even save lifes. One more analogy: **Theoretically, you can create pathways on paper like a road map, but** only by conversion into computer format do they become part of a useful, case-specific tool for everyday use.

For diagnostic pathways, the counterpart to road plans are the various directives, guidelines and recommendations, for which the relative levels of medical and legal liability can be summarized as follows.

> Directives must be followed, guidelines should be followed, and recommendations can be followed.

Often, diagnostics are given short shrift in guidelines and directives, or they are far from state of the art. In such a case, a diagnostic pathway is needed to close the gap, in which a consensus – evidence-based to the extent possible – is sought between the affected departments. This is the approach that has been followed in this book: For each of the pathways published here, an interdisciplinary working group has been established, consisting of clinicians and laboratory diagnosticians, and their recommendations are developed by consensus.

The most important technical terms are defined below as they shall be understood within the context of this book (German Medical Association, 1996 and 2006; Hart, 2000; Eckardt, 2006).

Directives are regulations that are binding on actions or omissions to which a legally authorized institution has agreed upon, set down in written form and published. Failure to comply therewith triggers defined sanctions, especially relating to social law and laws relating to professions. The best-known directive on laboratory diagnostics in Germany is the one of the German Medical Association (RiliBÄK), which governs the implementation of quality management.

Guidelines are systematically developed decision-making aids for specific cases of appropriate medical procedures. They are scientifically based, but are not binding. Rather, they represent practical "leeways for decisions and measures", from which one can or even must deviate in certain justified cases.

The Working Group of the Association of German Scientific Medical Societies (AWMF) was established in 1992 as the institution for creating medical guidelines. It has already posted more than 1,000 guidelines at its web site (www.awmf.org/leitlinien/leitlinien.html), which are divided into the categories S1 to S3:

- S1: Treatment recommendations from experts
- S2k: Consensus-based guidelines
- S2e: Evidence-based guidelines
- S3: Evidence- and consensus-based guidelines

The AWMF strives to ensure that its guidelines reflect the current state of scientific knowledge, which cannot always be guaranteed given the huge number of guidelines and rapid medical progress. Nevertheless, the AWMF guidelines guarantee greater quality and safety in medicine, and also take economic factors into consideration.

Recommendations and comments are intended to draw the attention of the medical profession and the general public to issues that are noteworthy or require modification.

A **memorandum** containing comprehensive information and explanation serves this purpose; its content will reflect the current state of knowledge, and possibly also outdated knowledge that is of use to physician in formulating opinions.

Clinical Pathway: A clinical pathway, by way of contrast, is a framework for the interdisciplinary description and control of all medical services during a hospital stay. Here, the individual steps must therefore not only be scientifically justified, but responsibility also assigned specifically to certain groups of people, such as physicians or nursing staff, and arranged in proper chronological order (German Medical Association, 2006). The Joint Commission on Accreditation of Healthcare Organizations explicitly states, "... that a clinical pathway can never replace the professional judgment of the respective qualified specialist for an individual situation ...". Currently, the scope of applicability for many clinical pathways extends to pre- and post-inpatient services and rehabilitation; these are then referred to as integrated pathways (Eckardt, 2006).

Diagnostic Pathway: A diagnostic pathway describes the entire process from the initial question, from the medical or organizational perspective, through to the findings. It consists of test indications (WHAT) for defined questions (WHAT

FOR) with the technical rationale (WHY) and the timing (WHEN).

In contrast to treatment processes, however, timing plays an ever diminishing role in modern laboratory diagnostics: With the appropriate implementation of information technology (IT), a comprehensive clarification of the initial question can be achieved in a very short time with (what appears to be) a single ordering step. Behind the scenes, of course, complex steps and decisions take place that require high levels of clinical laboratory expertise in addition to IT support. In the ideal case, this has no practical significance for the requestor. Important technical prerequisites for this ideal case are that a diagnostic pathway embodies algorithms to ensure the approval of all the necessary test materials at the point of electronic order entry, and to trigger automatic reflex testing when a pattern of abnormal values is recognized.

In addition to greater certainty in the process documentation and faster diagnosis, there are other reasons for the use of diagnostic pathways:

- Processes are more transparent and weaknesses are identified;
- Services are standardized, with concomitant lowering of costs; and,
- Their explanatory component broadens the knowledge of the users.

Ultimately, the development of diagnostic pathways brings even faster progress in laboratory medicine by providing a consistent motivation to explore the practical usefulness of innovative tests and – when the time is right – to introduce these into routine practice by consensus with other disciplines.

1.1.1 Legal Rulings

The number of liability lawsuits in the United States has risen sharply in recent years. This development is also evident in the Federal Republic of Germany; a similar trend is seen, although not as pronounced. The case law is based on the professional judgment of individual experts or expert bodies, which in turn are aligned with directives and guidelines to justify major decisions. It must indeed be made clear that guidelines as such have the effect of neither providing grounds for liability nor exemption from liability, but these guidelines can be observed to affect case law under a judiciary that is increasingly oriented toward authoritative texts (Ulsenheimer, 2008). How the diagnostic pathways are to be evaluated in the future regarding this discussion remains to be seen.

Walter G. Guder

1.2 Historical Development

The study of body fluids was employed in ancient times for deriving diagnoses, monitoring therapies, and sometimes even the prediction of diseases. Around the year 1700, the predominantly mystical-alchemical mindset of medieval times was replaced by the natural science perspective of chemistry. An example is the discovery of a white precipitate in acidified urine (Dekkers, 1695), known as the "dense substance similar to boiled egg" (albumen) that could soon be ascribed to nephrotic syndrome.

With the first chemical analysis of defined molecules – in the above case, albumin in urine – the early 19th century saw the birth of clinical chemistry (Päuser, 2003). Justus von Liebig became famous for many things, among them his lectures during the 1840/41 winter semester on "Organic chemistry in its relation to physiology and pathology" (Liebig, 1840). The rapid scientific and technological development during the 20th century has continuously extended the spectrum of potential investigations (▶ Figure 1.2). Contributions include those from new immunochemical, chromatographic and luminometric methods, which have extended the measurement range from millimolar down to femtomolar concentrations. Mass spectrometry can now be used to detect 500 different proteins in a sample of urine in a single analytical run, and over 3000 in blood. With high-throughput sequencing, it is now possible to analyze even a complete genome within one to two days.

In view of such technical possibilities, it is conceivable for the first time to conduct a complete analysis of a particular class of substances in a body fluid such that not only can all the molecules contained therein be detected, but also assayed quantitatively with defined accuracy and precision. With the technical and analytical possibilities of the future, the number and nature of investigations are likely to be even less limited than before.

The diagnostician will then not only be confronted with an almost unlimited abundance of technically possible investigations, but also with

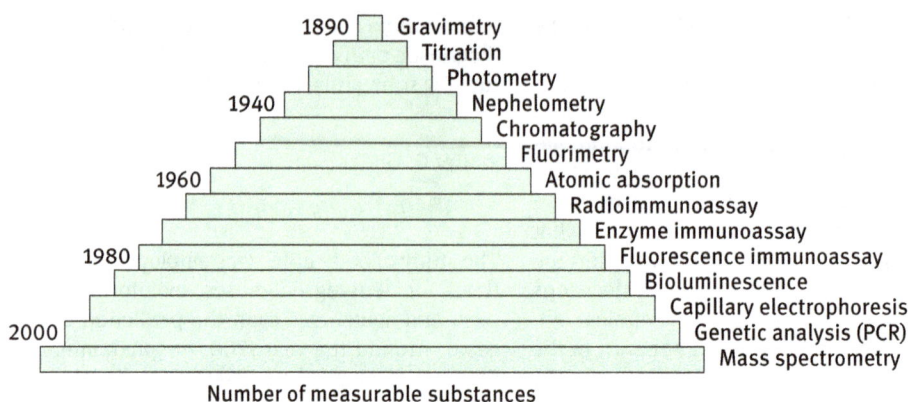

Number of measurable substances

Figure 1.2 Development of laboratory diagnostic procedures (amplified from Guder 1983). Over the course of the 20th century, the number of measurable substances in the human body rose from approximately 10^1 to more than 10^6, while the detection sensitivity was lowered from about 10^{-1} mol/L to below 10^{-12} mol/L (1 mole is equivalent to 6×10^{23} molecules; PCR = polymerase chain reaction).

an increasing number of economic, legal and ethical challenges to overcome. The final word, however, is the medical indication; that is what determines that any investigation should be undertaken only if it promises diagnostic, therapeutic, or prognostic utility. This requirement is currently defined as a "validation of the evidence of an investigation, as measured by the medical benefit" (Price, Christenson, 2003). This evidence is understood in the sense of the expression "evidence-based medicine".

Diagnostic pathways are an important tool for making the proper decision in the balancing act between the aforementioned challenges. A well-known illustrative example is the following: For over 100 years, creatinine has been used to prove or rule out impaired glomerular filtration in the kidney. However, the test is responsive only to severe renal impairment, and is also affected by tubular secretion and lower creatinine production with decreased muscle mass. Particularly in the elderly, falsely normal values can be camouflaged, and thus serious kidney damage overlooked. In 1985, cystatin C was proposed as a more sensitive marker unencumbered by these disadvantages, but this test currently (2013) is compensated at the flat rate of €11.66 according to German Scale of Medical Fees (GOÄ) compared with € 2.33 for the creatinine test. The pure reagent price for creatinine, and also the remuneration rates from the German Statutory Health Insurance (GKV), are in the euro-cents range. So, the inex-

pensive but less suitable creatinine remains the preferred renal marker in the clinic still today as 100 years earlier. By comparison, and depending on the institution, the number of cystatin C orders is in the tenths of a percent to single-digit percent range (private surveys). When considering these competing medical and economic requirements, an evidence-based pathway should specify for which questions and under what conditions is one or the other marker the better alternative. Even after more than 25 years, the lack of suitable studies means there is still no consensus among specialists: pediatricians recommend cystatin C as the test of first choice, while by contrast geriatricians and nephrologists do not.

In the interests of quality assurance, the directives of the German Medical Association (RiliBÄK, Bundesärztekammer 2008) stipulate that pre-analytical criteria such as the best time for collection, the proper sample material, etc. (Guder et al., 2015) must be considered. These stipulations must be incorporated into diagnostic pathways the future, because the ward personnel who order or perform blood draws still seem to be barely aware of them in spite of their medical and legal importance. This is true even for such frequently requested laboratory tests as potassium, for example (Wisser and Knoll, 1982). Due to hormonally controlled diurnal rhythms, values from samples drawn in the afternoon are 0.3 to 0.4 mmol/L higher than in the morning. By collecting serum instead of heparin plasma, the measured value increases by an average of 0.3 mmol/L due to the disintegration of thrombocytes; the error can amount to 1 mmol/L with massive thrombocytosis, so that the serum test is nearly worthless for the detection of hypokalemia (Guder and Hoffmann 1992).

This manual is the latest contribution to the development of laboratory diagnostic pathways. The multi-year effort on this work has shown how satisfying it can be to have brought colleagues from different specialties and schools to a consensus, from which this book and the electronic versions (Chapter 2.3) were created. As the examples show, medical knowledge is evolving quite rapidly now, so that some of the recommendations made in the first edition had to be revised only one year later. The editors and authors will have a continuing responsibility to check periodically that the book is still up to date. The fact that the work accomplished so far requires continuous follow-up speaks to its lasting value.

Georg Hoffmann, Walter G. Guder,
Johannes Aufenanger

1.3 Diagnostic Strategies

Diagnosis ("dia" = through, "gnosis" = knowledge) comes from Greek words meaning a "combing through" of symptoms with the aim of "gaining knowledge". More precisely, it is about recognizing and naming a disease based on a medical history, physical examination and other findings, in particular from laboratory tests. A correct diagnosis is a precondition for targeted therapy; it thus comes both at the end of a chain of logical inference as well as at the beginning of a chain of treatment activities.

Diagnoses are not made only in the field of medicine; in the broader sense, auto mechanics, stockbrokers or astrologers must also be described as diagnosticians. According to the general definition, each diagnosis is a consolidation of individual phenomena into a class of similar cases, which one can call by a common name. It is immaterial whether this "class" is based on a theoretical concept or not. The process can also be referred to as "classification", and the road that leads to the diagnosis would then be a "classifier". Mathematicians and computer scientists refer to such a clearly describable problem-solving approach as an "algorithm".

For diagnostic problems of average complexity, the decision tree is the most popular representation in the medical field. In the example shown in ▶ Figure 1.3a, chest pain, a normal ECG (ST elevation: "no"), and increased troponin leads to the NSTEMI class (non ST elevation myocardial infarction). Comprehensive etiological and patho-

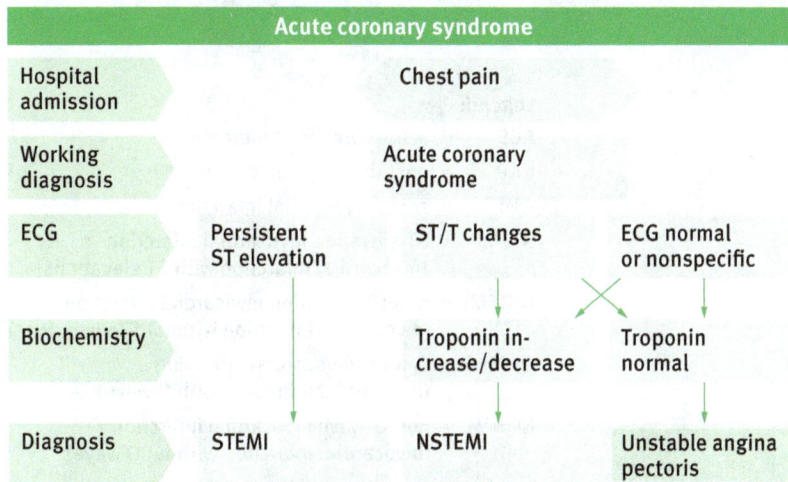

Acute coronary syndrome			
Hospital admission		Chest pain	
Working diagnosis		Acute coronary syndrome	
ECG	Persistent ST elevation	ST/T changes	ECG normal or nonspecific
Biochemistry		Troponin increase/decrease	Troponin normal
Diagnosis	STEMI	NSTEMI	Unstable angina pectoris

Figure 1.3a A simple clinical pathway for acute coronary syndrome (ACS) in accordance with the guideline from the European Society of Cardiology (ESC) 2012 (Achenbach, et al., 2012). For implementation as a diagnostic pathway, the diagram must be extended and revised in light of the most recent guideline (pp. 8–9). For abbreviations, see Figure 1.3b.

Stepwise diagnosis with a suspected acute coronary syndrome (ACS)

Symptom

Acute chest pain lasting
longer than 20 min

**rapidly as
possible**

12-lead ECG

No ———— Changed — Yes ——▶ Inverted T — No ———

Yes

**Immediately
and after 3 h**

hs-troponin

hs-troponin

Elevated

Elevated

No   Yes

No   Yes

Diagnosis

Possible
UAP

AMI/UAP

Possible
UAP

AMI/UAP

**Counter-
measures**

**After
1–2 days**

Diagnosis

Legend:

ACS   = acute coronary syndrome

UAP   = unstable angina pectoris

AMI   = acute myocardial infarction

STEMI   = ST-elevation myocardial infarction
                (myocardial infarction with ST elevations)

NSTEMI = non-ST-elevation myocardial infarction
                (myocardial infarction without ST elevations)

QwMI   = Q-wave myocardial infarction
                (myocardial infarction with Q wave)

NQwMI = non-Q-wave myocardial infarction
                (myocardial infarction without Q wave)

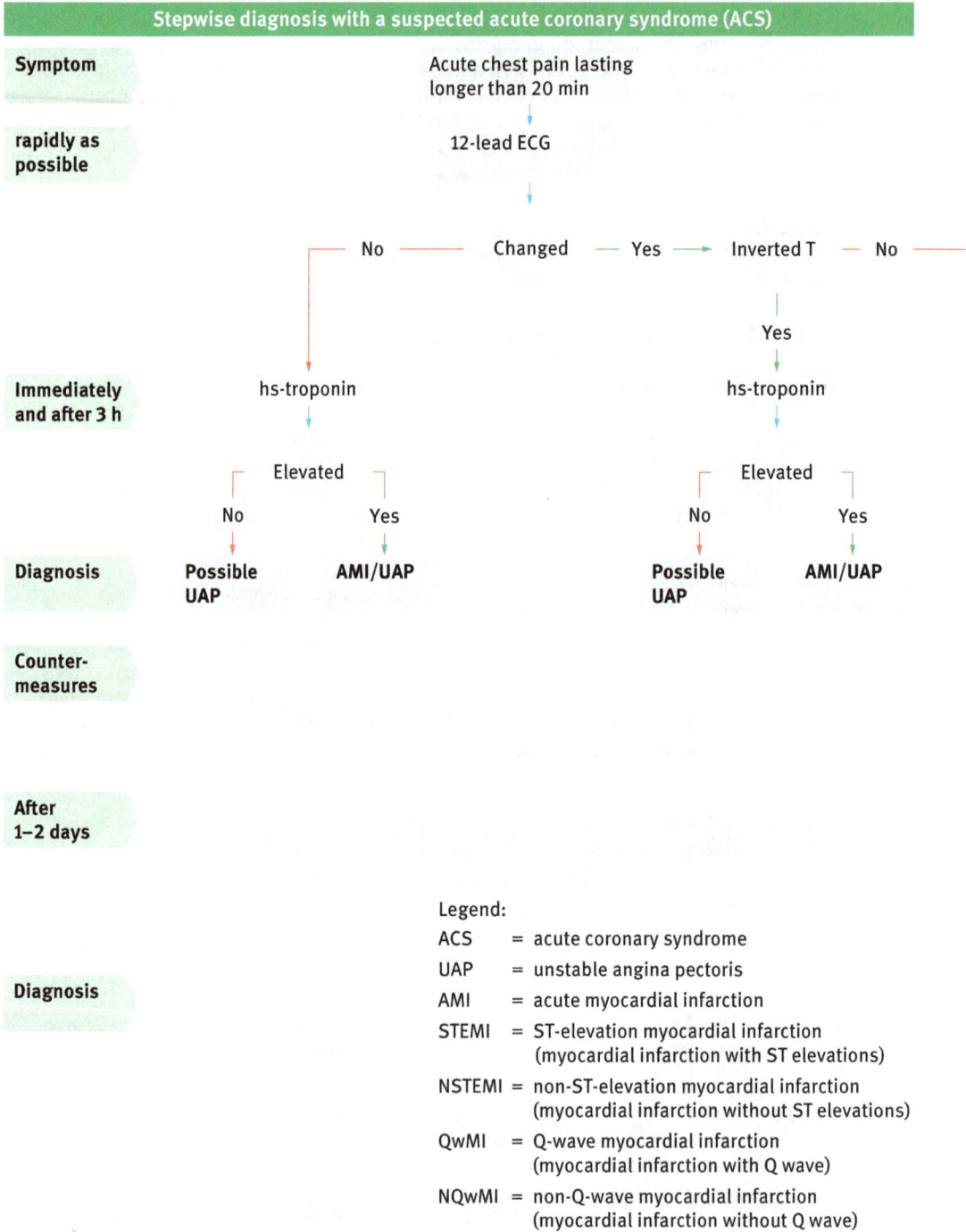

Figure 1.3b A simple clinical pathway according to the criteria of this book and the guideline from the European Society of Cardiology (ESC) 2012 (Achenbach, et al., 2012).

ST elevation ——————— Yes ——┐
         │   │
         No   │
         │   │
    hs-troponin   │
         │   │
      Elevated   │
   ┌─────┴─────┐   │
   No   Yes   │
   │   │   │
 UAP   **NSTEMI**   **STEMI**
   │   │   │
 Coronary   Immediate
 angiography   reperfusion
   └─────┬─────┘   │
         │   │
        ECG ─────────────────┘
         │
      Q peak
   ┌─────┴─────┐
   No   Yes
   │   │
 NQwMI   **QwMI**
 Non-transmural Transmural
 myocardial   myocardial
 infarction   infarction

Table 1.1 Possible origins of elevated troponin that are not due to an acute coronary syndrome (Achenbach, 2012).

- Chronic or acute renal failure
- Severe heart failure, acute or chronic
- Hypertensive crisis
- Tachy- or bradyarrhythmias
- Pulmonary embolism, severe pulmonary hypertonia
- Inflammatory diseases, e.g., myocarditis
- Acute neurological diseases, e.g., apoplexy or sub-arachnoid hemorrhage
- Aortic dissection, aortic valve disease, or hypertrophic cardiomyopathy
- Cardiac contusion, ablation therapy, pacemaker stimulation, cardioversion, or endomyocardial biopsy
- Hypothyroidism
- Stress cardiomyopathy
- Infiltrative myocardial diseases such as amyloidosis, hemochromatosis, sarcoidosis, and scleroderma
- Drug toxicity, e.g., adriamycin, 5-fluorouracil, herceptin, and snake venoms
- Burns that affect more than 30 % of the body surface are rhabdomyolysis
- Critically ill patients, especially with respiratory failure and sepsis

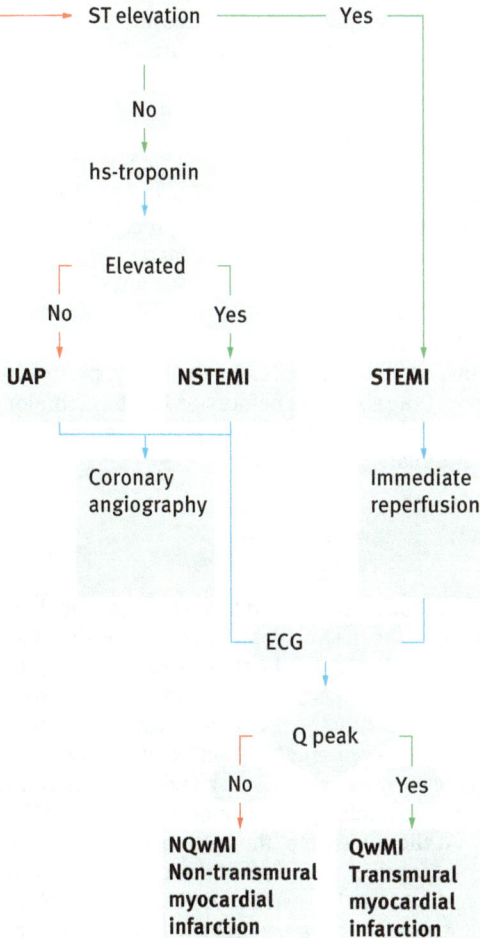

genetic concepts and a therapeutic treatment procedure are implied by this abbreviation, which is different from other similar medical scenarios, such as STEMI (Heidt, 2006).

Simple decision trees can be drawn out on paper with a few symbols, and are understood immediately by knowledgeable medically viewers. Such a tree is shown in ▶ Figure 1.3a, based on a guideline from the German Society of Cardiology (Achenbach 2012). Implementation as a complete diagnostic pathway according to the criteria of this book makes the picture significantly more complex, but also more correct from the perspective of laboratory diagnostics and information technology (▶ Figure 1.3b.): An alternative is given for every decision, and proposed timing also appears in the left margin. This corresponds to the guideline, but can be adapted to a specific department or institution. Thus, the optimal timing for troponin determinations depends on the available method in each case: For example, if a high-sensitivity troponin (hs-troponin) determination cannot be made because only a simple troponin rapid test is available, a negative value below the detection limit can qualify as "not increased" within the meaning of ▶ Figure 1.3b only after 6 to 9 hours, and not after only 3 hours.

For medical and economic reasons, it might also be useful to include other additional laboratory tests in a pathway even if they are not included in the specialty-specific guideline. Thus, there are a number of origins for elevated troponin that are not attributed to an acute coronary syndrome (▶ Table 1.1). If these are frequent in the relevant patient population, and possibly life-threatening, they must routinely be eliminated with appropriate tests.

However, what is critical for the development of diagnostic strategies is not only the approach *per se*, but also its efficiency and effectiveness. What is meant by this, in a given everyday situation, is both "doing the proper thing" as well as "doing the thing properly". Thus, it can make sense in private medical practice first to perform an ECG, while generally the first step in a hospital admission is to draw blood samples and order a series of lab tests (including for troponin).

The diagrams published in this book testify to the efficiency of processes, but usually not on the effectiveness thereof. Thus, one can glean from the diagrams which are the "proper" lab tests to perform for a particular diagnosis, but not, for example, whether it is "proper" to order them all at one time or successively. This latter decision depends on many factors: how much time is available, which tests can be run from the same blood sample, and which tests must be sent to a specialized laboratory? The definition of the diagnostic strategy, and the ultimately of the obligatory pathway, thus remains the province of the organization in which the pathway is to be used.

There are two basic strategies in laboratory diagnostics: profile diagnostics and stepwise diagnostics. In the second half of the last century, analyses have become increasingly automated so that ten or twenty analyses can easily be carried out in parallel from a single sample. Out of enthusiasm for what had become technically feasible, starting in the 1960s, clinicians began to order everything that was measurable. This strategy has had the advantage of quickly providing a good overview, especially in initial diagnoses, but marginal, poorly interpretable findings more often resulted in uncertainty rather than diagnostic knowledge. The main reason for this was that reference ranges have been defined as 95 percent ranges, which means that on average, a completely healthy person has at least one false positive value within a typical "Chem 20" profile. This can then result in a bundle of additional, more expensive follow-up tests.

Thus, for medical and economic reasons, the practice of using such untargeted profiles soon reached a limit. The preferred laboratory diagnostic strategy changed in the 1980s, away from profile testing and toward stepwise diagnostics. This latter entails obtaining an overview of which diseases to consider by starting off with a few symptom-oriented laboratory tests. The number of possible diagnoses is then gradually narrowed through further testing.

Each step within such a stepwise diagnostic scheme must therefore be based on a medical indication. The first step often proceeds from the clinical symptoms, medical history and physical examination alone, without any laboratory tests. A typical example is rheumatoid arthritis (▶ Fig. 4.52): Here, clinical signs such as swelling, effusion and morning stiffness must be present for more than six weeks before starting the laboratory diagnostics for rheumatoid factor, antibodies to citrullinated peptides, etc.

1.3.1 Stepwise Diagnosis or Profile Diagnosis?

Even though stepwise diagnostics form the basis of this book, it should not be concluded that diagnostic pathways for the stepwise narrowing of the focus on a suspected disease are the only proper diagnostic strategy. Obvious advantages include the clear representation, with a structure that is also clearly recognizable to laypersons and readily implementable by programmers (▶ Chapter 2.3).

At the same time, these strengths also constitute the major weakness of decision trees, for the "yes" and "no" arrows convey a false sense of certainty that – as in all other medical and biological sciences – belie the fallibility of laboratory diagnostics used in this way. Such algorithms only operate correctly if all the associated decisions made are 100 % correct.

On the other hand, if all the yes/no decisions within a diagnostic pathway have only a 95 % probability of being correct, for example, the probability of error grows rapidly. As shown in ▶ Figure 1.4, after more than 15 steps, it is not only cheaper but even more accurate to trust in the validity of a coin toss (with a 50 % probability of er-

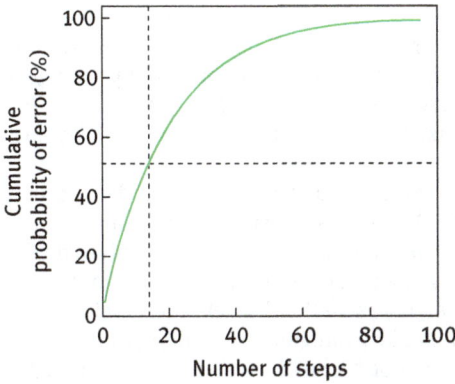

Figure 1.4 Probability of an incorrect decision when using decision trees with many individual steps. If each individual step is subject to an error of only 5 %, the probability of an incorrect diagnosis after about 15 steps is greater than 50 %. Error probabilities are generally even higher than 5 % (see Chapter 1.3.2).

ror) than to work through such a long diagnostic pathway.

A work-around can be to use range information instead of hard limits in the decision trees, for example, differentiated consideration of the glomerular filtration rate in kidney diseases.

▶ Figure 4.23 defines thirteen age-related ranges for making decisions on how to proceed (urine test strip, sediment, protein differentiation, and biopsy). Another example is shown in ▶ Figure 4.5 for the stepwise diagnostics in the case of diabetes mellitus (Kerner, et al., 2010). An HbA1c value of greater than 48 mmol/mol Hb confirms diabetes, while this is ruled out with a value below 39. For values in the gray area in between, an additional oral glucose tolerance test is recommended.

In summary, one can say that decision trees with their strict yes-no decisions are primarily suitable for relatively simple situations. For more complex problems, the completion of a more extensive laboratory profile can be superior. This is especially true for multimorbid patients, which tend to be the rule rather than the exception in, for example, the emergency rooms of acute care hospitals. In those cases, profiles provide the doctor an overall picture in less time, and they are less susceptible to individual mistakes.

Since it is difficult for the human eye to process large quantities of numbers, many doctors highlight all the pathological values with a marker, and focus their attention on these. It is better if one lets a computer do this: It can color pathological values with an intensity that varies according to

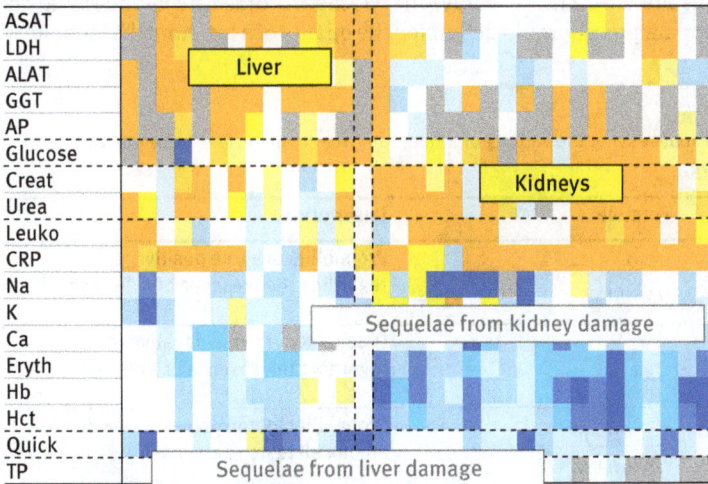

Figure 1.5 Clustering procedures draw the eye to the essential points in profile testing. Each vertical row represents a real patient from the emergency room of an acute care hospital. Increased laboratory values are yellow to orange, decreased values are light to dark blue. The computer sorts all the laboratory values by color; the "hot spots" immediately indicate to the viewer typical clinical situations that require various interventions: In the left half of the Excel spreadsheet, for example, are gathered patients with liver diseases who have decreased Quick values, while on the right side are patients with kidney diseases who have renal anemia (Hoffmann, 2011).

the degree of deviation from the norm (Haeckel, et al., 2010), and the patients can then be sorted into disease categories according to the color patterns (▶ Figure 1.5). This procedure is called clustering: It clusters similar colors into what are called "hot spots", and in this way automatically consolidates the reported findings (Hoffmann, et al., 2010).

A description of the various methods for evaluating profile testing is beyond the scope of this book. However, several chapters refer to computational methods that provide a consolidation of several laboratory values. In general, these involve simple summations, for example, the 4T score for detecting heparin-induced thrombocytopenia (HIT). (▶ Fig 4.44): The points assigned for individual findings (platelet count, kinetics of the platelet count decrease, etc.) are added up just as in a game of golf or in a ski jump competition: More than 4 points means an HIT diagnosis is likely, and requires a stepwise diagnostic clarification with antibody and function tests. An example of a complex score, which in addition to the cholesterol value takes into consideration patient sex, smoking, and blood pressure, can be found in ▶ Figure 4.11.

1.3.2 Diagnostic Quality Criteria

In addition to the economic and organizational aspects, statistical considerations are most critical for selecting the most appropriate procedure:

How likely is it that the patient has the disease in question *a priori*, i.e., regardless of test results? Moreover, how does this probability change if the test comes out positive? How many of the test results are correct, and how many are false positives?

In statistics, a false positive is defined as a result that makes a healthy person appear to be sick. For example, a measurement value can frequently be just outside the reference range, i.e., in the gray zone that by definition includes 5 % of all healthy individuals (▶ Chapter 1.3). Such a value is not "false" in the analytical sense, but can easily be misinterpreted when flagged with an asterisk by the computer. Other causes of false positive results are methodological interferences (for example, due to drugs), physiological factors such as circadian rhythms, and pathological conditions that alter a laboratory value in the same direction as would the disease in question. For the same reasons, one can also encounter false negative results, which make a sick person appear to be healthy.

The five basic statistical concepts that play a role in this context are summarized in ▶ Table 1.2. The *a priori* probability in medicine is referred to as *prevalence*, and means the proportion of patients with the disease in the population under study. The two metrics of *sensitivity* and *specificity* determine the quality of a test from the laboratory

Table 1.2 Key statistical measures for assessing the validity of a test; tp = true positive, fp = false positive, tn = true negative, fn = false negative.

Name	Formula	Description
Sensitivity	$\dfrac{rp}{rp+fn}$	Probability of a true positive result regarding the presence of a disease
Specificity	$\dfrac{rn}{rn+fp}$	Probability of a true negative result regarding the absence of a disease
Prevalence	$\dfrac{rp+fn}{rp+rn+fn+fp}$	Probability for the presence of a disease among all tested persons
Positive predictive value	$\dfrac{rp}{rp+fp}$	Probability for the presence of a disease with a positive test result
Negative predictive value	$\dfrac{rn}{rn+fn}$	Probability for ruling out a disease with a negative test result

perspective, while the positive and negative *predictive* values are the decisive indicators for the treating physician. Computer programs for calculating these factors are freely accessible on the internet (e.g.: www.medcalc.org/calc/diagnostic_test.php) in addition to being available as a smart phone app (www.medequations.com).

The sensitivity is the proportion of true positive results with a disease present, while the specificity is the proportion of true negative results among healthy individuals. Values for an acceptable test will be around 90 %, and over 95 % for a good test (▶ Table 1.3). However, one can "turn" the set screw of the limiting value to improve one of the two parameters at the expense of other. If the limit is lowered so that the test is more sensitive, more positive results are obtained. At the same time the test will also become less specific: more false positives will necessarily be obtained.

A very low limit should be chosen to avoid overlooking any patients with a disease; for example, blood donors who must not under any circumstances be infected with HIV. Conversely, the limit should be set relatively high when specificity is more important than the sensitivity, for example, to avoid any confusion with false positive results for healthy screening participants. However, turning the limit value set screw is always a balancing act; ultimately, medical laboratory practice must aim to employ tests with both high sensitivity and high specificity.

Sensitivity and specificity are determined retrospectively for persons who are known from the outset to be either healthy or sick. The determination of these two quality criteria is left to developers and laboratory technicians during the introduction phase of a new test. However, the criteria have little significance for the treating physician since the laboratory test would not be performed if the patient were already known to have the disease in question.

Rather, it is the opposite question: If the test comes out positive, how high is the probability that the patient has the disease in question? Moreover, how certain can one be that the disease is not present when the test result is negative? To make the calculation, not only are the sensitivity (sens) and specificity (spec) needed, but also the prevalence (prev):

Table 1.3 Sample calculation for a sensitivity and specificity of 95 % each and a prevalence of 5 %; D+ = disease present, D− = disease absent; T+ = positive test, T− = negative test; Σ = sum.

	T+	T−	Σ
K+	475	25	500
K−	475	9.025	9.500
Σ	950	9.050	10.000
Sensitivity			95.0 %
Specificity			95.0 %
Prevalence			5.0
Pos. predictive value			50.0 %
Neg. predictive value			99.7 %

Positive predictive value (pPV) =

$$\frac{sens \cdot prev}{sens \cdot prev + (1 - spec) \cdot (1 - prev)}$$

Negative predictive value (nPV) =

$$\frac{spec \cdot (1 - prev)}{spec \cdot (1 - prev) + (1 - sens) \cdot prev}$$

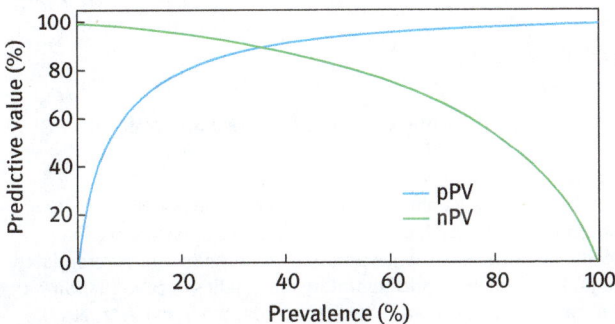

Figure 1.6 Calculation of the predictive values pPV and nPV for a laboratory test with 95 % specificity and 80 % sensitivity as a function of prevalence. The predictive value of this test is highest when the disease in question is present in about every third patient (prevalence of 30–40 %).

The best predictive value for a diagnostic test is found for an average disease incidence (▶ Figure 1.6). If the disease is quite rare (i.e., the prevalence is very low), the pPV drops dramatically while the nPV increases. This latter is not surprising, because if essentially none of the patients examined has the disease, then one can predict a negative outcome with high probability even without actually performing the test. More serious is a high number of false positives (poor pPV) because they result in expensive follow-up exams and worry the patient needlessly.

1.3.3 Stepwise Diagnosis during Screening of Clinically Unremarkable Persons

Especially when screening clinically unremarkable persons, it is important to have the best possible pPV and consequently a high specificity, for example, in breast cancer screening. Here, the specificity is 95 %, and the sensitivity is 80 %, exactly as is shown in ▶ Figure 1.6.

Most patients – and many doctors – believe the predictive value of such a test would be somewhere between 80 and 95 %; if the test is positive, then they assume that breast cancer is present. Since the prevalence in the target population is approximately 2 %, though, inspection of the

blue curve in ▶ Figure 1.6 shows that the pPV is only 25 %. This means that of every four women in whom a suspicious node is found, three do not have breast cancer. For the statistical layman, that sounds like low predictive value, but in reality it is a very good result: The prevalence of breast cancer in the group of women with a positive mammography result is no longer 2 %, but now 25 %.

In the course of stepwise diagnosis, if another test with similar sensitivity and specificity is then performed (e.g., a fine needle biopsy), the above curve shows a pPV of more than 80 %. Moving ahead to a third such test, the hit rate for a positive result is close to 100 %. This statistical regularity forms the rationale for why the stepwise narrowing of a disease suspicion is usually more accurate and more economical than untargeted "shotgun" diagnostics.

Screening tests without a medical indication not only generate additional costs, but can also result in bad decisions being made. An often-cited example is what is referred to as the "Quick/PTT Reflex" (Peetz, 2012) to rule out a significant bleeding tendency prior to surgery (Figure 4.42a: Diagnostic Pathway – Bleeding Tendency 1). The two global tests still form part of the routine preoperative program in many hospitals, although approximately ten studies conducted from 1986 to 2000 on

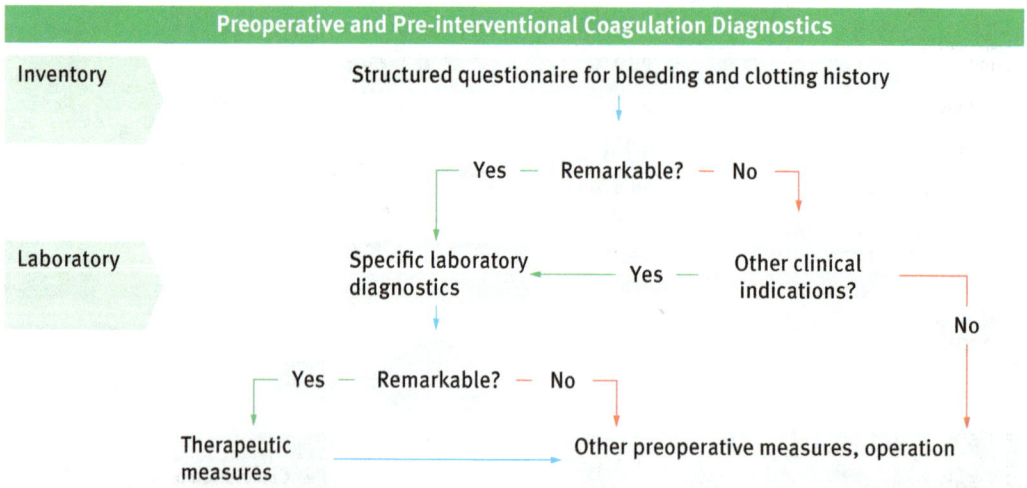

Figure 1.7 A guideline-based diagnostic pathway for preoperative and pre-interventional coagulation diagnostics includes as the first step a structured medical history (clinical symptoms, previous interventions, anticoagulant drugs, family medical history). Only a reasonable suspicion of increased bleeding or other clinical indications, such as the presence of a liver disease, will warrant the performance of differentiated hemostatic laboratory diagnostics in coordination with a coagulation specialist (adapted from Peetz, 2012).

more than 12,000 patients showed no significant benefit from untargeted coagulation tests with respect to the occurrence of intra- and postoperative bleeding complications arose (Chee, et al., 2008). The most common hereditary bleeding disease, the von Willebrand syndrome (vWS), is not generally recognized by global tests; conversely, there are numerous (clinical as well as methodological) origins of pathological PT and aPTT values that do not restrict suitability for an operation.

Therefore, a guideline-based prediction of postoperative bleeding does not include laboratory screening, but rather is based on a structured bleeding and clotting history. This includes, for example, questions about nosebleeds, the duration of menstrual bleeding, history of previous operations, medications, familial bleeding tendency, etc. Coagulation diagnostics are conducted only when a clinical suspicion is present.

Figure 1.7 is deliberately kept simple to highlight the proper sequence of steps: "indication → diagnostics → therapy". All the details of the specific laboratory diagnostics that follow a reasonable suspicion of bleeding tendency can be found in ▶ Chapter 4.6.

Walter Hofmann, Johannes Aufenanger, Georg Hoffmann

1.4 Outlook

With the comprehensive description of diagnostic pathways as a subset of clinical pathways, the authors, editors and publisher were breaking new ground – at least in German-speaking countries – because this is the first time the complex knowledge of (laboratory) diagnostics has been standardized and consistently represented in the form of decision trees. It is not the underlying algorithms that are novel, but rather the systematics that this book has applied to the task.

As is explained in detail in Chapter 1.1, the pathways featured here as examples are neither recommendations, guidelines nor directives, but rather constitute a standalone management tool. They aren't meant to be comprehensive or have universal validity. **Following publication of the first edition, it was reported that economists and other non-medical personnel used the book as a pretext to deny reimbursement for any laboratory tests that were not included in the Figures. As explained in Chapter 1.3, this is an unacceptable simplification of medical diagnostics and constitutes an abuse of this book.**

The editorial team has set itself the future goal of moving beyond laboratory diagnostics and integrating additional diagnostic pathways from other medical disciplines, such as pathology and microbiology, endoscopy and radiology. All told, these will certainly provide a substantially better representation of the decision-making processes used to develop a diagnosis under actual clinical conditions. However, we feel that at the initial stage, laboratory diagnosis – and here again mainly clinical chemistry – is complex and demanding enough.

It will become obvious in the future whether the simpler pathways summarized here will provide support to doctors and nurses, IT professionals, and medical cost controllers in their daily work and thus gain wide acceptance, not least among the ones who pay the bills, i.e., patients and health insurance companies.

If these diagnostic pathways are implemented properly, any concerns about possible restrictions on diagnoses, the freedom to choose therapies, or tying the physician's hands, will be unfounded, but such issues must be taken seriously and discussed in the appropriate forums: academic societies, professional associations, medical associations, etc. The concerns of the health insurers must likewise be addressed, in which cost increases are coupled with sophisticated discussions of quality. If the pathways reflect the current state of knowledge, the opposite will be the case: As set out in Section 2.2, these pathways help both to avoid superfluous investigations and also not to overlook other important investigations.

In choosing the examples, we have focused on pathways for common problems and simple, recurring processes, without completely excluding the rare and more complex cases. The choice was not easy, and certainly still needs supplementation: several major clinical pictures that are widespread and important from the laboratory diagnosis perspective, such as cancer or dementia, have received only cursory attention and were not dealt with in detail.

It became clear during the preparation of the graphics that not all pathways, even those that are frequent or important, are reducible to the form of simple decision trees. The more complex the problem, the greater the need for either a specialist's expertise or a doctor's experience and intuition – otherwise, one can only have faith that the rapid development of information and communication technology in this post-genomic era will provide us with entirely new tools for pattern recognition and machine learning.

Literature

Achenbach S, Stardien S, Zeymer U et al. Kommentar zu den Leitlinien der Europäischen Gesellschaft für Kardiologie (ESC) zur Diagnostik und Therapie des akuten Koronarsyndroms ohne persistierende ST-Streckenhebung. Kardiologie 2012; 6: 283–301

Bundesärztekammer: Ärztliche Leitlinien – Definitionen, Ziel, Leitlinie ACS 2012, Implementierung in BAÄ, KBV, AWMF (Hrsg): Ärztliches Qualitätsmanagement, Texte und Materialien der BÄK zur Fortbildung und Weiterbildung. 1996; 10: 177ff.

Bundesärztekammer: Richtlinien der Bundesärztekammer zur Qualitätssicherung laboratoriumsmedizinischer Untersuchungen. Dtsch Ärztebl 2008; 105: C301–15

Bundesärztekammer: Verbindlichkeit von Richtlinien, Leitlinien, Empfehlungen und Stellungnahmen, Stand 01. 06. 1998, letzte Änderung 24. 11. 2006 (www.Bundesaerztekammer.de)

Chee Y, Crawfor J, Watson H, Greaves M. Guidelines on the assessment of bleeding risk prior to surgery or invasive procedures). Brit J Haem 2008; 140: 496–504

Dekkers: Exercitationes practicae circa medendi methodum (V), Boutestein, Leiden, 1695 p. 338

Eckardt J, Sens B: Praxishandbuch Integrierte Behandlungspfade. Economica Verlag, Heidelberg, 2006, ISBN 978-3-87081-430-4

Guder WG, Fiedler GM, da Fonseca-Wollheim F et al. Quality of Diagnostic Samples. 4th edition 2015 BD-Diagnostics, Oxford

Guder WG: Indikation und Beurteilung klinisch-chemischer Untersuchungen. Med Klin 1983; 78: 524–528.

Guder WG, Hoffmann GE. Analytische und medizinische Aspekte der flammenphotometrischen Elektrolytbestimmung. Lab Med 1992; 15:14-8.

Haeckel R, Wosniok W, Hoffmann G. Standardisierung von Laborergebnissen: Ergebnisquotient. J Lab Med 2010; 34: 95–98

Hart D: Ärztliche Leitlinien. Z ärztl Qualitätssicherung und Fortbildung 2000; 94: 65–69

Heidt M: Leitliniengerechte Herzdiagnostik. Trillium Report 2006; 4: 68

Hoffmann G. IT-Werkzeuge zur Auswertung großer labordiagnostischer Datensätze. KCM 2011; 42: 124–127. Download unter www.dgkl.de

Hoffmann G, Zapatka M, Findeisen P, Wörner S, Martus P, Neumaier M. Data Mining in klinischen Datensätzen. J Lab Med 2010; 34: 227–233

Kerner W, Brückel J. Definition, Klassifikation und Diagnostik. Diabetologie 2010; 5: 109–112

Liebig J: Die Organische Chemie in ihrer Anwendung auf Physiologie und Pathologie. Braunschweig F. Vieweg 1840

Päuser S (Ed.). Senses, Sensors and Systems. Editiones Roche, 2003

Peetz D. Präoperative und präinterventionelle Gerinnungsdiagnostik: Wider den „Quick-PTT-Reflex". Trillium-Report 2012; 10: 218–219 (Download unter www.trillium.de)

Price CP, Christenson RH: Evidence Based Laboratory Medicine. AACC Press, 2003

Renz H: Praktische Labordiagnostik. Walter de Gruyter, Berlin, 2009, ISBN 978-311019576-7

Ulsenheimer K, Biermann E: Leitlinien und Standard. Anästh Intensivmed 2008; 49: 105–106

Wisser H, Knoll E: Tageszeitliche Änderungen klinisch chemischer Messgrößen. Ärztl. Lab 1982; 28: 99–108

2 Implementation

Walter Hofmann, Georg Hoffmann

2.1 Organizational Requirements in the Hospital

For diagnostic pathways to be established successfully in everyday life, the user must be convinced of the benefits. One must not make the mistake of wanting to represent every problem and process in clinical practice. Approaching the process of developing a diagnosis too comprehensively can lead to a complete rejection, and thus the failure of the project. This is possibly the reason for the result from many national and international studies (Cleland, 2002; Schneider, 2005; Steel, 2008) that even long-established guidelines are only put into practice to a small extent.

It is therefore better to confine the effort to frequent and rather simple decisions. As is true in many areas of management, the Pareto principle, also known as 80/20 rule, is also valid here. By this rule, 80 percent of the desired results can be achieved with 20 percent of the total effort expended, while the remaining 20 percent requires the majority of the work (Koch, 1998). This principle goes back to the statistical calculations made by the Italian scientist Vilfrede Pareto (1848–1923), and can be derived without substantial mathematical effort: one begins by listing all the diagnoses made within a given period, and determines their number. The Table thus generated is then sorted by frequencies and graphed (▶ Figure 2.1 a, b). The cumulative sums of the percentages show at a glance how many diagnoses cover 80 percent of all patients. This number is frequently even less than 20 percent, and it is on these that the effort to develop pathways should then focus.

Even if the formulation of diagnostic pathways is restricted to only the ten main diagnoses in a ward or department, their introduction is not straightforward. Thus, while processes such as blood draws or requests for functional tests were previously initiated by a person, these are suddenly now triggered by computer. It can also occur that a test ordered while a physician is doing rounds will, according to the pathway, require a prior stepwise diagnosis and must be justified in

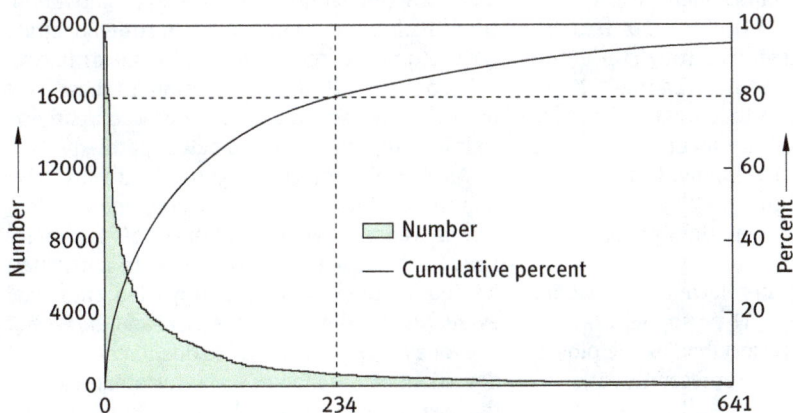

Figure 2.1a Frequency distribution of main diagnoses at German hospitals in 2008 (Source: DRG browser www.g-drg.de). 80 percent of all cases were covered by 12.3 percent of all assigned ICD codes (intersection of the two dashed lines). There are an additional 1,269 diagnoses beyond the right-hand border of the graph, but these account for only five percent of the cases. Over one hundred of them were only assigned once among the hospitals reviewed in 2008.

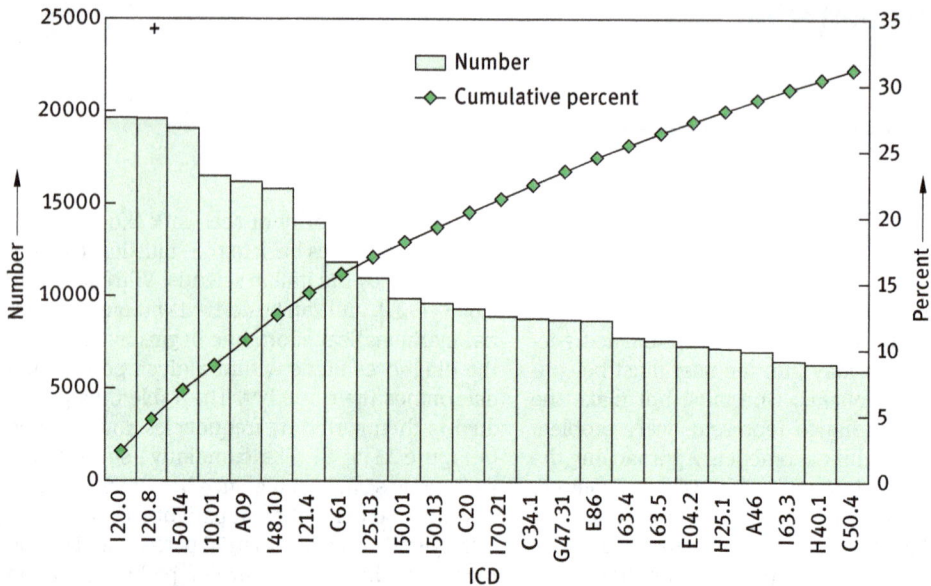

Figure 2.1b The 25 most common ICD codes cover nearly one-third of all hospital cases in Germany. The most frequent are cardiovascular diseases (initial letter I), followed by cancers (first letter C) and intestinal infections (A09).

writing. Hospital administrators must appreciate that the introduction of pathways represents an intrusion into established structures and practices, and can call traditional hierarchies into question.

The implementation of such changes in hospital operation requires measures that are known collectively as "change management" in the business administration field (Kirchner, 2001; Leoprechting, 2005). Without going through the entire toolbox of relevant procedures (Baumol, 2008) at this point, several items that are important for pathway implementation are mentioned below. Briefly, the three crucial elements in the initial acceptance of responsibility are:
- Assignment for implementation by the hospital management;
- Early involvement of all relevant professional groups (doctors, nurses, IT personnel);
- Support by the supervisory bodies (employee organizations, personnel representatives).

As with all major projects in a hospital or clinical group, management must be squarely behind the implementation. In the face of high costs, anticipated resistance, and long time frames, half-hearted support will doom such a project. It is particularly important in this context to bring all the stakeholders onboard from the outset, and where possible to anchor the successful implementation in agreed objectives with the responsible employees (management by objectives).

Striking a balance among the strategic considerations of the hospital management within the local structure requires a high level of motivation, coordination and communication. To demonstrate the usefulness of the venture and achieve rapid results, one should start with a "simple" diagnostic pathway and schedule ongoing accompanying training programs with competent partners.

As with all projects, diagnostic pathways also require continuous training of staff and developers, as well as ongoing analysis of discrepancies between targets and performance. In particular, it is important to conduct IT-supported, statistical evaluations of the number of users and the type of use for every pathway, and to document frequent deviations. If too many exceptions are identified, the users must be asked why they don't use either the pathway as a whole, or at least certain of its components. In this way, any vulnerabilities or outdated rules can be identified. A select group of people – usually the senior physicians and head nurses – should ensure that the content of the diagnostic pathways is continuously upgraded to reflect medical requirements and ongoing technical developments.

In most cases, however, any adjustments made relate less to the pathways themselves and more to the implementation mechanisms. Not infrequently, the relevant projects founder for lack of organizational effort, and ultimately from resistance by the medical, nursing, or IT staff. Optimal IT support is the crucial factor in keeping the manual effort for performance requirements and documentation as low as possible. What must be kept in mind is that:

- The use of computer programs only makes sense if the processes have previously been logically structured and completely described – that is, are IT-ready;
- All users of the system must be technically networked so as to have access at all levels to the process data – "from request to findings" – at a glance;
- All performance requirements must be implemented in paperless format, and automated to the extent possible with "intelligent" (i.e., rule-based) algorithms (order entry).

Diagnostic pathways generally improve the process flow, but this can vary from department to department, even concerning the same problem. Thus, the guidelines for pediatric surgery differ from those for adults (for example, in the clarification and treatment of hypogastric pain). Nevertheless, surgeons focus during their diagnosis on establishing whether the patient is a candidate for surgery, regardless of age. By contrast, the pathway created by a conservative specialist will focus on clarification of the hypogastric pain through non-invasive procedures that play no role in determining readiness for surgery. Nevertheless, the steps involved in clarifying an acute abdomen must not differ fundamentally depending on the ward in which the patient is present. The skill of the project manager is in flexibly representing the individual needs of the various users and still making the resulting pathway as a whole generally usable.

Finally, a word on costs: New projects are always hard on the budget because they entail substantial up-front costs. In the case of diagnostic pathways, the introduction cannot be covered by petty cash. Therefore, the necessary financial and human resources must be defined and agreed to

in advance so as not to jeopardize a successful implementation from the start. Only with a budget secured at all levels (programming and technical implementation, maintenance and further development, monitoring and documentation) will the project meet with success.

Johannes Aufenanger, Georg Hoffmann

2.2 Economic Impacts

An international meta-analysis of 27 trials involving over 11,000 participants (Rotter, 2010) confirmed in principle the positive impacts of clinical pathways outlined in the previous chapter. In addition to improving the documentation, the Cochrane study group primarily found a reduction in the length of stay and rate of complications. As to the question of whether clinical pathways truly reduce the overall cost per case or only shift costs to other sectors, the authors were unable to answer with confidence.

There are no such systematic studies on diagnostic pathways, which is not surprising considering that the subject is relatively new and the rate of penetration to date is still low. For many German hospitals, the proximate motivation for introducing clinical pathways was the establishment in 2003 of a remuneration system based on diagnosis-related groups (DRGs). This created tension between revenue assurance and cost reductions on the one hand, while at the same time increasing quality as much as possible. Every country so far that has introduced DRGs has consistently reported the use of clinical pathways to improve the effectiveness (▶ Table 2.1) and efficiency (▶ Table 2.2) of treatment processes. For hospitals in the DRG system, both of these often translate into the issue of economic survival (Schlüchtermann, 2005). This puts the value chain of structured service processes increasingly in the foreground.

In a study entitled: "The significance of Laboratory Testing for the German Diagnose Related Group System", it was determined that 62 % of all compensation-related secondary diagnoses in Germany were exclusively or primarily developed from laboratory values (Hoffmann, 2004). When the associated ICD codes were automatically communicated from the laboratory information system to the requester, the coding quality improved: In one hospital in southern Germany where this

Table 2.1 Effectiveness Increases.

Strategic target	Target achievement
Acceleration of the treatment process and improvements in treatment outcomes	Reliable laboratory diagnostics Rapid sample transport Timely transmission of findings
Reducing investigations	Evidence-based diagnostic pathways, standardized requests
Effective therapies and therapy monitoring	Timely, reliable laboratory diagnostics based on clinical guidelines6666

Table 2.2 Efficiency Increases (modified from Bruni, 2007).

Strategic target	Target achievement
Rapid formulation of the main diagnosis	Through better case management based on faster and more reliable clinical lab findings when patient admitted
Comprehensive formulation of secondary diagnoses	Evidence for secondary diagnoses and reasons for case severity
Increased coding quality	Proposed ICD coding by the laboratory based on a putative secondary diagnosis
Reduction in administrative effort	Correct and above all comprehensive coding, thereby revenue assurance
Avoidance of overtreatment	Simpler order entry, if possible via the order entry system, automatic incorporation of treatment monitoring
Reduction in patient length of stay	Interdisciplinary coordination of diagnostic pathways
Increase in continuity of care	Reduction in turnaround time
	Laboratory as the Center of Competence in the hospital

was implemented, for example, the coding frequency for *Pseudomonas* infections (ICD B96.5) increased by approximately 70 % (Brown, 2005).

In this DRG era, laboratory diagnostics must above all fulfill the criteria of accuracy, affordability, and rapidity. While the first two points have always been essential criteria for economic success, short lead times have become an important factor under DRG conditions. With the daily nursing rates that were customary in Germany until 2003, this aspect had been largely ignored; quite the contrary, there was often money to be gained through delays in the process. In a fee-per-case system, by contrast, the turn-around-time (TAT) from sample collection to when the analysis results are transmitted or the therapeutic measures implemented must be reduced as much as possible to shorten the length of stay (Aufenanger, 2011).

However, diagnostic pathways do not promote revenue optimization or improved bed occupancy rates in the DRG system, but rather serve primarily for quality improvements and the elimination of any interfering factors in the process flow. Thus, the lack of treatment-relevant laboratory values or the doctor waiting to receive findings can have economically significant consequences, including the cancellation of planned operations or delayed patient discharge. Ideally, the length of stay can be shortened considerably merely by speeding up diagnostic processes during the first days after admission, and additional charges reduced to a minimum. This saves on the cost per patient and at the same time increases revenue based on the higher numbers of patients. However, even if this is not the case, simply the higher transparency in workflow management from the point of initial examination will improve employee and patient satisfaction, as well as improving the reputation of the hospital (Greiling, 2006).

Moreover, the clinical and thus also diagnostic pathways will enable compliance with the statutory provisions. The medical care provided must correspond to the current state of scientific knowledge, and be of the quality required by professional standards (German Social Security Code V, § 135 a (SGB V)). For services that are not necessary or not economical, the insured cannot file a claim, the service provider must not provide, and health insurance companies will not approve (SGB V, § 12). According to HGrG (German Budgetary Principles Act) § 53, processes must furthermore be structured in such a way that the risk of diagnostic or treatment mistakes, or of giving incorrect medical advice, is as low as possible.

Laboratory results document the success of treatments in black and white. They thus fulfill in a special way the commitment to risk management, which protects the hospital and staff on civil rights claims and criminal consequences (Lohfert, 2006).

When a hospital decides to make its service processes visible and accessible to all participants in the form of diagnostic pathways, this is especially beneficial to internal quality assurance. Transparency and traceability enable

- Diagnoses to be formulated according to established and uniform quality standards that take the entire process into consideration across sectors;
- Interdisciplinary communication between all participating professional groups (doctors, nurses, IT, cost control, etc.) to be improved;
- Deficiencies and potential improvements in diagnostics to be identified;
- The nature and scope of resources to be enumerated precisely;
- Specialist departments to receive effective and valid data for process control and employee training; and,
- A broad framework of legal certainty to be created.

Without diagnostic pathways, the scope and nature of the particular diagnostic measures to be employed are left to the subjective judgment of the individual physician. In particular, with a heightened need for protection, younger professionals tend to overcompensate to cover themselves even in the absence of a medical indication. This results in too many expensive tests being ordered.

More so than ever before, the overall costs for the patient are under scrutiny in the DRG system. Thus, it is no longer simply an isolated consider-ation of the laboratory costs, but rather the extent to which this contributes to the value chain in the overall hospital economics (Aufenanger, 2010). In a diagnosis-based payment system, the quality of diagnosis and particularly of the laboratory test results naturally determines success or failure in medical and economic terms (Aufenanger, 2011). From the business economics perspective, this already operates at the admissions desk and in the emergency room to determine the composition of the case mix; further along it governs numerous internal patient care processes, and ultimately the complete coding of all diagnoses in discharge letters also contributes to adequate compensation.

Diagnostic pathways that are confined to the laboratory medicine, taken alone, are certainly no guarantee of business success, but as a relatively simple introduction to the complex interplay of diagnostic departments from pathology and microbiology, through radiology, and all the way to endoscopy and functional diagnosis, they make a substantial contribution to the success of comprehensive pathways initiative. This book should thus be understood as a guide to modern disease management in a world of increasing demands and finite resources. Pathway-controlled laboratory diagnostics bridges the gap between medical and economical needs in hospitals (Lohfert, 2006), and is in the vanguard of other technical and clinical departments that will be involved – either directly or indirectly – in diagnostics.

Georg Hoffmann

2.3 Implementation of Information Technology

After the organizational and economic aspects of diagnostic pathways, the third major remaining challenge is the implementation of IT programs. Project execution is divided into three phases:

- Creation of the organizational, technical and financial requirements;
- Visual representation of the pathways on paper (diagrams, text, tables); and,
- Translation of content into an IT environment.

The essential aspects of the first point were already described in the preceding chapters: a clear mandate must be given, a working group must be

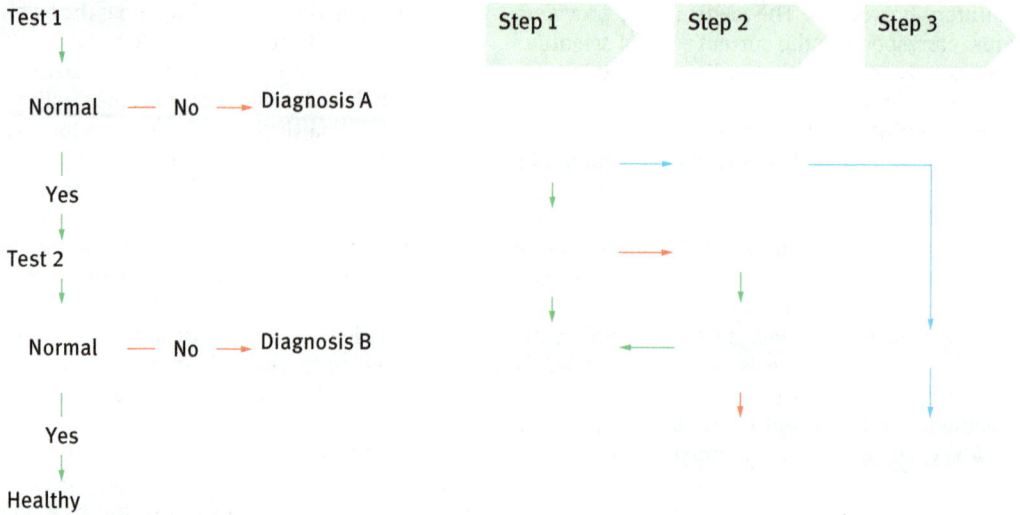

Figure 2.2 The pathways are suitably represented by decision trees (left) or combinations with flowcharts, such as what are known as "swim lanes" (right).

established, and a budget of financial and human resources must be provided.

There are various possibilities for the visual presentation of clinical pathways, and the choice depends on the objective. While it is decisions that drive the formulation of diagnoses, in treatments it is rather the responsibilities and timing that play the dominant role. Thus, decision trees are the basis for diagnostic pathways, while for treatment pathways it is mainly flowcharts, which can also be combined with decision trees (▶ Figure 2.2).

Note the use of standardized symbols for actions (e.g., rectangles or block arrows), decisions (mostly diamonds with arrows), process endpoints (circles), diagnoses (document icon), etc. The examples in ▶ Figure 2.2 are most easily created using the "AutoShapes" feature in MS Office. More professional, but less widespread, is MS Visio, and elaborate tools for IT-based process modeling, such as Adonis, Aris or Sycat, can also be used for complex clinical pathway projects. However, paper and pencil work fine when just starting out.

To integrate the decision trees presented in this book into a comprehensive clinical pathway, one needs what are known as "event-driven process chains" (EPC) that assign an activity to each event, an actor to each activity, and allocate the necessary resources or organizational means to each actor. This type of modeling is used, for example, in the design concept that ensures the compatibility of various IT systems for the healthcare telematics (i.e., data telecommunications) infrastructure in Germany (Becker, 2006), but is not necessary for the construction of simple diagnostic pathways.

The third step of the project involves the decision trees conceived for the human eye being translated into the computer environment. All IT system manufacturers (HIS; LIS) now offer tools for the creation of computer-readable rules, but the physicians or technical assistants are usually left with the task of achieving the technically correct conversion of graphical decision trees into algorithms. A contribution to an article series for the 2009 DGKL Annual Convention, entitled "You are the doctor", reported on a pilot project covering the IT implementation of diagnostic pathways (Aufenanger, 2009).

At this meeting, four different laboratory information system manufacturers indicated that the technical prerequisites for implementing diagnostic pathways are already in place. Most often, these are sets of rules of the "if/then" type, which

```
Bilirubin                Order:
determination            TBIL
      ↓
>21 µmol/L  — No →  NAD   IF TBIL >21
                         THEN Jaundice
                         ELSE End
      |
     Yes
      ↓
Jaundice                 IF jaundice
                         THEN Order:
                         Profile H 4711
      ↓
Hepatitis
diagnosis
```

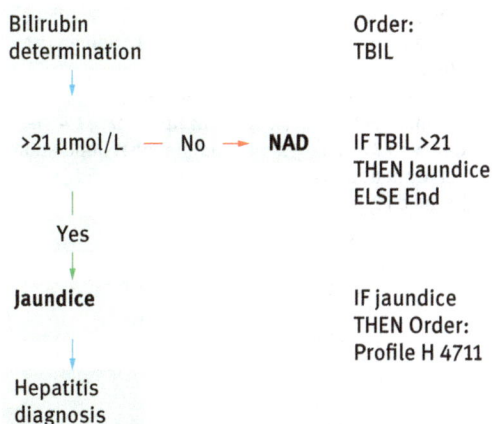

Figure 2.3 Implementation of a decision tree in a computer program. Shown here are two actions (orders), a decision (IF TBIL > 21 THEN…), an end point (NAD = no abnormality detected, no further action), and a diagnosis (Hepatitis).

have long been in routine use in doing medical validation or submitting paperless laboratory test requests via an order entry system. They are usually created and maintained by the users themselves, after receiving appropriate training, and do not require special computer science knowledge (▶ Figure 2.3).

In the simplest case, all the arrows in a diagram are converted into sentences, such as 'IF bilirubin > 21 µmol/L THEN jaundice ELSE unremarkable'. The concatenation of many such sentences ('IF bilirubin > 21 µmol/L THEN jaundice, IF jaundice THEN specific hepatitis diagnostics') creates a rule-based system that, with a complexity of as few as 100 rules, can definitely give a user the impression of artificial intelligence. However, increasing the scope of the system likewise increases its complexity, and thus makes it more prone to error.

It is the responsibility of the manufacturer to ensure the maintainability of the rule-based system through automatic rule generators, visual aids, program-based warnings, and the like. The corresponding proposals had already been announced as the second German edition went to press (2013), but it will still take several years until the use of easily manageable IT products or "downloadable pathways" becomes routine in the hospitals and laboratories.

Literature

Aufenanger J: Helfen diagnostische Pfade das ökonomische Ergebnis eines Krankenhauses zu verbessern? Eine Betrachtung aus Sicht der Laboratoriumsmedizin. J Lab Med 2011; 35: im Druck

Aufenanger J: IT-gestützte Diagnostikpfade (mit Beitragen von E. Kotting, U. Schenk, H. Baur und F. Neuhaus). Trillium Report 2009; 7: 121–125 (www.trillium.de)

Aufenanger J, Schernikau E, Wieland E: Die zukunftige Rolle des Krankenhauslabors. J Lab Med 2010; 34: 271–277

Baumol U: Change Management in Organisationen – situative Methodenkonstruktion für flexible Veränderungsprozesse. Gabler, Wiesbaden 2008 (www.fernuni-hagen.de/bima/publikationen/ Change Management_Methodenkonstruktion_ 2008.shtml)

Becker K: Prozessanalyse Integrierter Behandlungspfade. In Eckhardt und Sens (Hrsg). Praxishandbuch Integrierte Behandlungspfade, S. 65–79. Economica, Heidelberg, 2006

Braun S: Gezielter anfordern und richtiger kodieren. Trillium Report 2005; 3: 14

Bruni K: Welche Bedeutung gewinnt die Labormedizin mit der Einführung der SwissDRG 2009–2011. Diplomarbeit Universitätsspital Zurich 2007

Bruni K: Welche Bedeutung gewinnt die Labormedizin mit der Einführung der SwissDRG 2009–2011. Diplomarbeit Universitätsspital Zurich 2007

Cleland JG, Cohen-Solal A, Aquilar JC, Dietz R, Eastaugh J, Follath F et al.: Management of heart failure in primary care (the IMPROVEMENT of Heart Failure Programme): an international survey. Lancet 2002; 360 (9346): 1631–1639

Greiling M, Muszynski T: Pfade zu effizienten Prozessen. Prozessgestaltung im Krankenhaus. Baumann Fachverlage, 2006

Hoffmann G, Schenker M, Kammann M, Meyer-Luerssen D, Wilke MH: The significance of laboratory testing for the German diagnosis-related group system. Clin Lab. 2004; 50: 599–607

Kirchner H, Kirchner W: Change Management im Krankenhaus – Strategische Neuorientierung für Non-Profit-Unternehmen. Verlag W. Kohlhammer 2001

Koch R: Das 80/20-Prinzip. Mehr Erfolg mit weniger Aufwand. Campus, Frankfurt/M.; New York, 1998

Leoprechting G von, Hoffmann G: Change Management im Krankenhaus – Sehnsucht nach Veränderung. Trillium Report 2005; 3: 32–33 (www.trillium.de)

Lohfert C, Kalmar P: Behandlungspfade: Erfahrungen, Erwartungen, Perspektiven. Internist 2006; 47: 676–683

Rotter T, Kinsman L, James EL, Machotta A, Gothe H, Willis J, Snow P, Kugler J: Clinical pathways: effects on professional practice, patient outcomes, length of stay and hospital costs. Cochrane Database of Systematic Reviews 2010, Heft 3,1–166

Schlüchtermann J, Sibbel R, Prill M: Clinical Pathways als Prozesssteuerungsinstrument im Krankenhaus, in: Peter Oberender (Hrsg.): Clinical Pathways: 2005 Stuttgart, Berlin, Koln: Kohlhammer, 43–58

Schneider F, Mwenke R, Harter M, Salize HJ, Janssen B, Bergmann F et al.: Sind Bonussysteme auf eine leitlinienkonforme haus -und nervenärztliche Depressionsbehandlung übertragbar? Nervenarzt 2005; 76: 308–314

Steel N, Bachmann M, Maisey S, Shekelle P, Breeze E, Marmot M et al.: Self report receipt of care consistent with 32 quality indicators: national population survey of adults aged 50 or more in England Br. Med J 2008; 337: a 957

II: Specialist Section

3 Practical Examples for Screening Examinations

Johannes Aufenanger

3.1 Internist Admissions Screening

One of the most important and optimizable processes in a hospital is the patient admission. What occurs at this outpatient-inpatient interface sets the course for an efficient treatment workflow, and thus governs revenues and costs. The first hours spent by the patient in a clinic are critical to the

- Economic efficiency of the treatment processes;
- Effort expended by clinical staff; and,
- Patient satisfaction.

Admission is the "moment of truth" for patients and their families in terms of building confidence, the experience of quality, and willingness to cooperate in the hospital. There is no second chance to make a good first impression, especially if the patient has an appointment, doesn't have any acute injuries, and is in full command of his/her faculties (Klinikarzt, 2006). In this area, sample logistics, reliable laboratory diagnostics, and the timely submission of findings are particularly important factors in increasing treatment effectiveness and efficiency (▶ Chapter 2.2). At the patient admissions stage, diagnostic pathways trigger reliable diagnostics in a targeted manner, helping to avoid unnecessary investigations and contributing significantly to the reliability of costing procedures.

In the emergency or main admissions room of a hospital, decisions regarding the further workflow concerning the patient must be made within the shortest possible time. Organizationally, it is not always possible for a patient to be seen at first by the physician on duty. Rather, for economy of time, assistants will often be authorized to schedule pre-agreed diagnostic measures, the results of which will guide the physician on duty in further diagnostic strategies. The triage nurse or triage doctor will use the diagnostic pathways as an effective decision-making tool to optimize patient admission.

While organ-related laboratory profiles (heart, liver, kidney profiles) routinely used to develop the admission diagnosis at many hospitals, the pathways presented in this section are based on cardinal symptoms. This is not about rigid procedures that serve as a type of cookbook medicine to restrict a physician's freedom of decision. Rather, they posit accepted, defined courses of treatment for the diagnosis in a patient with a describable symptom or disease picture, and offer latitude for nuanced decisions (alternative pathway branches, or sub-pathways). The profile can be modified depending on the conditions in the medical history. Through agreements with the submitters, the laboratory is authorized to undertake further differential diagnostic clarification for the given constellation of symptoms.

Ideally, practical implementation of this system should involve an electronic request system (order entry). The requester merely selects the problem or symptom complex according to the clinical symptoms, and automatically obtains an order ticket for the clinical laboratory (▶ Figure 3.1).

The example shown in Figure 3.2 is of a patient presenting in a hospital emergency room with dyspnea and chest pain. Based on the symptoms, an initial differential diagnosis will consider myocardial infarction and/or pulmonary embolism. The requester is immediately presented with a default order combination based on consensus by the responsible specialist departments of the hospital, which can be changed or supplemented at any given time according to medical history information obtained. Even a trained assistant is thus able to call up the initial important information relating to laboratory tests, and thus facilitate the differential diagnosis decision to be made by the physician on duty. This can contribute to a greatly improved internal workflow for the hospital, and a more efficient organizational structure in emergency room admissions: the length of the patient's emergency room stay is significantly reduced, the patient's continuity of care is increased, administrative costs for doctors, nurses and laboratory

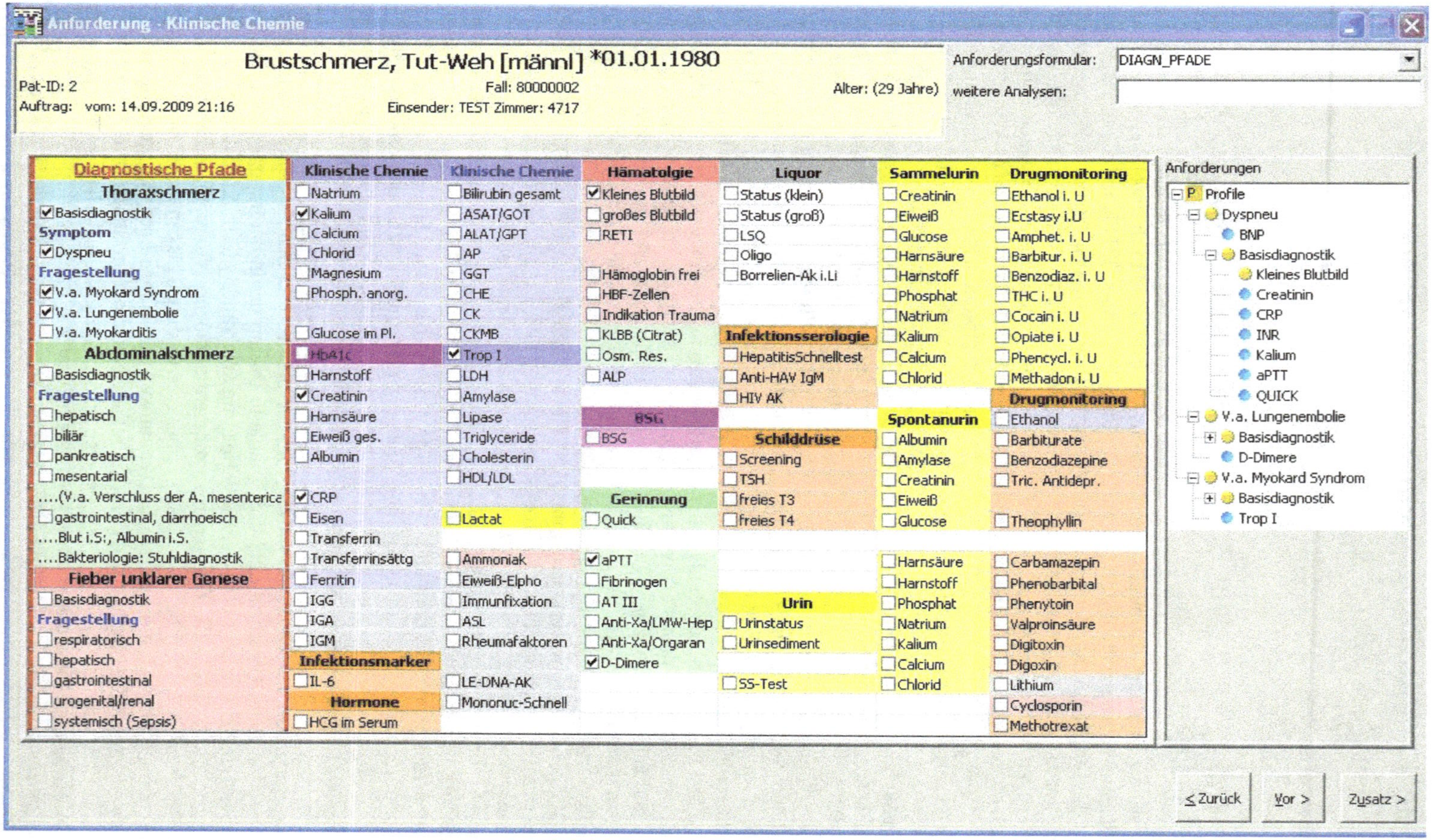

Figure 3.1 Integration of the symptom-oriented problem into the laboratory test order. Depending on the question, a diagnostic pathway can be supplemented and modified at any time using the form shown in the example. In modern IT systems, the layout and content can be adapted by the user at any time.

staff are reduced, and last but not least, communications between the laboratory and the recipients are improved.

Once supplied by the laboratory the results will be digitally communicated to the requester either as a confirmation or exclusion according to the guideline consensus interpretation, with the option of recommending additional diagnostic measures. This "initial result" thus represents the basis for further differential diagnostics and laboratory analysis measures. As in the above case, expanded thrombophilia diagnostics the emergency room already contributes to triggering a targeted therapy.

The pathways proceed from one basic clinical symptom (▶ Figure 3.3) or a simple question, which can also be detected by medical assistance personnel (e.g., triage nurse).

In terms of an initial screening, a timely formulation of the basic diagnostic approach can be a determining factor from which the physician on duty can proceed to further differential diagnosis. This makes it possible to avoid time delays in the procedure for admitting a patient, while at the same time making preliminary differential diagnostic decisions available to the admitting hospitals and wards, which helps to speed up the patient management workflow significantly.

In the latter case, various procedures are presented using the example of acute abdominal pain. While the suspected diagnosis in ▶ Figure 3.4a is inferred from the origin of pain, the diagnostic pathway in ▶ Figure 3.4b derives from the pain localization. The first case shows the simpler approach, which can be addressed by the medical assistant staff, while the approach using pain localization requires contact with a physician, but then leads more decisively to the diagnosis. Both approaches depend on the respective host organization in the corresponding hospitals.

Literature

Wirtschaftlichkeit im Krankenhaus – Effizienzreserven schon bei der Patientenaufnahme nutzen. Klinikarzt 2006; 35, S. XVI–XVII

Pravention, Diagnose, Therapie und Nachsorge der Sepsis, Revision der S-2k Leitlinien der Deutschen Sepsis-Gesellschaft e. V. (DSG) und der Deutschen Interdisziplinaren Vereinigung für Intensiv- und Notfallmedizin (DIVI), 2010; http://www.uni-duesseldorf.de/AWMF/

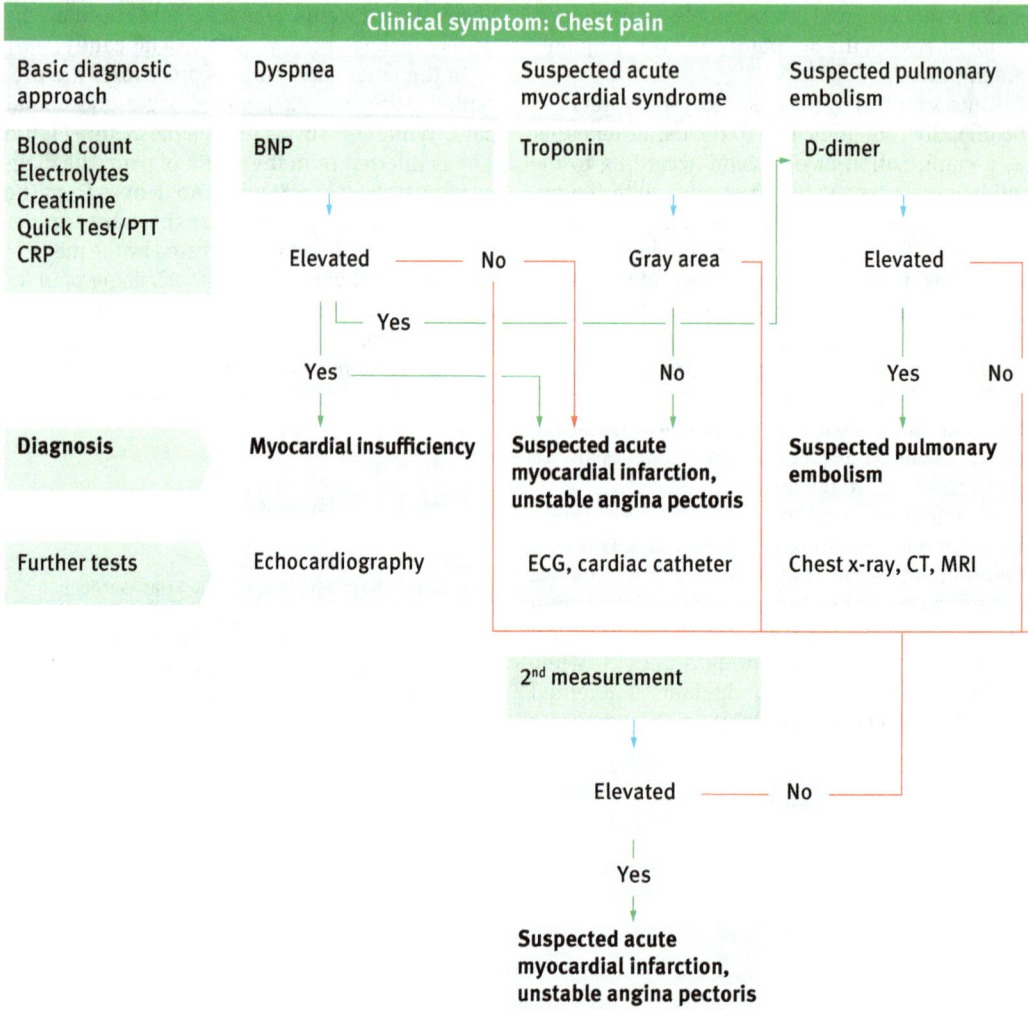

Clinical symptom: Chest pain

Basic diagnostic approach	Dyspnea	Suspected acute myocardial syndrome	Suspected pulmonary embolism

Blood count
Electrolytes
Creatinine
Quick Test/PTT
CRP

BNP   Troponin   D-dimer

Elevated —— No —— Gray area   Elevated

Yes

Yes   No   Yes   No

Diagnosis   **Myocardial insufficiency**   **Suspected acute myocardial infarction, unstable angina pectoris**   **Suspected pulmonary embolism**

Further tests   Echocardiography   ECG, cardiac catheter   Chest x-ray, CT, MRI

2nd measurement

Elevated —— No

Yes

Suspected acute myocardial infarction, unstable angina pectoris

Suspected myocarditis   DD
Chest pain

Troponin

       Gray area ————— No ———

No remarkable
changes in the
second measurement

Suspected myocarditis

Cardiotropic viruses,   Diagnosis:
antibodies   epigastric pain

2nd measurement

      Elevated ————— No ———

        Yes

Suspected myocarditis

Cardiotropic viruses,
antibodies

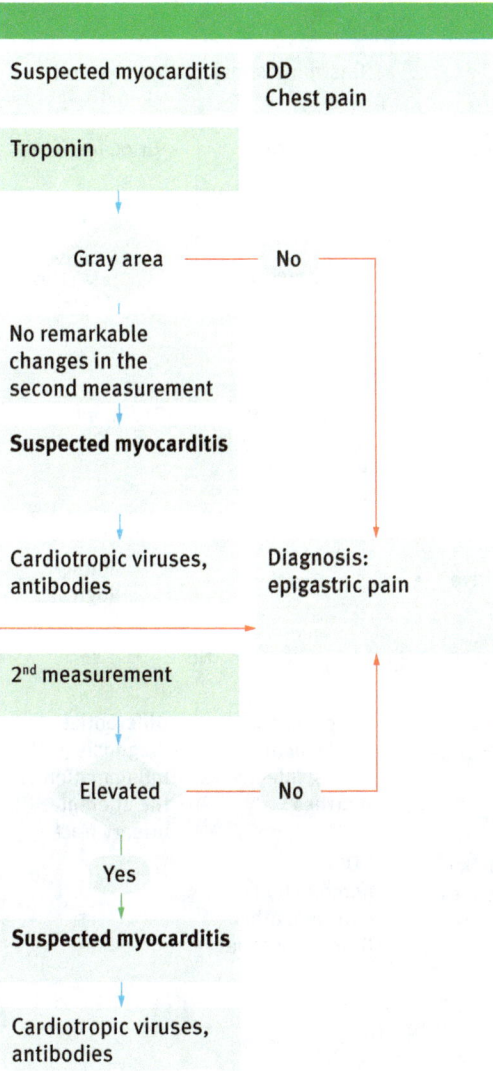

Figure 3.2 Diagnostic Pathway: acute chest pain.
The basic diagnostic approach is combined with specific analyses, each of which is evaluated according
to symptom/question during the decision-making
processes. Example: an elevated BNP together with
elevated D-dimer leads to a presumptive diagnosis of
pulmonary embolism.

Clinical symptom: Fever of unknown origin			
Basic diagnostic approach	Respiratory	Hepatic	Gastrointestinal	Urogenital Renal

Blood count **Differential blood count** **Creatinine** **CRP** **Immunoglobulins** **IL-6 (esp. in infants)**	Blood gas analysis	ALT	Electrolytes	Urine test strips

Respiratory: Blood gas analysis → Patho-logical — No → ... Yes ↓ Chest x-ray, tracheal secretion, sputum for germs

Hepatic: ALT → Elevated — No → ... Yes ↓ Hepatitis serology ↓ Positive — Yes ↓ Suspected hepatitis / No → DD re other liver diseases

Gastrointestinal: Electrolytes → Lowered — No → ... Yes ↓ Temperature, stool analysis for germs, viruses, parasites ↓ Positive — Yes ↓ Suspected appendicitis, colitis, infect. diarrhea / No → DD re noninfectious diarrhea, other GI tract diseases

Urogenital/Renal: Urine test strips → Positive "test strip sieve" — No → Yes ↓ Sediment ↓ Patho-logical — Yes ↓ Differential diagnosis (DD) Inflammation of the efferent urinary tract

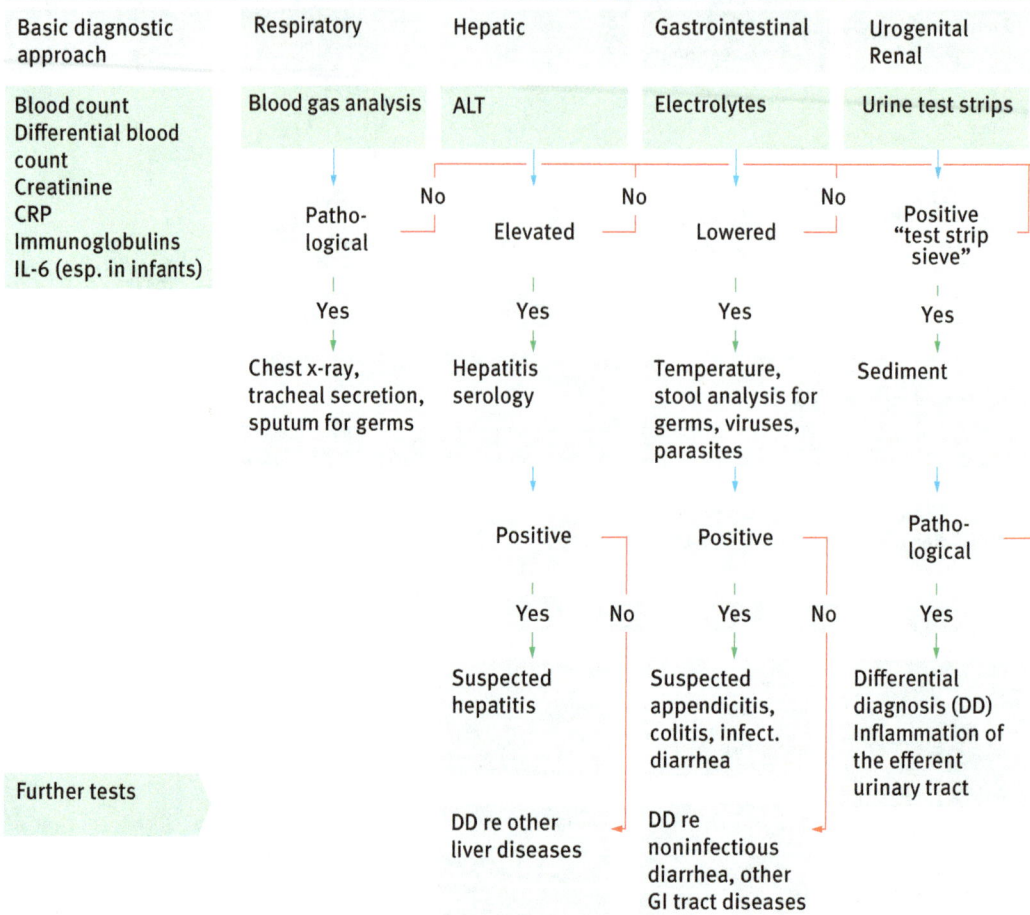

Further tests

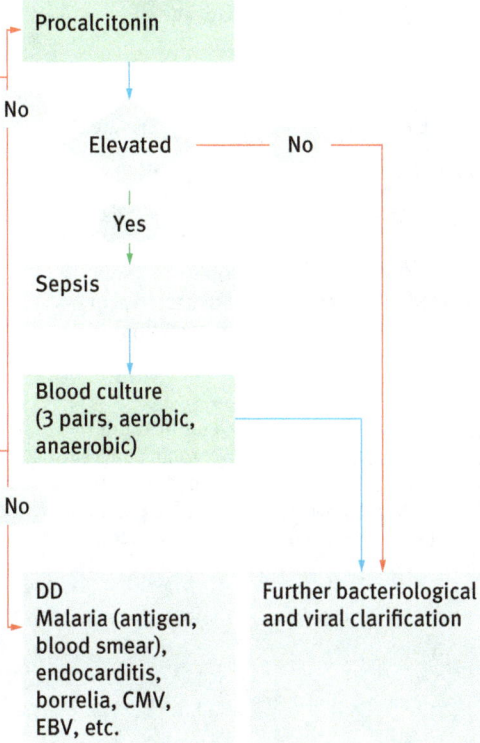

systemic	DD Fever of unknown origin

Procalcitonin

No

Elevated —— No

Yes

Sepsis

Blood culture
(3 pairs, aerobic,
anaerobic)

No

DD
Malaria (antigen,
blood smear),
endocarditis,
borrelia, CMV,
EBV, etc.

Further bacteriological
and viral clarification

Figure 3.3 Fever of unknown origin.

Clinical symptom: Abdominal pain		
Basic diagnostic approach	Hepatic	Biliary	Pancreatic

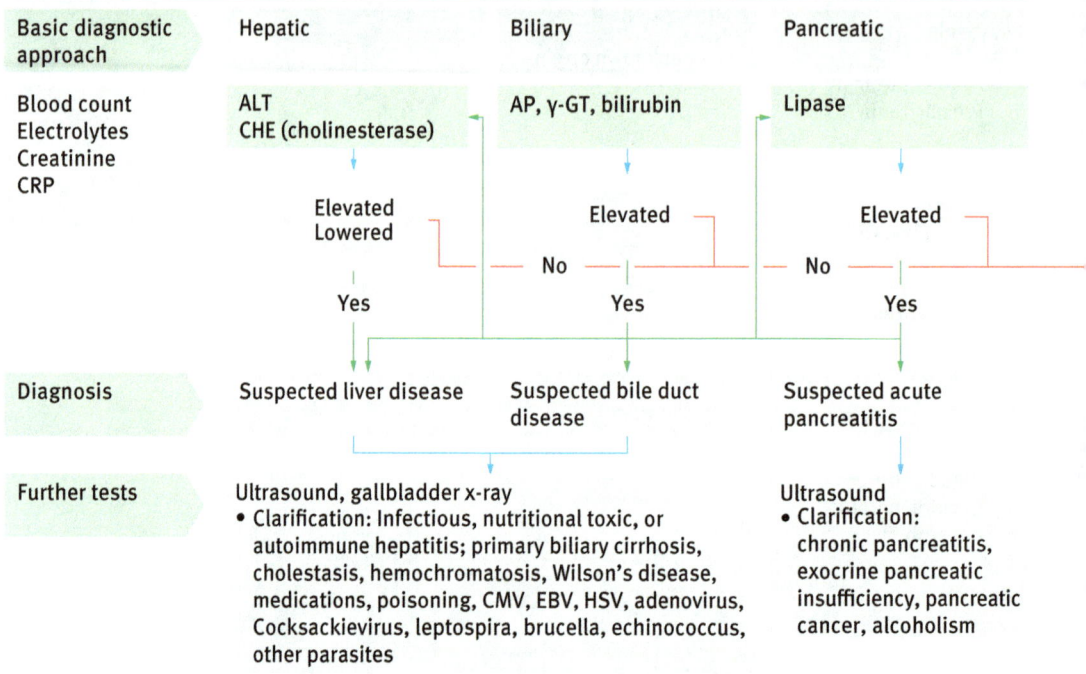

Blood count Electrolytes Creatinine CRP	ALT CHE (cholinesterase)	AP, γ-GT, bilirubin	Lipase
	Elevated Lowered	Elevated	Elevated
	— No —	— No —	— No —
	Yes	Yes	Yes

Diagnosis

	Suspected liver disease	Suspected bile duct disease	Suspected acute pancreatitis

Further tests

Ultrasound, gallbladder x-ray
- Clarification: Infectious, nutritional toxic, or autoimmune hepatitis; primary biliary cirrhosis, cholestasis, hemochromatosis, Wilson's disease, medications, poisoning, CMV, EBV, HSV, adenovirus, Cocksackievirus, leptospira, brucella, echinococcus, other parasites

Ultrasound
- Clarification: chronic pancreatitis, exocrine pancreatic insufficiency, pancreatic cancer, alcoholism

| Mesenteric | Diarrheal Gastrointestinal | Differential diagnosis, abdominal pain |

Lactate

Elevated

No ———————— Stool for blood, albumin, germs, and parasites ——— No

Yes

Blood for IL-6, and if necessary LBP (lipopolysaccharide-binding protein)

Suspected mesenteric infarct

Ultrasound Angiography

Intestinal x-ray
• Clarification: infectious diarrhea, colitis, Crohn's disease, polyposis, gastric ulcers, carcinomas, helminthic diseases

Further DD, e.g., acute porphyria, hypogastric pain

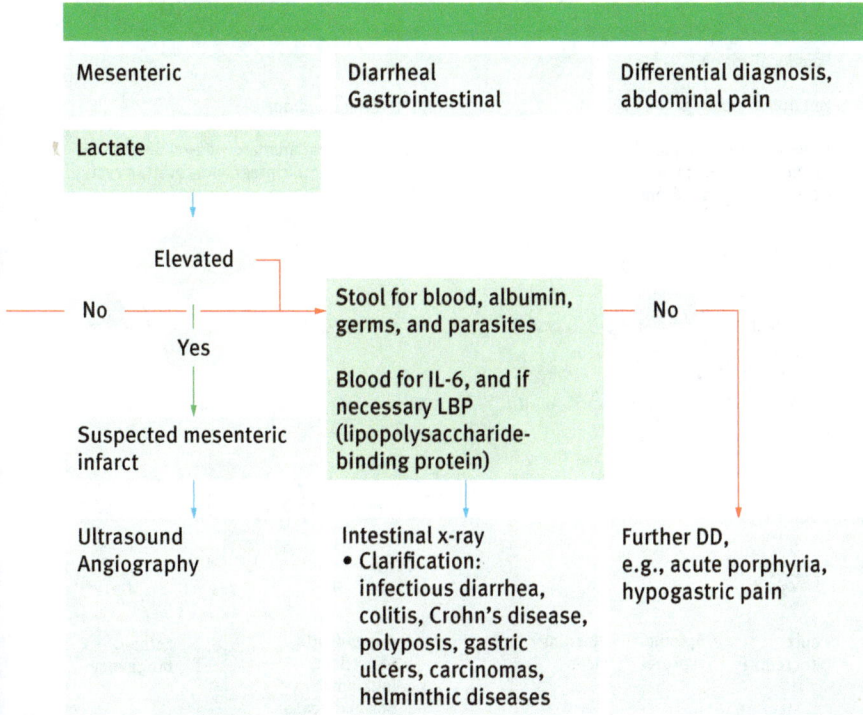

Figure 3.4a Abdominal pain and acute abdomen.

Abdominal Pain Differential Diagnosis by Pain Localization: Acute Abdomen

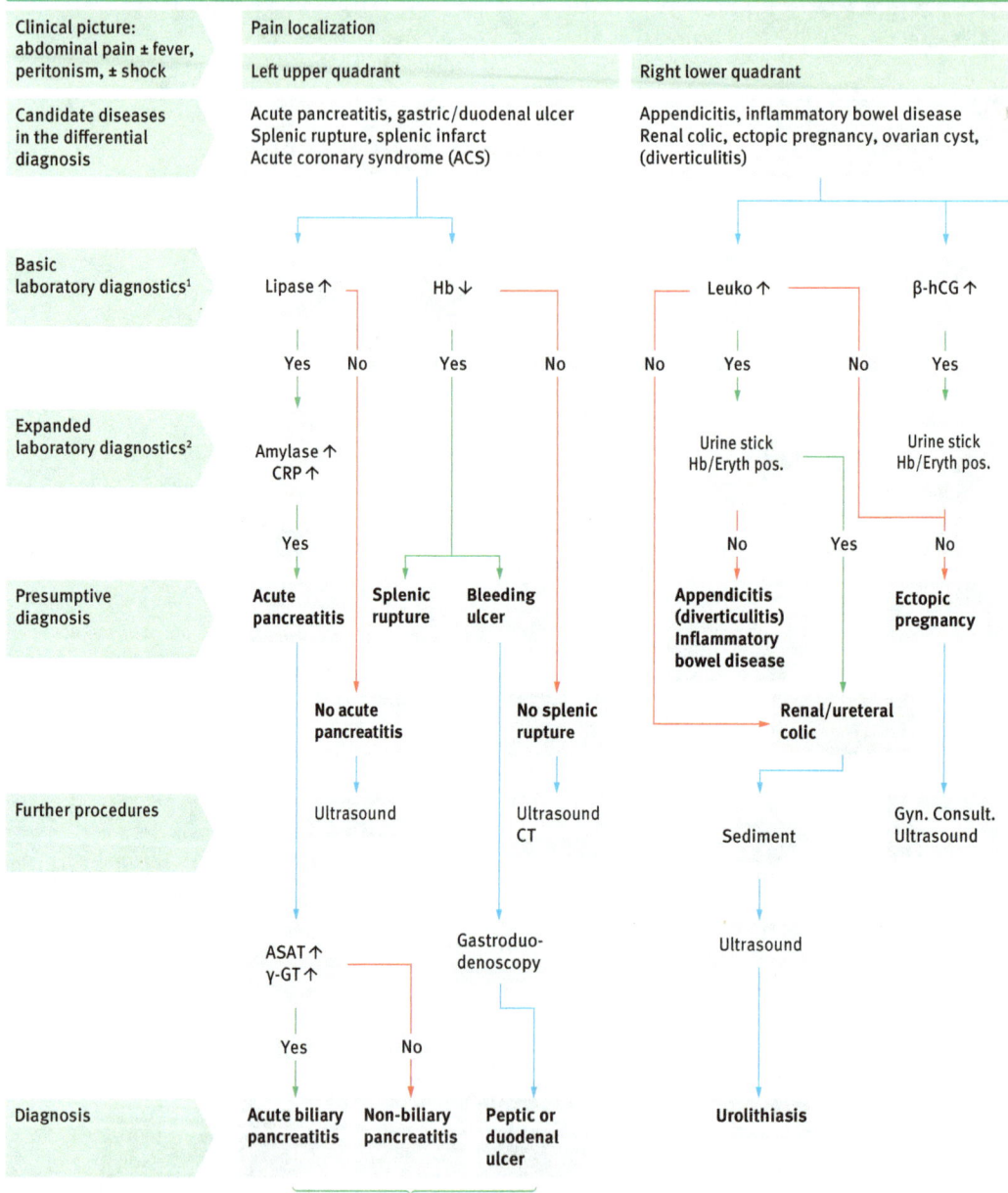

Clinical picture: abdominal pain ± fever, peritonism, ± shock

Pain localization

Left upper quadrant	Right lower quadrant

Candidate diseases in the differential diagnosis

Acute pancreatitis, gastric/duodenal ulcer
Splenic rupture, splenic infarct
Acute coronary syndrome (ACS)

Appendicitis, inflammatory bowel disease
Renal colic, ectopic pregnancy, ovarian cyst,
(diverticulitis)

Basic laboratory diagnostics[1]

Lipase ↑   Hb ↓   Leuko ↑   β-hCG ↑

Yes   No   Yes   No   No   Yes   No   Yes

Expanded laboratory diagnostics[2]

Amylase ↑
CRP ↑

Urine stick   Urine stick
Hb/Eryth pos.   Hb/Eryth pos.

Yes

No   Yes   No

Presumptive diagnosis

Acute   **Splenic**   **Bleeding**
pancreatitis   **rupture**   **ulcer**

Appendicitis   **Ectopic**
(diverticulitis)   **pregnancy**
Inflammatory
bowel disease

No acute   **No splenic**
pancreatitis   **rupture**

Renal/ureteral
colic

Further procedures

Ultrasound   Ultrasound
                  CT

Sediment   Gyn. Consult.
                  Ultrasound

ASAT ↑   Gastroduo-
γ-GT ↑   denoscopy

Ultrasound

Yes   No

Diagnosis

Acute biliary   **Non-biliary**   **Peptic or**
pancreatitis   **pancreatitis** **duodenal**
                                      ulcer

Urolithiasis

see **acute pancreatitis** diagnostic pathway ↗

[1] (Lactate), creatinine, Quick, aPTT, blood test and leukocytes, CRP, Lipase, ALAT, γ-GT, urinalysis, [in women of childbearing age: β-hCG]
[2] AP, ASAT, (GLDH), LDH, blood gas analysis, porphobilinogen

Figure 3.4b Abdominal pain and acute abdomen.

Pain localization

Right upper quadrant	Left lower quadrant	diffuse generalized, intense
Cholecystitis, choledocholithiasis Cholestasis, liver disease Acute coronary syndrome (ACS)	Diverticulitis, inflammatory bowel disease Renal colic, ectopic pregnancy Ovarian cyst	Mesenteric infarct, Mesenteric venous thrombosis, perforation, Subileus/ileus, peritonitis, porphyria

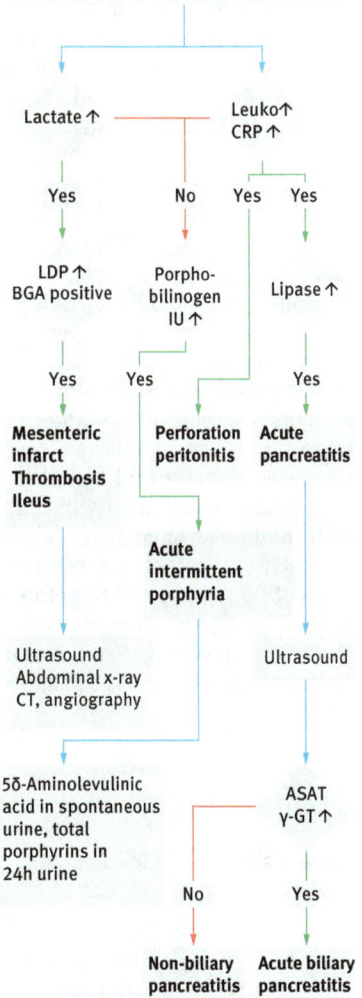

Right upper quadrant

γ-GT ↑ — ALAT ↑

Yes — No — Yes

AP ↑ Bilirubin ↑ / ASAT ↑ (GLDH) ↑

Yes / Yes

Cholestasis Biliary disease / **Liver disease with hepatocellular necrosis**

No cholestasis No acute liver disease

Ultrasound / Ultrasound Hepatitis serology Ruling out toxic damage

ECG Troponin ↑

Yes

Acute coronary syndrome

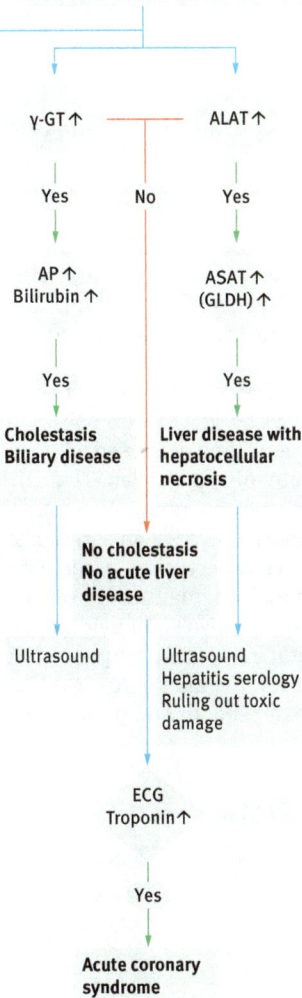

Left lower quadrant

Leuko ↑ — γ-hCG ↑

No — Yes — No — Yes — No

Urine stick Hb/Eryth pos. / Urine stick Hb/Eryth pos.

No / No

Diverticulitis Inflammatory bowel disease / **Ectopic pregnancy**

Renal/ureteral colic

Sediment / Ultrasound CT Endoscopy / Gynecol. consult., ultrasound

Ultrasound / Ruling out ovarian cyst through ultrasound (Gynecol. Consult.)

Urolithiasis

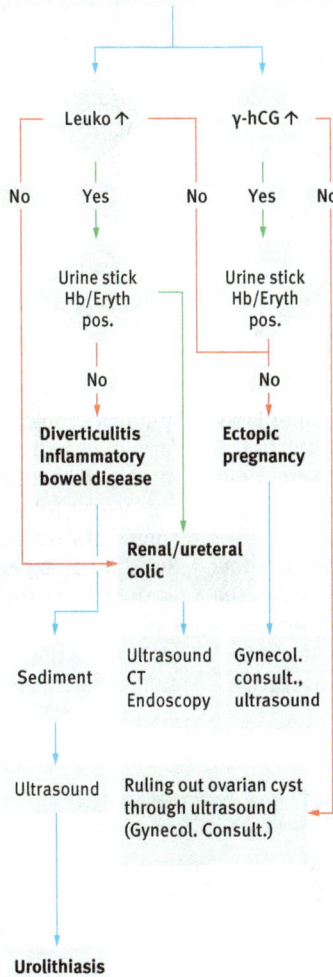

diffuse generalized, intense

Lactate ↑ — Leuko ↑ CRP ↑

Yes — No — Yes — Yes

LDP ↑ BGA positive / Porpho-bilinogen IU ↑ / Lipase ↑

Yes / Yes / Yes

Mesenteric infarct Thrombosis Ileus / **Perforation peritonitis** / **Acute pancreatitis**

Acute intermittent porphyria

Ultrasound Abdominal x-ray CT, angiography / Ultrasound

5δ-Aminolevulinic acid in spontaneous urine, total porphyrins in 24h urine

ASAT γ-GT ↑

No — Yes

Non-biliary pancreatitis / **Acute biliary pancreatitis**

see **acute pancreatitis** diagnostic pathway ↗

Jürgen Hallbach, Fritz Degel, Herbert Desel,
Norbert Felgenhauer

3.2 Acute Poisoning

Acute intoxication in adults in Germany and other European countries is most commonly caused by alcohol and medications (e.g., psychotropic drugs, hypnotics, sedatives, analgesics), but can also be caused by recreational drugs. While deliberate ingestion predominates in adults, the majority of poisonings in children, and particularly in young children, is accidental.

Toxicological analysis is essential for exposure assessment (▶ Figure 3.5). The exposure assessment is the basis for an early and reliable diagnosis and specific therapy decisions in poisoning cases.

Simple toxicological studies along with non-poison-specific basic diagnostic tests should be possible in any emergency laboratory, while more comprehensive toxicological studies usually requires a specialized laboratory (regional laboratory center). In complicated cases with clinical necessity, difficult and complex investigations should be possible at any time, and should normally require no more than 3 hours.

Specific symptoms are present only in a few types of poisoning, and therefore it is rather the clinical toxidrome that provides a rationale to clarify the poisoning. Several examples are presented below that should be adapted to local conditions.

Quantification is not necessary in every case of poisoning because it often does not contribute to clarifying the severity and need for therapy in a toxidrome. However, quantification is indispensable in cases of poisoning in which the blood levels determine the use of specific, expensive and possibly risky treatment measures. Examples of such toxins include: iron, paracetamol, lithium, salicylic acid, carbamazepine, theophylline, phenobarbital, valproate, and digoxin/digitoxin.

In the presence of clinical indications or remarkable preliminary investigations (e.g., osmotic gap, unexplained acidosis, and anion gap), additional noxious substances such as ethylene glycol, glycol, methanol, 4-hydroxybutyric acid (GHB), amanitins, doxepin, amitriptyline, trimipramine, carboxyhemoglobin (COHb) and methemoglobin (MetHb) should also be quantified.

In serious cases, the toxicological analysis findings should always be shared with poison information center experts, and discussed with and interpreted by the attending physician. Thus, the poison control center (poison information center) should always become involved at an early stage. Substantial experience is necessary, particularly in the proper estimation of quantitative results, since the relative timing between individual toxicokinetics and therapeutic/toxic ranges is difficult to assess; moreover, therapeutic/toxic ranges are often procedure dependent and present only

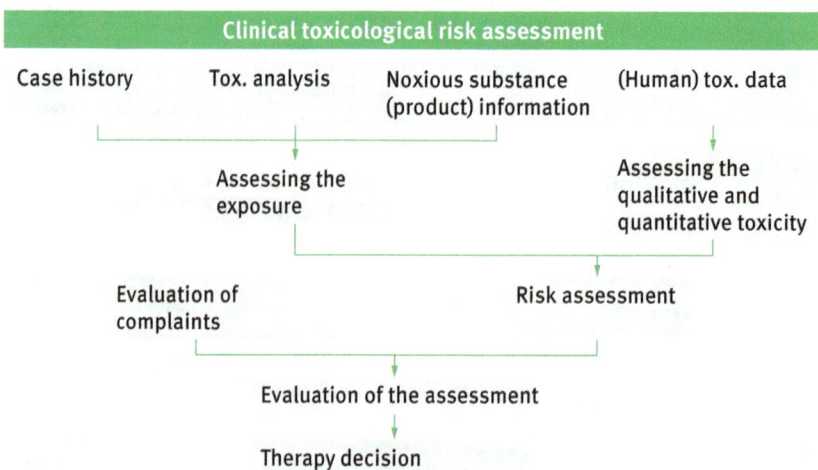

Figure 3.5 Exposure assessment in poisoning cases.

a rough indication of the intoxication risk assessment.

> In immunoassays, the result is positive when it is above a predetermined cut-off value. In Germany, however, there is no commonly agreed definition of these cut-off values. It is therefore necessary to use the respective laboratory cut-off values depending on the specifications of the manufacturer.

> In chromatographic investigations, a positive result means the reliable identification of the corresponding substance. In the case of mass spectrometry, this is done by using retention times and analysis of the mass spectrum. In SIM (single ion monitoring) methods or LC-MS/MS, at least 3 mass traces must be analyzed, i.e., two qualifier ions.

3.2.1 Acute Drug Intoxication

3.2.1.1 Forms and Origins of Acute Drug Intoxication

A drug intoxication can be an accidental overdose, or can be parasuicidal or suicidal. Most of these overdoses are observed in patients with multiple drug abuse. Since the toxicological analysis results are generally not yet available at the primary care stage, targeted and safe antidote treatment will not be possible at that point in time, and only symptomatic treatment can be provided initially. Heroin, methadone, benzodiazepines, alcohol and doxepin (as an often overdosed concomitant medication in the medical treatment of addiction diseases), which all exhibit central nervous system sedative effects, are the most common. These drugs are also sometimes combined with central nervous system stimulating substances, such as cocaine or amphetamines. In terms of drug emergencies, hallucinogenic drugs such as LSD and hallucinogenic mushrooms play a rather subordinate role. A still increasing role in emergency and addiction medicine is being played by gamma-butyrolactone (GBL) and gamma hydroxybutyrate (GHB) (active ingredients in "liquid ecstasy").

Drug Detection Decision Tree

Drug screening (▶ Figure 3.6) usually involves immunochemical analysis of substance groups and individual substances in the urine, and should always be supplemented by a creatinine determination. The lowest possible cut-off values should be selected for the "positive/negative" decision, corresponding to a high sensitivity, and the use of automated immunoassay systems is preferable. According to international directives and recommendations, all positive results must be verified by a second method that is more specific and more sensitive, usually gas chromatography/mass spectrometry. Since these investigations are targeted to specific substances, it is also referred to as "targeted" analysis. In immunoassays, manipulations must necessarily be excluded. At least urinary creatinine should be measured in parallel (indication of dilution), and so-called manipulation tests should be performed if available.

The identification of substances that are undetectable by immunoassay can only be done by an untargeted analysis using chromatography, preferably GCMS. Due to the somewhat limited specificity and sensitivity of immunoassays, a chromatographic investigation should also be carried out even with a negative immunoassay result in cases of persistent suspicion.

In general, quantitative blood test findings hardly ever correlate with the severity of a drug intoxication, while they can be quite valuable in assessing the course. Alternatively, quantification in the urine relative to creatinine can be done for use in assessing the course, wherein the concentration of the identified individual substances must be used as the basis, because depending on metabolism and cross-reactivity of the metabolites, immunochemical group tests can give measurement results indicating an increase even in the absence of renewed consumption. The identified metabolites can also ultimately contribute to the course assessment as, for example, in the metabolism of diamorphine (diacetylmorphine, or heroin) via monoacetylmorphine (MAM) into morphine. If, in addition to diamorphine or its metabolites, small quantities of codeine (-acetylated) are also found in the test sample, this indicates the inclusion of a product made from raw opium (mainly in illegal street heroin). Another example of the importance of detecting metabolites that bears mentioning is that while taking di-

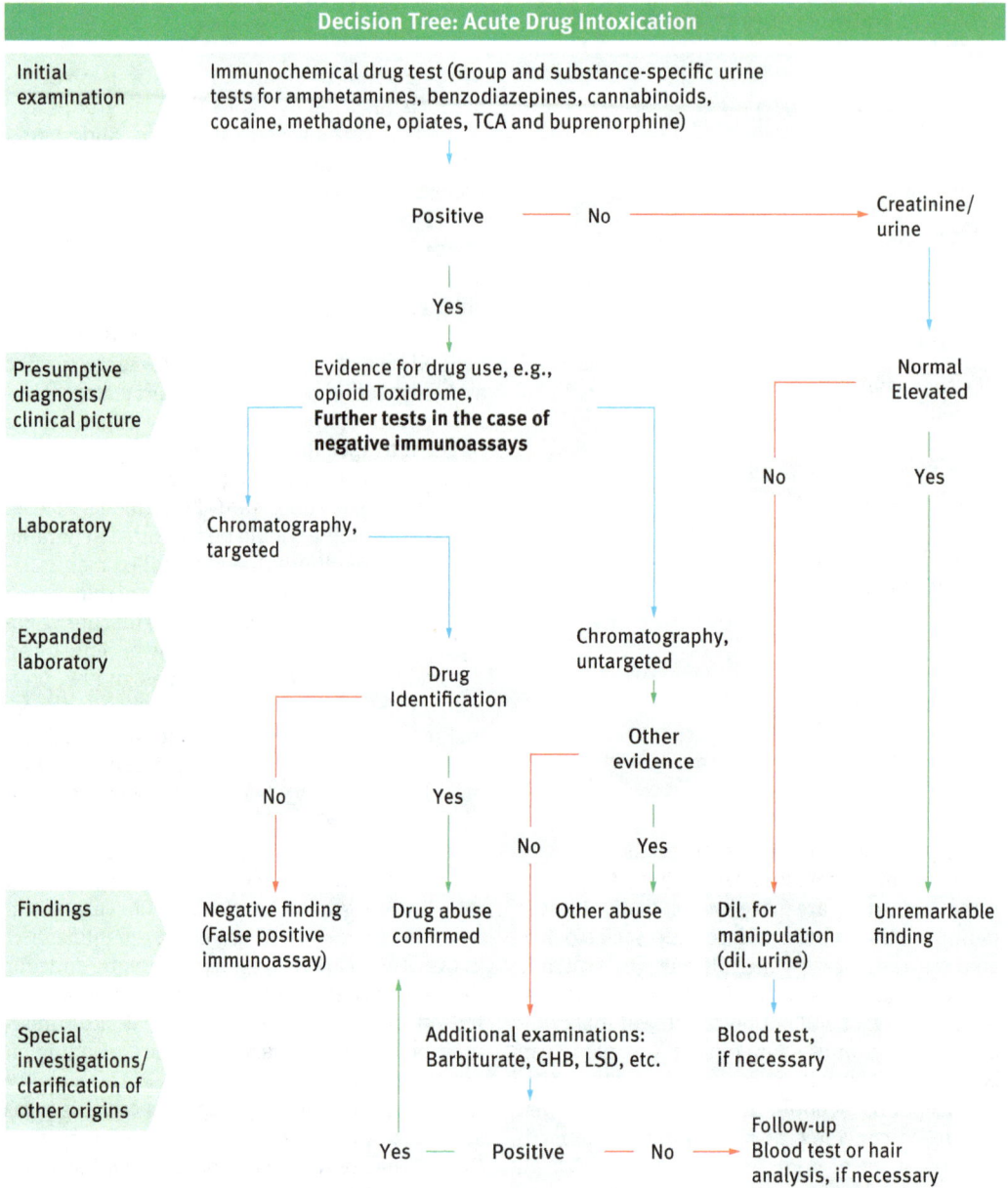

Figure 3.6 Decision Tree: Acute Drug Intoxication.

azepam, nordazepam, oxazepam and temazepam are initially detected as metabolites in the urine, while it is only oxazepam later in the course.

Hair analysis, which can be done with extreme sensitivity today, can also provide evidence of a longer drug history. Thus, in cases of acute drug intoxication, if necessary, it is possible on forensic grounds to distinguish between one-time drug use and prolonged consumption, even after a few weeks.

3.2.2 Toxidromes

Poisoning can lead to a more or less characteristic symptom complex, which is called a toxidrome. This has superseded the formerly used term "cardinal symptoms". Toxidromes usually constitute medical emergencies. Caution is required, however, since mixed drug intoxications can mask typical toxidromes and, *inter alia*, systemic infections can also lead to symptom complexes that closely resemble toxidromes. Thus, general unknown screening should be conducted in all cases of poisoning of unknown origin.

3.2.2.1 Anticholinergic Toxidrome

Forms and origins of the anticholinergic toxidrome

Symptoms: mydriasis (dilated pupils), visual disturbances, somnolence up to coma (delirium), decreased bowel sounds, dry skin, fever, ileus, myoclonus, psychosis, convulsions, and urinary retention ("blind, mad, red, hot, dry, the bowel and the bladder lose their tone, and the heart runs alone").

Complications: hypertension, hyperthermia, tachycardia.

Triggers: antihistamines, phenothiazine antipsychotics, antidepressants, anticholinergic anti-Parkinson agents such as biperidine, scopolamine-containing herbal drugs such as *Brugmansia* (Angel Trumpet).

A very frequently occurring substance from this compound class is diphenhydramine, which is obtainable without a prescription and is used as an antiallergic agent, sleep-inducing drug, and anti-emetic. Typical symptoms of intoxication are dry mouth and mydriasis (as with atropine) and the previously mentioned signs of anticholinergic syndrome (agitation and delirium, tonic-clonic convulsions, hyperthermia, respiratory stimulation followed by paralysis, circulatory collapse, and coma). The central nervous system effects of diphenhydramine are significantly intensified by alcohol and other drugs. Therapeutic measures include pharmacotherapy treatment of the decreased seizure threshold with diazepam, antidote therapy with physostigmine, and supportive intensive care.

Decision tree for anticholinergic toxidrome

There are no specific immunological screening methods for the substances that can lead to an anticholinergic toxidrome. However, due of their cross-reactivity diphenhydramine and doxylamine can often be detected by immunoassays for tricyclic antidepressants, but care must be taken because of quite different cross-reactivities of the individual substances in the available test systems (▶ Figure 3.7).

The validation and differentiation of positive findings, as well as expansion of the analysis with a negative immunoassay, requires chromatographic screening to be performed, preferably on urine and serum. Among the substances that lead to an anticholinergic syndrome, there are fortunately no representatives that evade detection under general unknown screening.

To the extent that it is necessary for making treatment decisions, the screening should also be oriented toward the quantification (semiquantitative examination) of the substances found.

3.2.2.2 Cholinergic Toxidrome

Forms and origins of the cholinergic toxidrome

Symptoms: salivation, bronchial exudation, bronchospasms, diarrhea, defecation, vomiting, miosis, muscle cramps, and central convulsions.

Complications: bradycardia, hypothermia, need for mechanical ventilation.

Triggers: organophosphates (only alkyl phosphates: insecticides and nerve agents), carbamates (only insecticides, usually methyl substituted active ingredients), muscarine (fungal toxin from the red-staining inocybe).

Decision tree for cholinergic toxidrome

A simple preliminary test for organophosphates and carbamates is the determination of cholinesterase (CHE) in the serum or plasma (▶ Abb. 3.8). Serum cholinesterase is similar to the toxicologically relevant target molecule of these agents, acetylcholinesterase (AChE), and is significantly inhibited. A remarkably lower CHE can corroborate suspected intoxication through measurement of the erythrocyte ACHE in dilute, hemolyzed whole blood. The CHE and hemoglobin (Hb) must be determined simultaneously.

Decision Tree: anticholinergic toxidrome

Initial examination

Symptomatic or immunochemical detection of tricyclic antidepressants inter alia (Note: maprotiline is poorly detectable)

Positive ⸺ No

Yes

Presumptive diagnosis/ clinical picture

Persistent anticholinergic toxidrome even with a possibly negative immunoassay result ⸺ Yes

Laboratory

No

Chromatography/urine, semiquantitative determination in serum if necessary

Untargeted chromatographic screening in the urine

In the toxic range ⸺ Positive

No · Yes · No · Yes

Expanded laboratory

Quantitative follow-up study if necessary

Semiquantitative determination in serum

In the toxic range

Yes · No

Findings

No indication of poisoning/ long-standing poisoning

Anticholinergic syndrome in poisoning with...

Other poisoning with...

No ⸺ Persistent unclear symptoma- tology ⸺ Yes

Substance detection without toxicity

Special examinations/ clarification of other origins

Expanded toxicological screening, poison control center, regional toxicological laboratory; Note: continuous ECG monitoring necessary, early contact with poison control center

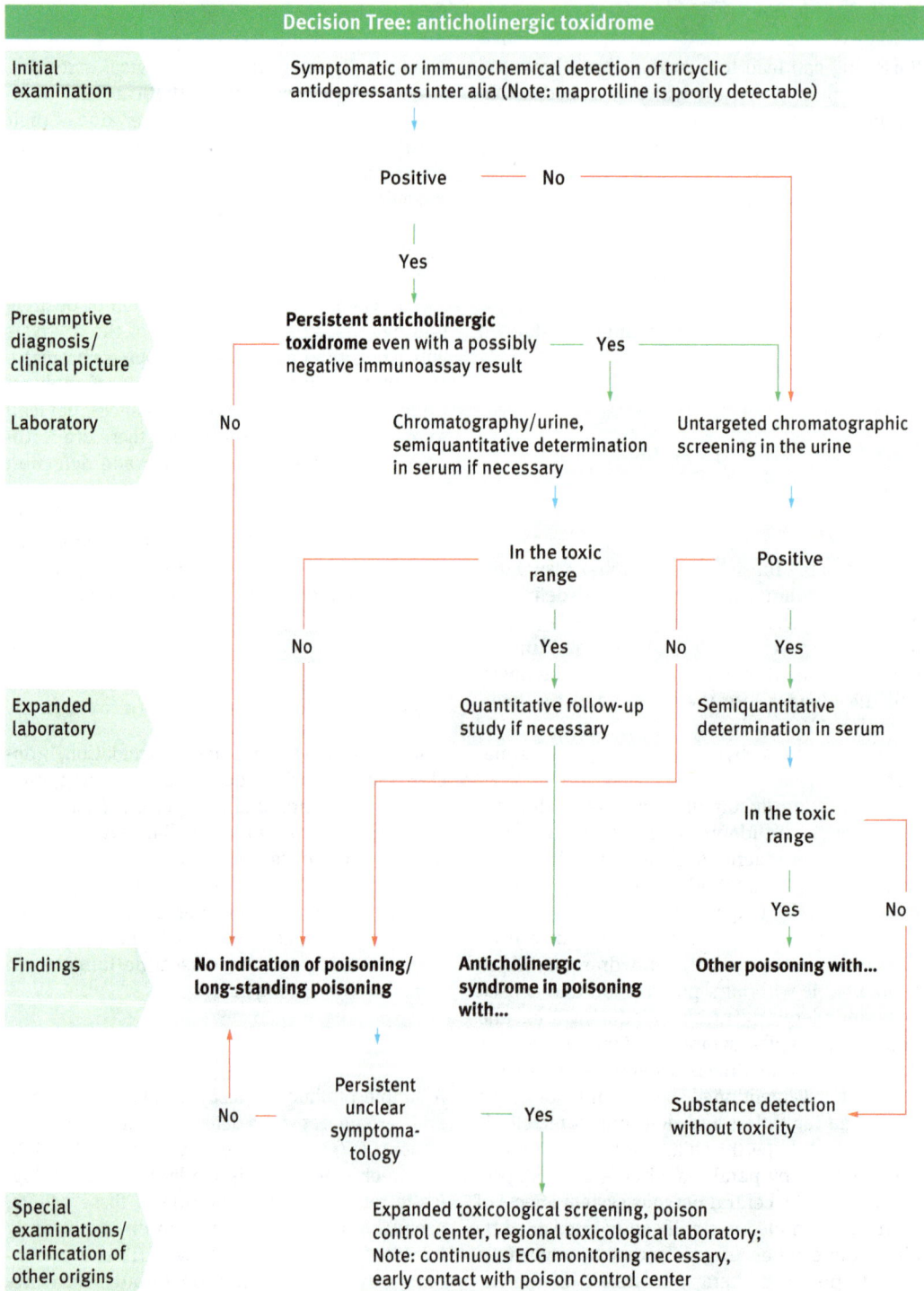

Figure 3.7 Decision Tree: anticholinergic toxidrome.

| Decision Tree: Cholinergic toxidrome. |

Initial examination

Serum cholinesterase

Positive —— No

Yes

Presumptive diagnosis/ clinical picture

Persistent cholinergic toxidrome even with a possibly normal CHE result —— Yes

Laboratory

No

Targeted chromatographic screening

Untargeted chromatographic screening in the urine

No

Positive

Positive

Yes

No

Yes

Expanded laboratory

Semiquantitative determination in serum

In the toxic range

Yes   No

Findings

No indication of poisoning/ long-standing poisoning

Cholinergic syndrome in poisoning with...

Other poisoning with...

No —— Persistent unclear symptomatology —— Yes

Substance detection without toxicity

Special examinations/ clarification of other origins

Expanded toxicological screening, chemical warfare agent verification (*vide supra* , poison control center, regional toxicological laboratory; Note: Early contact with poison control center

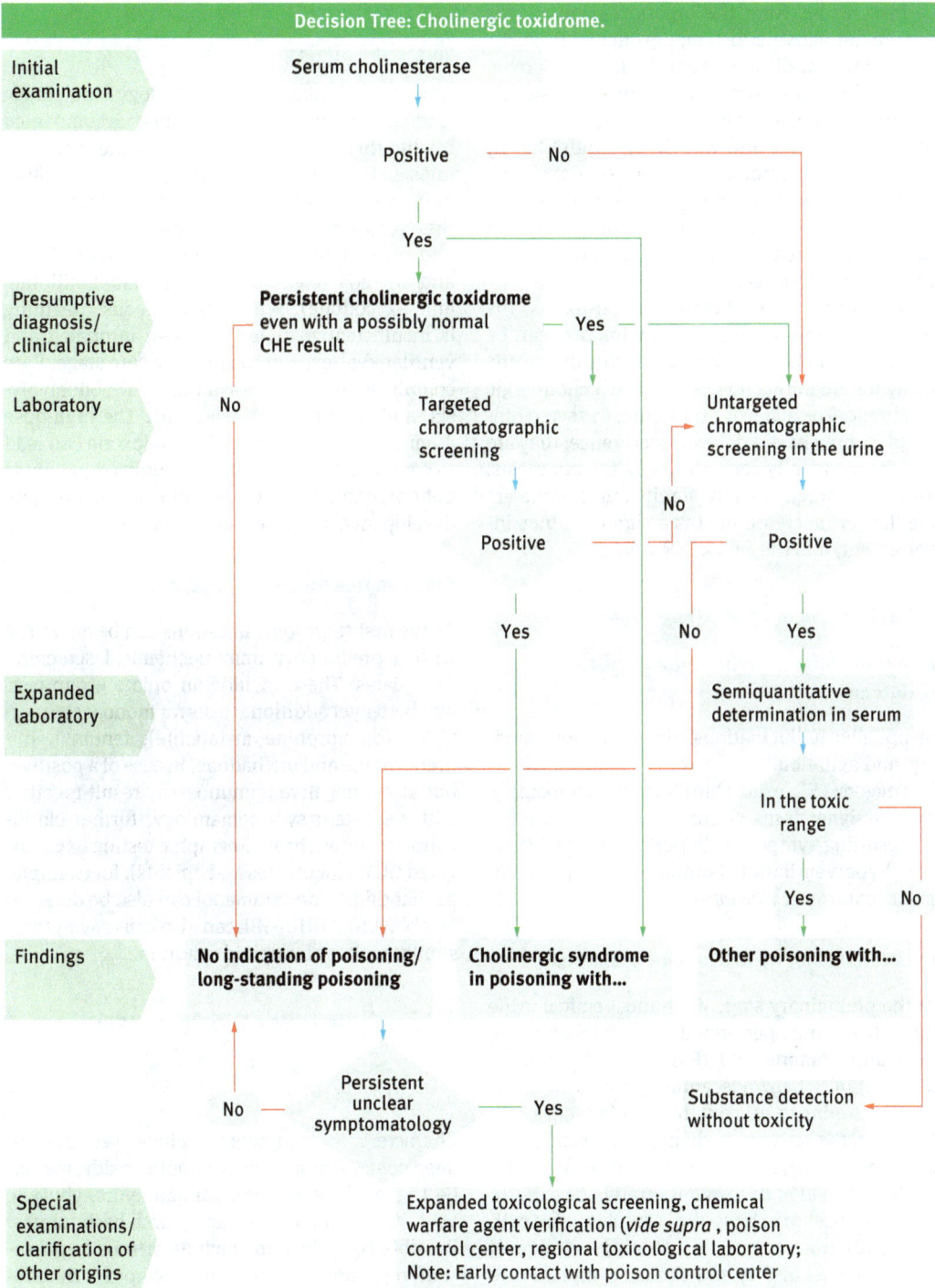

Figure 3.8 Decision Tree: Cholinergic toxidrome.

Insecticides from the organophosphate and carbamate active substance groups can be detected quite well by General Unknown Screening, while the measurement of chemical warfare agents in biological samples is a substantial analytical challenge and will likely require highly specialized laboratories. The detection of chemical warfare agents in biological samples is used only infrequently for therapeutic purposes, and rather more often for the verification of possible chemical warfare agent use.

Nota bene: In the field of fungal toxins, the only amanitin-related fungal toxins that can be detected in an ELISA-based laboratory diagnostic assay for amanitins do not occur in a cholinergic syndrome. The signs of liver failure in severe fungal poisoning have a delayed occurrence; they are not diagnostically relevant, only for prognosis. Thus, the prognostically significant parameters are the serum creatinine (as a sign of kidney involvement) and the Quick INR value.

3.2.2.3 Hallucinogenic Toxidrome

Forms and origins of the hallucinogenic toxidrome

Symptoms: hallucinations, disorientation, anxiety, and agitation.

Triggers: LSD, psilocybin ("magic mushrooms"), some designer drugs, cocaine.

Resulting symptoms: hypertension, tachycardia, hyperventilation (similar to sympathomimetic toxidrome, *vide infra*).

Decision tree for hallucinogenic toxidrome

At the preliminary stage, immunochemical urine drug tests are performed for amphetamine, methamphetamine and derivatives, cocaine or its metabolite benzoylecgonine, and LSD, along with creatinine to rule out dilution (▶ Figure 3.9). However, the active ingredients of hallucinogenic mushrooms (psilocybin) or even mescaline cannot be detected in this way. It is rarely possible to detect psilocybin in biological samples, even with the aid of chromatographic screening techniques, so the medical history and clinical symptoms are particularly diagnostically significant in this case. By contrast, it is a simple matter to detect the active substance residues in drug samples held for evidence.

3.2.2.4 Opiate/Opioid Toxidrome

Forms and origins of the opioid toxidrome

Opioid poisoning symptomatology can range from somnolence to deep coma, accompanied by life-threatening respiratory depression and miosis. Possible complications include pulmonary edema and circulatory shock. Triggers of this toxidrome include diamorphine (heroin) and other opiates (e.g., morphine and codeine) and opioids (e.g., fentanyl, tramadol, tilidine, and oxycodone). When spontaneous breathing is insufficient, patients are often intubated and ventilated already at the primary care stage. Rare complications include aspiration, rhabdomyolysis, and compartment syndrome. The high-dose administration of the antidote naloxone can lead to complications, because the addicted patient is not only rapidly awakened but can also abruptly develop an acute withdrawal syndrome.

Decision tree for opioid toxidrome

As the first step, some questions can be answered with a preliminary immunochemical screening for opiates. These include an opiate group test, and better yet additional tests for monoacetylmorphine (diamorphine metabolite), fentanyl, buprenorphine and methadone. In case of a positive, but also a negative immunoassay result together with persistent symptomatology, further clarification requires chromatographic testing (e.g., targeted GCMS for opiates and opioids), for example, so that tilidine and tramadol can also be detected (▶ Abb. 3.10). GHB/GBL can also cause symptoms similar to those for opioid syndrome.

3.2.2.5 Sedative/Hypnotic Toxidrome

Forms and origins of the sedative/hypnotic toxidrome

Characteristic symptoms include sedation to deep coma. The sedative/hypnotic toxidrome can be triggered by ethanol, gamma-hydroxybutyric acid (GHB), anticonvulsants, and barbiturates. Possible complications include arterial hypotension, respiratory depression up to apnea, rhabdomyolysis, and compartment syndrome.

Even benzodiazepines and benzodiazepine-like substances such as zopiclone, zolpidem and zaleplon frequently cause a sedative/

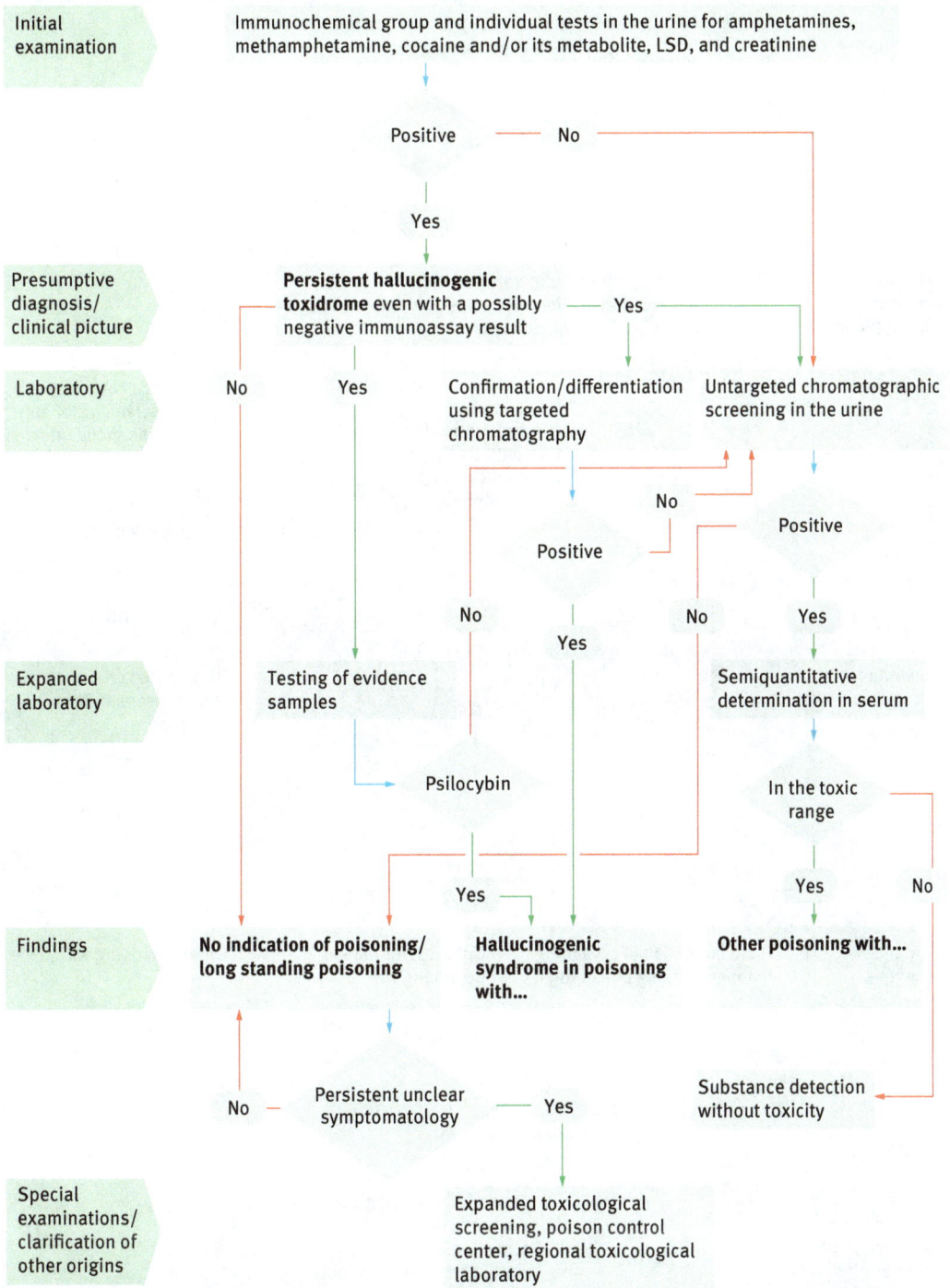

Decision Tree: Hallucinogenic toxidrome

Initial examination
Immunochemical group and individual tests in the urine for amphetamines, methamphetamine, cocaine and/or its metabolite, LSD, and creatinine

Positive — No

Yes

Presumptive diagnosis/ clinical picture
Persistent hallucinogenic toxidrome even with a possibly negative immunoassay result — Yes

Laboratory
No   Yes   Confirmation/differentiation using targeted chromatography   Untargeted chromatographic screening in the urine

No

Positive   Positive

No   No   Yes

Expanded laboratory
Testing of evidence samples   Semiquantitative determination in serum

Yes

Psilocybin   In the toxic range

Yes   No

Findings
No indication of poisoning/ long standing poisoning   Yes   **Hallucinogenic syndrome in poisoning with...**   **Other poisoning with...**

No —   Persistent unclear symptomatology   — Yes   Substance detection without toxicity

Special examinations/ clarification of other origins
Expanded toxicological screening, poison control center, regional toxicological laboratory

Figure 3.9 Decision Tree: Hallucinogenic toxidrome.

Decision Tree: Opioid toxidrome

Initial examination

Immunochemical group urine tests for opiates, fentanyl, buprenorphine, and methadone

Positive —— No

Yes

Presumptive diagnosis/ clinical picture

Persistent sedative/hypnotic toxidrome even with a possibly negative immunoassay —— Yes

Laboratory

No

Confirmation/ differentiation using targeted chromatography —— No

Untargeted chromatographic screening for opiates/opioids in the urine

Yes —— Positive

Yes

No

Expanded laboratory

Untargeted chromatographic screening in the urine

No —— Positive

Yes

Findings

No indication of poisoning/ long-standing poisoning

Opioid syndrome in poisoning with...

Other poisoning with...

No —— Persistent unclear symptomatology —— Yes

Special examinations/ clarification of other origins

Expanded toxicological screening, poison control center, regional toxicological laboratory; Note: Early contact of poison control center if possible

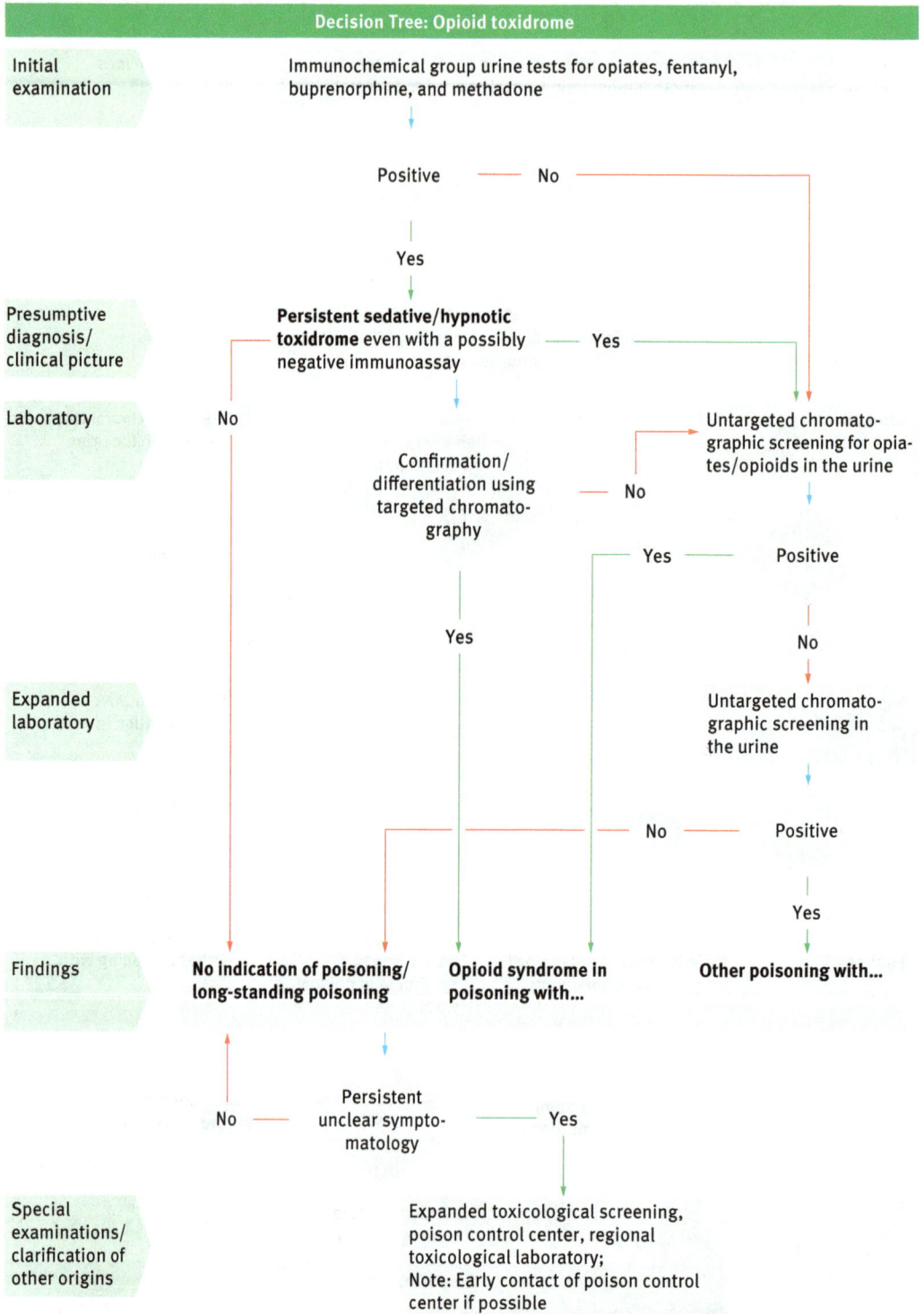

Figure 3.10 Decision Tree: Opioid toxidrome.

hypnotic toxidrome. However, with one-time and oral administration of these agents, the symptoms will almost always be limited to deep sedation.

Decision tree for sedative/hypnotic toxidrome

The most important initial examination is the enzymatic determination of ethanol in the serum (ADH method). In addition, it should be feasible in the first step to perform immunochemical group tests for barbiturates, especially for benzodiazepines in the serum and/or urine, and TDM tests for common anticonvulsants. It is important to note that some of benzodiazepines are detectable in the urine only after hydrolysis of the conjugated metabolites (▶ Abb. 3.11).

Targeted GCMS analysis is used to confirm the screening results, and if it is necessary to expand the investigation to other anticonvulsants. These studies, and an enzymatic preliminary investigation of GHB if deemed necessary, as well as their confirmations by GCMS, will be conducted at the regional laboratory center.

3.2.2.6 Sympathomimetic Toxidrome

Forms and origins of the sympathomimetic toxidrome

A sympathomimetic toxidrome can be indicated by hyperhidrosis, dehydration, hypertension, tachycardia, tremors, agitation, generalized seizures, coma, anxiety, confusion, hallucinations and mydriasis. The clinical appearance resembles an anticholinergic syndrome. However, there are significant differences in the sympathomimetic toxidrome, especially wet skin and profuse sweating. The responsible noxious substances include amphetamine or methamphetamine and analogs, phenylpropanolamines, cocaine, ephedrine and pseudoephedrine, as well as more recently cathinone and piperazine derivatives. Complications arise in the form of cardiac arrhythmias and acute coronary syndrome.

Decision tree for sympathomimetic toxidrome

As a first step, urine immunoassays can be run for amphetamine, methamphetamine and derivatives, as well as cocaine and/or its metabolite. However, a number of designer drugs, phenyl-propanolamines, and possibly also ephedrine/pseudoephedrine will not be detected in this way. Thus, a chromatographic analysis will be required at the earliest possible opportunity (▶ Figure 3.12).

3.2.3 Acute Poisoning of Unknown Origin

3.2.3.1 Forms and Origins of Acute Poisoning of Unknown Origin

Acute poisoning is a frequent reason for emergency room admissions in hospitals. The clinical approach begins with an investigation of the external circumstances and screening for toxidromes. However, restriction to toxidromes and frequently occurring poisons can lead to a misdiagnosis; careful consideration is necessary, and with possible reconsideration during the course. Thus, general unknown screening should be performed early on in any acute illness situation in question. Severe poisoning requires rapid and targeted action. However, the practice of emergency medicine is always caught in the dilemma that decisions must be made quite rapidly, often without sufficient information being available. The clinical course and prognosis are decisively influenced by the emergency measures taken, detection of the toxin, and prompt administration of the appropriate treatment. Qualitative blood and urine investigations can help to confirm toxin ingestion, although only for relatively few substances do specific therapeutic decisions require quantitative testing.

3.2.3.2 Decision Tree for Acute Poisoning of Unknown Origin

For toxicological analysis, serum/plasma (3 mL) and urine (10 mL), and possibly other evidence samples, should always be obtained (▶ Figure 3.13).

Analytics in acute care hospitals: in accordance with international recommendations, qualitative testing for cocaine, opiates, amphetamines, tricyclic antidepressants, paraquat and, if necessary, benzodiazepines and cannabinoids, should be possible in every hospital that receives poisoning patients (Hallbach, et al., 2009). Barbiturates, propoxyphene and phencyclidine, also referred to here, currently play only a minor role in Germany. Additionally, quantitative testing for

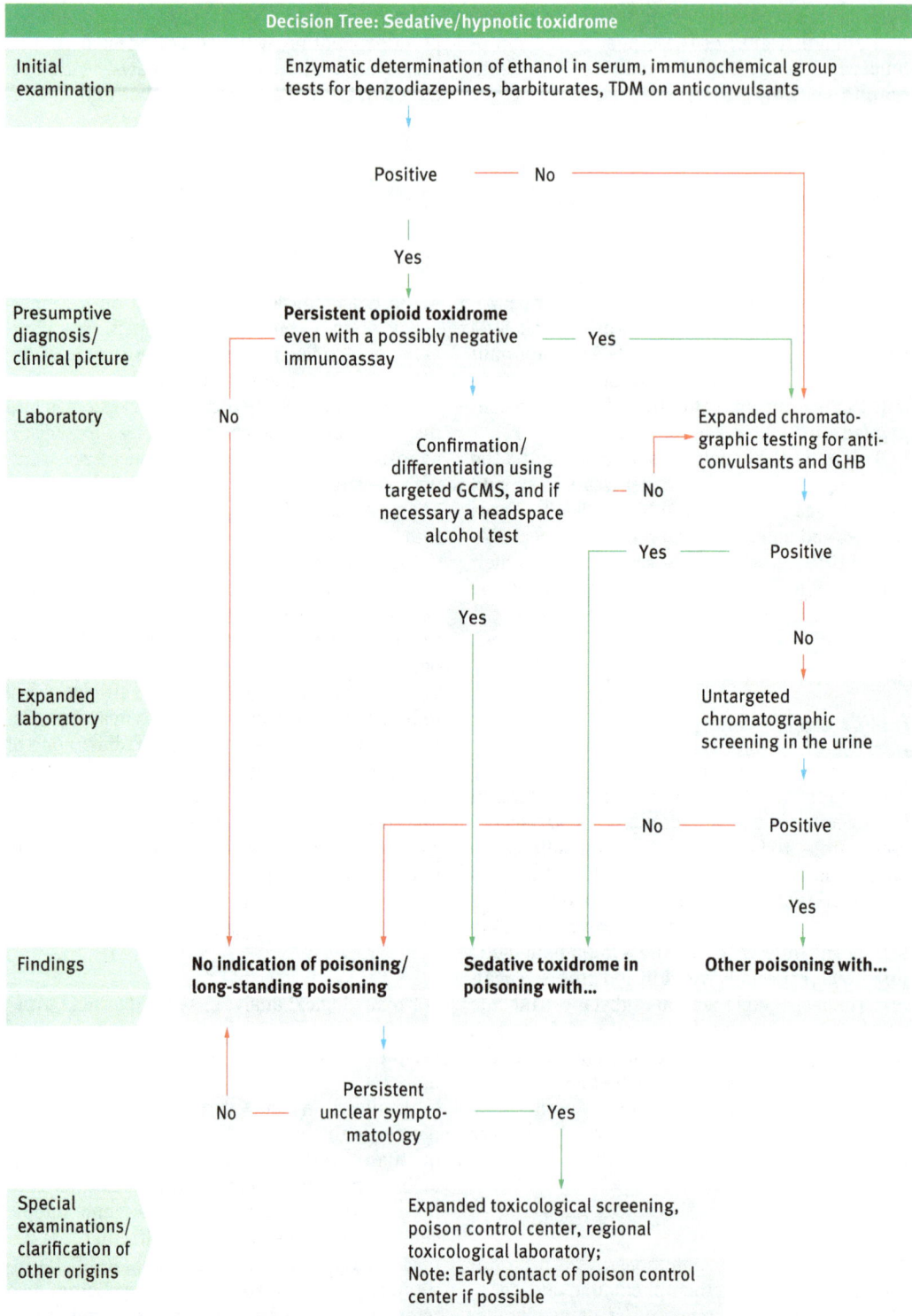

Figure 3.11 Decision Tree: Sedative/hypnotic toxidrome.

Decision Tree: Sympathomimetic toxidrome

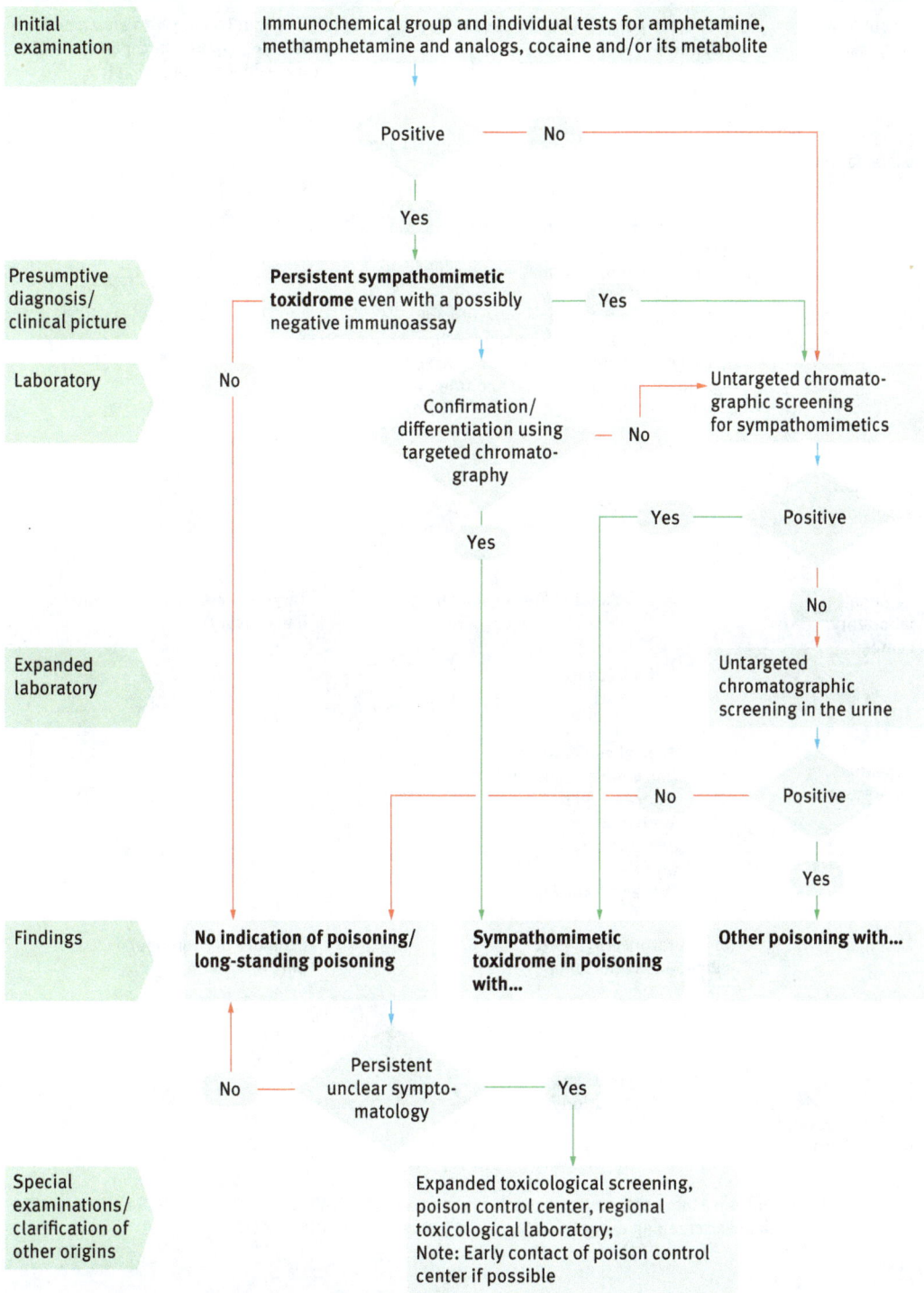

Initial examination

Immunochemical group and individual tests for amphetamine, methamphetamine and analogs, cocaine and/or its metabolite

Positive — No

Yes

Presumptive diagnosis/ clinical picture

Persistent sympathomimetic toxidrome even with a possibly negative immunoassay — Yes

Laboratory

No

Confirmation/ differentiation using targeted chromatography

— No

Untargeted chromatographic screening for sympathomimetics

Yes — Positive

Yes

No

Expanded laboratory

Untargeted chromatographic screening in the urine

No — Positive

Yes

Findings

No indication of poisoning/ long-standing poisoning

Sympathomimetic toxidrome in poisoning with...

Other poisoning with...

No — Persistent unclear symptomatology — Yes

Special examinations/ clarification of other origins

Expanded toxicological screening, poison control center, regional toxicological laboratory;
Note: Early contact of poison control center if possible

Figure 3.12 Decision Tree: Sympathomimetic toxidrome.

Decision Tree: Acute Poisoning of Unknown Origin

Presumptive diagnosis	**Suspected poisoning without specific indications**
	Suspected poisoning with substance-specific indications (third-party medical history, evidence samples, etc.)

Initial examination

a) Basic clinical chemistry laboratory

b) Qualitative testing for: cocaine, opiates, amphetamines, tricyclic antidepressants, paraquat, and possibly benzodiazepines and cannabinoids

c) Quantitative testing for: paracetamol, lithium, salicylates, COHb and metHb, theophylline, valproic acid, carbamazepine, digoxin, phenobarbital, iron and transferrin, as well as ethanol

If necessary, testing from c)

Persistent suspicion

Positive — Yes

No

Regional laboratory center

General unknown screening *

Targeted analysis (quantitative, if necessary)

If necessary

Positive

Positive

Expanded laboratory

Specialized testing (third-party laboratory, if necessary) for:
Methanol
GHB and GBL
Glycols
Oral antidiabetics

No

Yes

Yes

No

Findings

No laboratory diagnostic indications of poisoning

Evidence of overdose/ poisoning with...

Special examinations/ clarification of other origins

Prognostic parameters, e.g., lactate determination

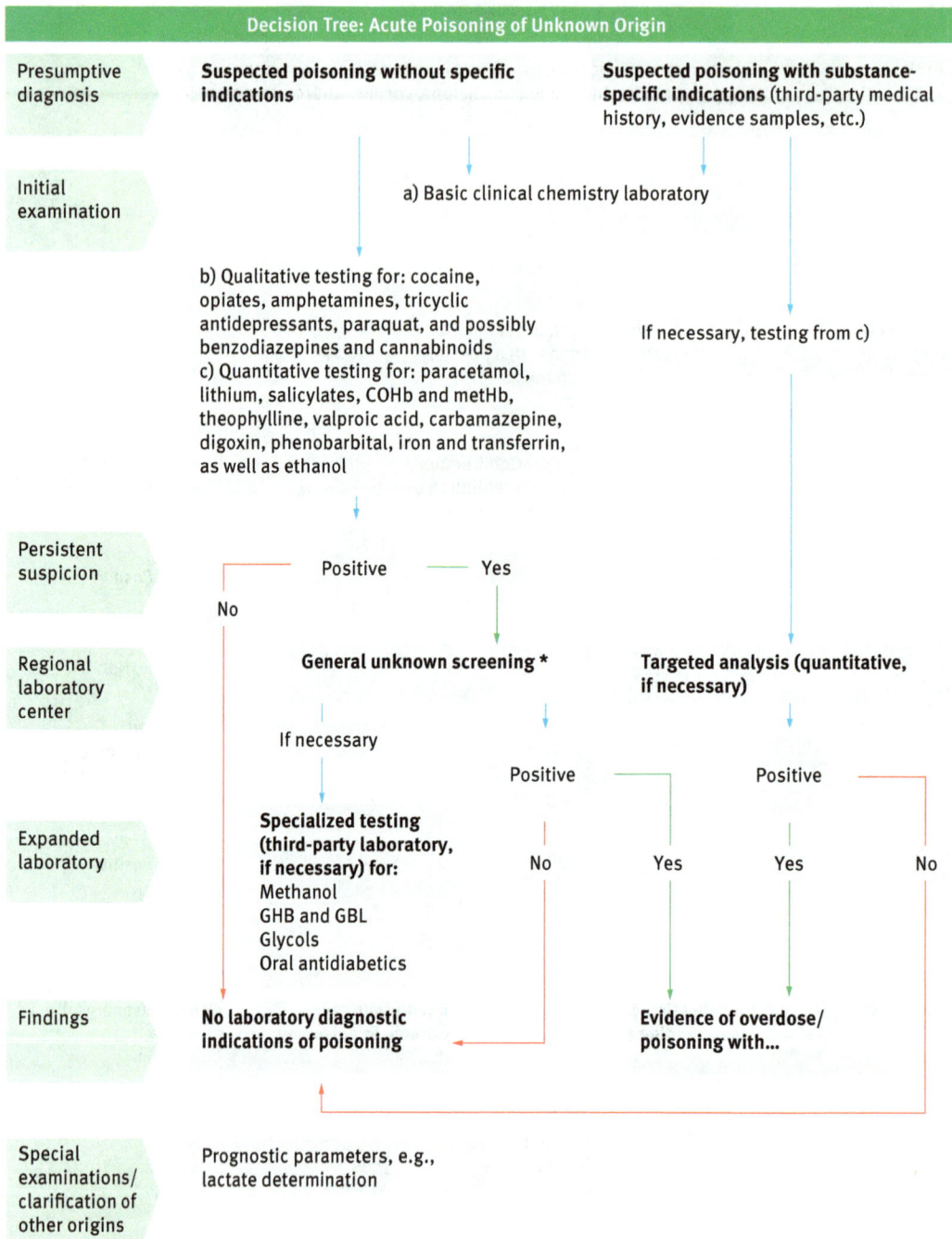

Figure 3.13 Decision Tree: acute poisoning of unknown origin; * General unknown screening using GC/MS and/or HPLC-DAD and/or HPLC-MS/MS and/or LC-MS (QTrap) and/or HPLC/MS-Q-TOF.

acetaminophen, lithium, salicylates, COHb and metHb, theophylline, valproic acid, carbamazepine, digoxin, phenobarbital, iron and transferrin, as well as ethanol, should be performed within one hour. It is desirable for this also to be done for methanol, GHB and GBL, and ethylene glycol, among other compounds. Unfortunately, though, this is currently not feasible everywhere, so that this testing must frequently be done at regional laboratories.

Analysis in a regional laboratory center: General unknown analysis is the real challenge in clinical toxicological analysis. It is indispensable in all severe cases, and in making high-risk treatment decisions. The general unknown screening method of choice is an untargeted, broadly based chromatographic approach that is capable of comprehensive testing for drugs and other substances in the urine and serum. The performance limits of the process must be known. The use of GCMS analysis is preferred based on the many years of experience and the availability of excellent and comprehensive spectral libraries. High-pressure liquid chromatographic methods (HPLC-DAD, HPLC-MS/MS, HPLC-MS (QTrap) and HPLC/MS-TOF) can be employed in a complementary manner, especially since they offer better detection, even of substances that are difficult to extract and thermolabile. These liquid chromatography/ mass spectrometry methods are now increasingly used in the first instance, since they can be performed with little sample preparation and smaller sample volumes, and additionally have higher identification power than does GC/MS analysis. For example, high-resolution mass spectrometry techniques such as HPLC-MS-TOF determine the exact molecular weight, and thus have particularly high identification power.

There are a few types of poisoning in the general unknown screening category that cannot be detected, but these cause relatively unique symptoms and on forensic grounds can be confirmed by at least qualitative tests. These include poisoning with cyanide, LSD, antidiabetics, hydroxycoumarins (superwarfarins), psilocybin, phosphine, botulinum toxin, ricin, and paraquat. Unfortunately, the tests required are only available in a few laboratories.

Any substance is a potential poison at some dose, and even the most modern chromatographic analysis systems cannot be expected to detect every conceivable substance. More important is the communication between the clinicians, poison control center staff, and analysts to enable the choice of a more targeted analytical strategy, possibly based on clinical indications for certain substances. Obviously, with very specific indications for a certain type of poisoning, a targeted and possibly quantitative analysis can rapidly provide useful guidance for treatment. Very rare or difficult special investigations (e.g., for oral antidiabetic drugs) should be delegated to the appropriate specialized laboratories where necessary.

Unlike in forensics or in drug screening outside the emergency medicine context, a confirmatory analysis is not always necessary before making diagnostic and treatment decisions. However, unconfirmed findings must be made clearly identifiable as such.

In evaluating the progression and making a prognosis, high expectations are frequently placed on monitoring blood levels, but the predictive power is often severely limited by missing information and various other factors, including the therapeutic measures performed. More prognostic significance can be found in the more general laboratory parameters that enable assessments of organ function and serve as more general outcome markers, such as creatinine (kidney function) or coagulation parameters (liver function), BNP (heart function), and especially lactate according to a recent study (Manini, et al., 2010).

Literature

Hallbach J, Degel F, Desel H and Felgenhauer N. Analytical role in clinical toxicology: impact on the diagnosis and treatment of poisoned patients. J Lab Med 2009; 33(2): 71–87 (online only).

Kuelpmann WR, editor. Clinical Toxicological Analysis. Wiley-Blackwell 2009.

Felgenhauer N, Hallbach J. Toxikologie, Vergiftungen, Drogenscreening. In: Praktische Labordiagnostik, H. Renz, Hrsg., de Gruyter 2009.

Manini A F, Kumar A, Olson D, Vlahov D and Hoffman R S. Utility of serum lactate to predict drug-overdose fatality. Clinical Toxicology 2010; 48: 730–736.

Table 3.1 Clinical findings for the analysis of extravascular fluids.

Material	Symptoms, findings, presumptive diagnoses
Cerebrospinal fluid fistula	Meningitis, brain abscess, dysosmia, cephalalgia
Pleural effusion	Dyspnea, chest pain, cough
Pericardial effusion	Retrosternal pain, progressive heart failure, cough
Chyle	Dyspnea, cyanosis, respiratory failure
Ascites	Increase in girth and weight, dyspnea, elevation of the diaphragm
Peritoneal dialysate	Abdominal pain, rebound tenderness, fever

Eray Yagmur

3.3 Extravascular Fluids

Physiologically speaking, the extravascular spaces contain only a few milliliters of liquid, so that in principle any extravascular fluid accessible by puncture can reflect a pathological process with clinical symptomatology (▶ Table 3.1).

Thus, laboratory examination of the aspirate or effusion contributes substantially to confirming the working clinical diagnosis and assessment of the therapeutic outcome. The identification of extravascular fluids also provides information on their place of origin and makes a further contribution to the clinical diagnosis. Furthermore, from the extravascular spaces can also be obtained analytical test samples that for therapeutic reasons had previously been installed in the extravascular space. Thus, the clinical chemical and cellular testing of drainage dialysate is a safe procedure for the early detection of life-threatening peritonitis in peritoneal dialysis (PD) patients. The analysis of aspirates/wound secretions, effusions, and drainage samples begins with a sensitive preanalysis, which will influence interpretation of the laboratory findings. A visual assessment of the color and visual appearance of the material should be made immediately upon receipt in the laboratory. The subsequent analytical phase can be divided into the clinical chemical analysis and cell/corpuscle analysis. Together with the assessment of sample appearance, the clinical chemical analysis of extravascular fluids from native samples facilitates the distinction between transudate and exudate. If necessary, a timely venous blood draw should be performed. Thus, to increase the diagnostic value of the analysis, the aspirate/serum quotient can be determined with whole blood used as an "internal standard" (e.g., for cerebrospinal fluid

(CSF) fistula diagnostics). Test samples for cellular analysis, in particular leukocyte cell line, red blood cells, and tumor cells, should be sent in EDTA tubes to the laboratory as soon as possible (within the 4 hours after the specimen being collected). Due to the unphysiological composition of the material resulting from accelerated cell death, longer periods can result falsely low cell counts and inaccurate cell differentiation. In modern laboratory analysis, there is a synergy between automated flow cytometry analytical methods and manual techniques (cell enrichment through cytocentrifugation, microscopic chamber counts, and established hematological staining methods) depending on the question and sample quality (cell-rich exudates vs. transudates with few cells, ▶ Figure 3.18a). Gram staining and further processing of blood cultures for pathogen cultivation serve to orient the microbiological diagnostics.

3.3.1 Cerebrospinal Fluid Fistula Diagnostics

Surgical intervention, trauma, a tumor or inflammatory disease in the immediate vicinity of the subarachnoid space boundaries can cause leakage of the cerebrospinal fluid (CSF). If undetected, this event, also known as a CSF fistula or CSF leak, can lead to fatal complications such as meningitis, a brain abscess, and dysosmia. A CSF fistula can be detected with higher certainty by laboratory tests. This requires only the collection of some of the suspected extravascular fluid. This fluid can, for example, be seen to drip from the nose (rhinoliquorrhea) or ear (otoliquorrhea), and should be collected in a sterile neutral tube. For non-visible outflows, cautious tamponade of, e.g., the nasal vestibule or the external auditory canal is recommended using a standardized or comparable cotton roll, e.g., Salivette® (Sarstedt). After collection, the soaked cotton plug is placed in the Salivette® container and centrifuged. Collection of suspect fluids along the vertebral column or from the cranium must be obtained through puncture. The material must be stored between 4 °C and 8 °C until being sent to the laboratory. To differentiate the suspected extravascular fluid from serum, it is necessary to collect a sample of venous whole blood simultaneously.

The highest diagnostic sensitivity for CSF detection is shown by β-trace protein and the CSF-specific β$_2$-transferrin. Increased β-trace protein concentrations (>1.0 mg/L) compared to the serum sample, or increased β-trace protein (extravascular body fluid/serum) ratios >2 are evidence of CSF admixture (Reiber, et al., 2003; Arrer, et al., 2004; Schnabel, et al., 2004; Kristof, et al., 2008). Our own internal laboratory investigation of 50 serum samples for β-trace protein has shown a benchmark value range in the 95th percentile of 0.40–0.93 mg/L. The additional evidence of the CSF-specific β$_2$-transferrin band from immunofixation electrophoresis increases the diagnostic sensitivity of the analysis, since this is absent from the serum. A careful visual assessment of sample appearance helps to avoid misinterpretations, since blood admixture can lead to falsely low β-trace protein concentrations and the absence of evidence of β2-transferrin due to a dilution effect (▶ Figure 3.14).

3.3.2 Peritoneal Dialysis Diagnostics

Catheter-associated inflammation in peritoneal dialysis (PD) patients is an alarming complication. Approximately 50 % of PD peritonitis cases are caused by skin germs such as *Staphylococcus epidermidis* and *Staphylococcus aureus* (Thodis, et al., 2005; Vargemezis and Thodis, 2005). The dialysis fluid is likewise a factor that contributes to infections, because its non-physiological composition leads to altered mesothelial function over time. In addition, the dilution effect can destabilize the local phagocytic system and the presence of cytokines (Selgas, et al., 1998).

According to the definition, PD peritonitis is likely if two of the following three criteria are present (Thodis, et al., 1998; Wanten, et al., 1996; Fried and Piraino, 2009):

1. Turbid outflow, more than 100 leukocytes/μL with > 50 % neutrophils
2. Abdominal pain with rebound tenderness, and fever
3. Evidence of microorganisms in the culture or from Gram staining

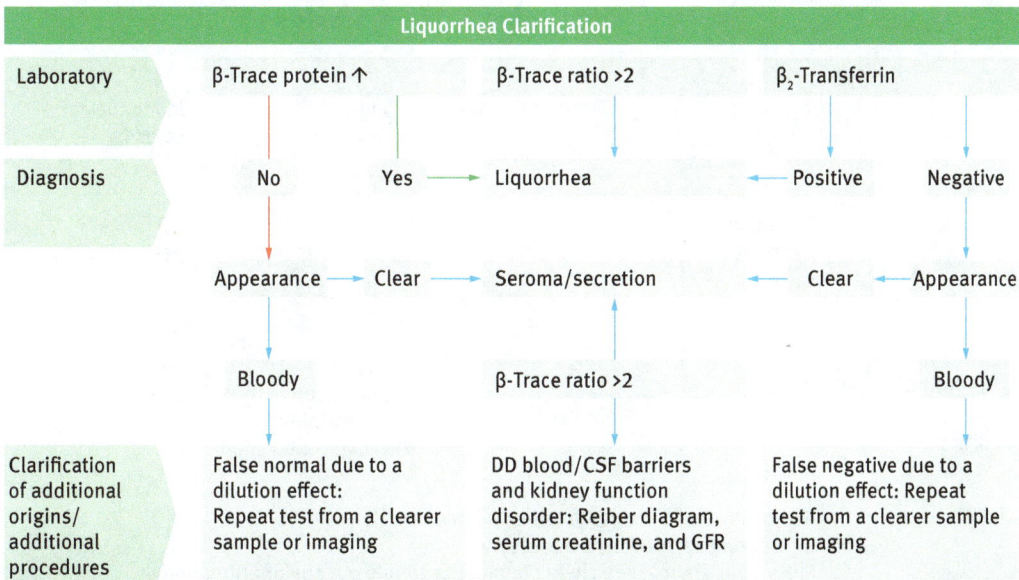

Figure 3.14 Liquorrhea clarification.

Turbid dialysate and cell counts above 100/µL with > 50 % neutrophils is considered pathological (Tranaeus, et al., 1998). Additional abdominal symptoms or detection of pathogens indicate an urgent suspicion of bacterial peritonitis, and antimicrobial therapy should be initiated. A major problem is the low pathogen density due to the dilution effect of large amounts of fluid.

In CAPD patients, cellular analysis of the drainage dialysate, leukocyte cell counts, and leukocyte differentiation contribute to a timely diagnosis and assessment of the peritonitis course. The diagnosis begins with the preanalysis. The drainage dialysate in EDTA tubes should be sent to the laboratory as rapidly as possible, within 4 hours of obtaining the test material (Fried und Piraino, 2009). The unphysiological osmotic composition of the test materials arising from the accelerated cell death that attends longer waiting times will result in falsely low cell counts and erroneous cell differentiation. Leukocytes and erythrocytes will

no longer be detectable. The color and appearance of the dialysate should be visually assessed immediately upon receipt in the laboratory. Next, leukocyte esterase and hemoglobin peroxidase should be tested using reflectance photometry (Fried and Piraino, 2009). The detection of these reactions with test strip coupled with unremarkable leukocyte and erythrocyte counts indicates a preanalytical error, and a new test sample is required. With leukocyte counts > 100/µL, the cell differentiation in the dialysate should be determined either via automated flow cytometry or microscopically after cytocentrifugation and subsequent panoptic staining. Neutrophils, eosinophils and mononuclear cells in the dialysate are taken into consideration.

Turbid to clear drainage dialysate with a leukocyte count < 100/µL and eosinophils > 10 % points to eosinophilic peritonitis. It develops relatively early after catheter placement, and is interpreted as an allergic reaction to the foreign material.

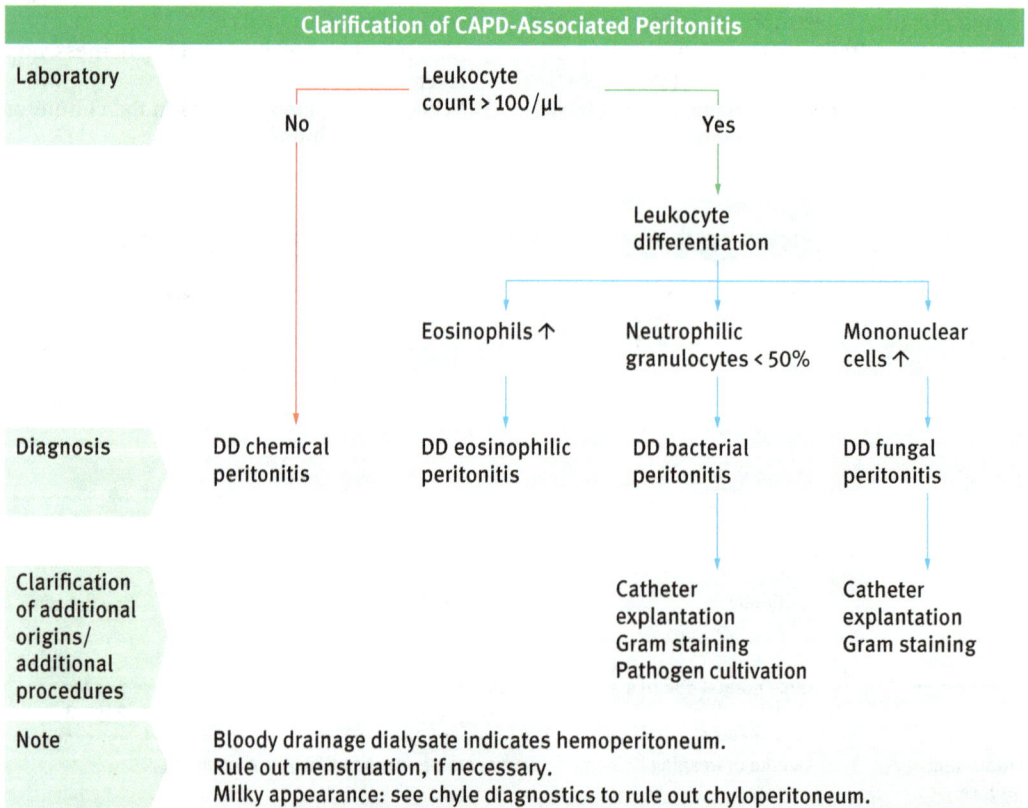

Figure 3.15 Clarification of CAPD-Associated Peritonitis.

With sterile cultures, local cortisone treatment can be carried out (sterile eosinophilic peritonitis). In principle, though, therapeutic intervention is not indicated. The differential diagnosis should also consider chemical peritonitis, which can be understood as hypersensitivity to the local drug therapy (Fried and Piraino, 2009).

Mononuclear cells are the predominant cell type in fungal peritonitis. Its symptomatology is similar to that of bacterial peritonitis, and catheter explantation is indicated (Thodis, et al., 1998) (▶ Figure 3.15).

3.3.3 Chyle Diagnostics

Lymph is normally a clear liquid, while milky, turbid lymph from the intestinal tract is defined as chyle, depending on dietary intake and/or the content of long-chain fats (Agrawal, et al., 2008). Samples need not appear milky and turbid, since chyle that is yellowish to serous can also be present (Skouras und Kalomenidis, 2010).

Chylothorax can be triggered by malignant diseases of the lymphatic system, and mediastinal metastases and tumors, as well as following thoracic surgery, cardiovascular surgery, or chest trauma (Doerr, et al., 2005).

In terms of the differential diagnosis, the milky appearance of the sample is important in distinguishing between pseudochyle and true chyle. The former occurs in chronic inflammatory diseases in rheumatic diseases, liver cirrhosis, and amyloidosis, the color/appearance of which is

determined by cholesterol-lecithin. Pseudochyle characteristically has a high cholesterol concentration and low triglyceride content.

Moreover, chyle can further be detected through lipoprotein electrophoresis and triglyceride concentration determination. Thus, the concentration of triglycerides is higher than that of cholesterol in the sample undergoing examination, and also higher than the triglyceride concentration in serum, since the fats obtained from the diet enter the bloodstream via the thoracic duct. Chylomicrons are detectable in lipoprotein electrophoresis (Skouras and Kalomenidis, 2010; Maldonado, et al., 2009). In pseudochyle by contrast, there is neither evidence of chylomicrons nor is the triglyceride concentration increased compared to serum and plasma. However, a high serum cholesterol concentration can be found in pseudochyle as compared with chyle. Chyle contains a high proportion of lymphocytic elements (Agrawal, et al., 2008; Maldonado, et al., 2009) (▶ Figure 3.16.).

3.3.4 Urine Leakage Diagnostics

Serous aspirates or fluid emerging from surgical wounds in the vicinity of the urinary tract can be reliably identified with a corresponding clinical chemistry examination with regard to their origin. Urine admixture in the aspirate results in significantly increased creatinine and urea concentrations that are several times higher than in serum. The phosphate concentration can also

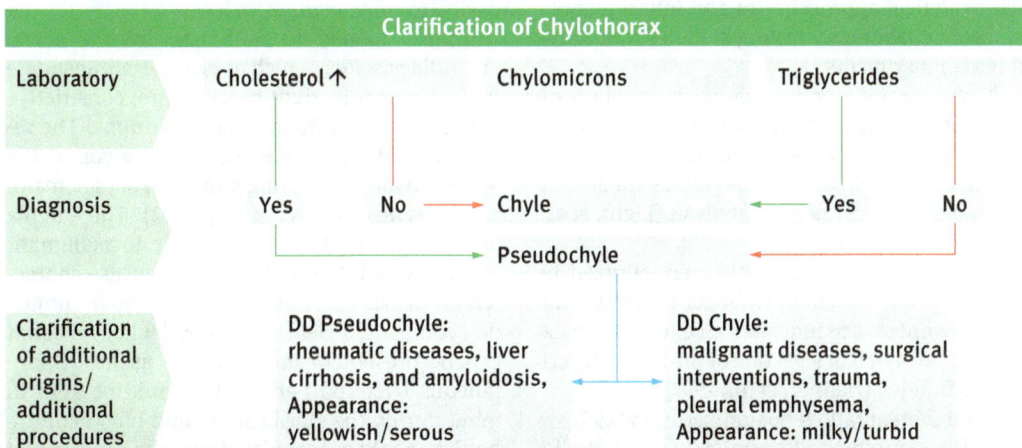

Figure 3.16 Clarification of Chylothorax.

Clarification of Urine Leakage				
Laboratory	Creatinine ↑ or urine ↑ or phosphate ↑			Glucose ↑ or total protein ↑

Diagnosis Yes No ——→ Secretion/seroma ←—— Yes No

Urine leakage ←————

Clarification of additional origins/ additional procedures

Confirmation through:
– Ultrasound
– Nuclear medical testing
– i.v. Indigo carmine excretion test:
   Indigo carmine detection

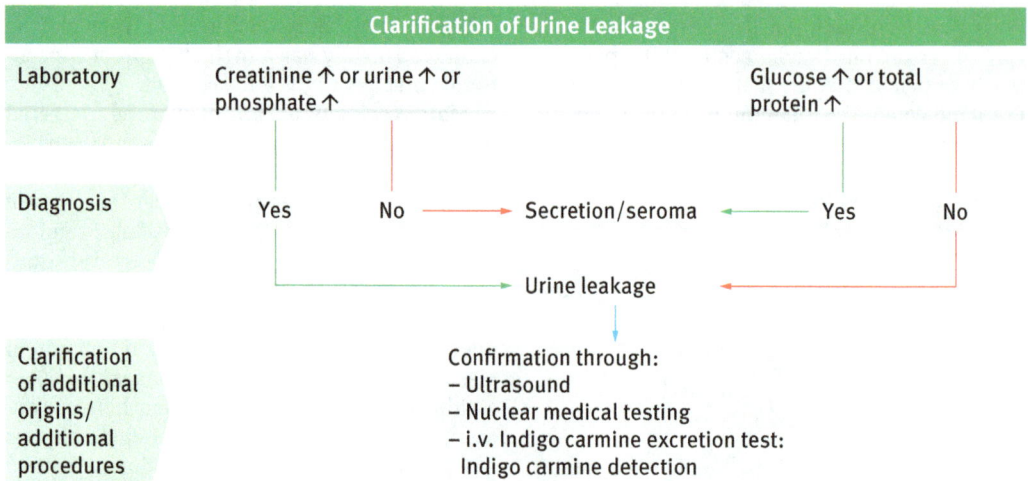

Figure 3.17 Clarification of Urine Leakage.

be significantly increased. Furthermore, the test material exhibits lower total protein and glucose concentrations than in serum. Diagnostic imaging is also carried out the laboratory analysis, in addition to ultrasound and/or nuclear medical examination (▶ Figure 3.17).

3.3.5 Effusion Diagnostics

Due to their common anatomical origin, the peritoneal, pleural and pericardial extravascular spaces have identical mesothelial linings (Ji and Nie, 2008). This explains the fundamentally similar analytical approaches to and interpretations of medical laboratory testing samples from these three compartments.

Thus, the differential diagnosis involves diagnostic sampling through ultrasound-guided aspiration to assess the color and appearance, laboratory examination to classify as transudate or exudate, and cytological analysis (Light, et al., 1972) (▶ Figure 3.18a).

A transudate is frequently characterized by its clear-yellowish color, whereas a more turbid, viscous appearance indicates an exudate. An exudate is present if at least one of the following criteria is fulfilled (Heffner, et al., 1997):
- Total protein ratio (effusion/serum) > 0.5
- LDH ratio (effusion/serum) > 0.6 (with malignant tumors, often > 1)

For the leukocyte determination and differentiation and the erythrocyte count, the aspirate should be collected in EDTA tubes. The clinical chemical analysis is carried out on native samples. In determining the effusion/serum ratios, an additional timely venous blood draw should be made.

3.3.5.1 Ascites

In addition to promoting collateral circulation and splenomegaly, portal hypertension triggered by pre-, intra- and posthepatic causes also leads to ascites (fluid accumulation in the peritoneal cavity) (Møller, et al., 2009).

Approximately 80 % of cases involve portal or cardiac ascites, which appears as a transudate in liver cirrhosis, right heart failure, constrictive pericarditis, and Budd-Chiari syndrome. The remaining 20 % are exudates, and most commonly appear in malignant, inflammatory, or pancreatogenic ascites (Moore, et al., 2003). The sample appearance is often hemorrhagic in malignant ascites. A high LDH concentration is also characteristic of ascites. Peritonitis with positive antigen detection and a clearly elevated leukocyte count can be present in inflammatory ascites. Spontaneous bacterial peritonitis should be kept in mind during the clarification, and blood culture bottles should be inoculated with the test material (Moore, et al., 2003; Rimola, et al., 2000).

Differentiation of Pathological Effusions			
		Transudate	Exudate
Visual checking upon receipt		Clear Yellowish	Turbid
Laboratory	Specific gravity	< 1.015	≥ 1.015
	Cell number	Elevated	Lowered
	Cell type	Lymphocytes	Neutrophilic granulocytes, tumor cells
	Albumin difference (serum/effusion)	< 11 g/L	11 g/L
	Total protein ratio (effusion/serum)	< 0.5	≥ 0.5
	LDH ratio (effusion/serum)	< 0.6	≥ 0.6
Etiology		benign, non-inflammatory	malignant, inflammatory

Figure 3.18a Differentiation of pathological effusions; albumin difference = serum-ascites albumin gradient (SAAG).

Increased amylase and lipase concentrations are typically found in pancreatogenic ascites. The basic diagnostic approach consists of determining the total protein concentration and the serum/ascites albumin ratio (EASL, 2010). The lower the total protein concentration and the higher the albumin ratio, the more likely the sample is a transudate (Moore, et al., 2003, Moore, et al., 2013).

Based on the two most common primary diseases with ascites, liver cirrhosis (80 %) and malignant tumors from peritoneal carcinomatosis (10 %), ascites is also differentiated into benign/portal and malignant types. This distinction is more accurate in the context of differential diagnosis, and consists of reviewing the cellular findings in combination with the total protein, albumin difference vs. serum, cholesterol, and carcinoembryonic antigen (CEA), along with amylase and lipase (▶ Figure 3.18b).

3.3.5.2 Pleural effusion

Pleural effusion often begins as cardiac effusion arising from decompensated heart failure. Moreover, malignant neoplasms and inflammatory events are frequently observed as causes of pleural effusion. In addition to imaging methods and the clinical symptomatology and medical history of the patient, laboratory testing can also provide information on the origin of the pleural effusion (Stanzel and Ernst, 2008).

Transudative effusions are found in 30 % of cases, and are accompanied by decompensated left heart failure, pulmonary embolism, liver cirrhosis, nephrotic syndrome or peritoneal dialysis (Lew, 2010; Kiafar and Gilani, 2008). The effusion event is exudative in about 70 % of cases, and is caused by malignant tumors and inflammatory processes (lung cancer, metastatic breast cancer,

Clarification of Ascites			
Laboratory	Albumin difference ≥ 11 g/L	Neutrophilic granulocytes ≥ 250/µL	Cholesterol ≥ 45 mg/dL
	Total protein ≥ 25 g/L		Amylase/Lipase ↑
	LDH ≥ 200 U/L		CEA ≥ 2.5 µg/L
Diagnosis	No Yes → Exudate		← Yes No
	→ Transudate		
		Neutrophilic granulocytes < 250/µL	
Clarification of additional origins/ additional procedures	DD Transudate (benign, non-inflammatory): Portal cardiac ascites, right heart failure, constrictive pericarditis, liver cirrhosis, Budd-Chiari syndrome, appearance: clear yellowish		DD Exudate (malign, inflammatory): Malignant tumors, pancreatogenic, spontaneous bacterial peritonitis
Note	Microbiological clarification: spontaneous vs. secondary bacterial peritonitis; cytological clarification with suspected malignant ascites		

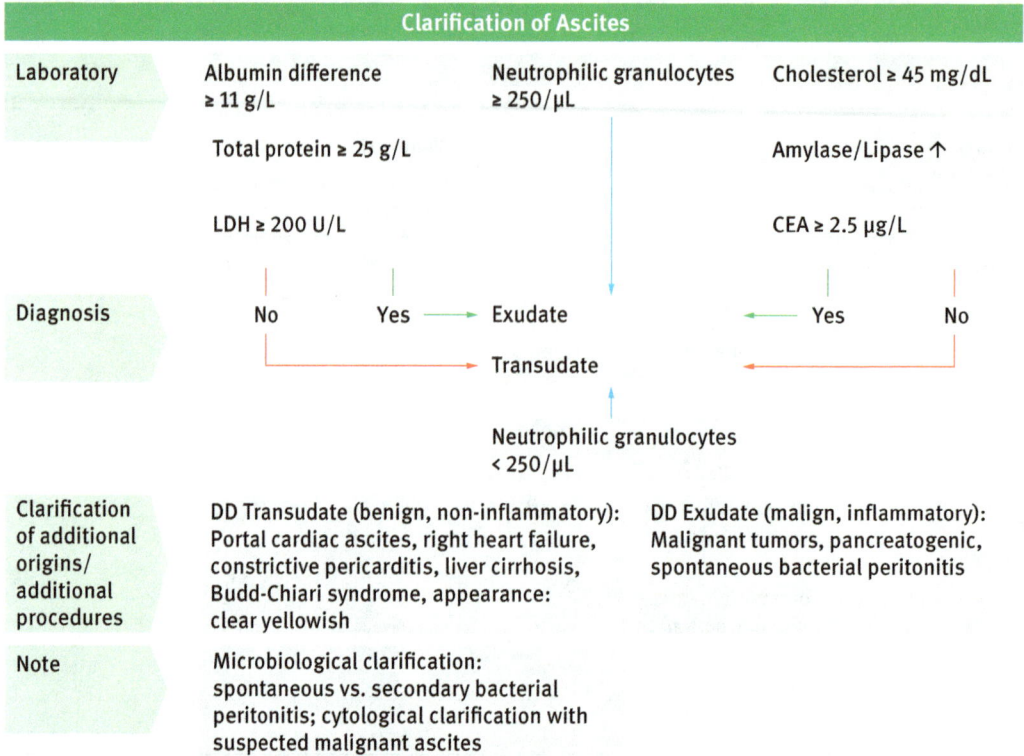

Figure 3.18b Clarification of ascites Additive determination of the LDH concentration can inform the decision of spontaneous vs. secondary bacterial peritonitis. 48 hours after beginning antibiotic therapy for bacterial peritonitis, the cell count should be repeated to help rule out spontaneous bacterial peritonitis if the cell count drops. A case of secondary bacterial peritonitis will exhibit an increasing cell count despite the antibiotic therapy. Additionally noteworthy would be 2 of 3 possible laboratory changes: total protein > 10 g/L, or LDH > 200 U/L, or glucose < 50 mg/dL (Runyon criteria) (Runyon, et al., 2013). The protein concentration in cardiac ascites = 25 g/L (SAAG ≥ 11 g/L, DD portal hypertension), and in cirrhotic ascites < 25 g/L.

malignant lymphoma and tuberculosis, pneumonia) (Loddenkemper, 1998) (▶ Figure 3.18c).

3.3.5.3 Pericardial effusions

Medical laboratory examination of pericardial fluid with effusion symptomatology can aid the diagnostic process and contribute information to the etiology. Patients often receive a diagnosis of idiopathic pericarditis without the benefit of prior differentiation through laboratory analysis (Sagrista-Sauleda, et al., 2000). Pericardial effusions can arise from a malignant process, as well as in cases of uremia from renal failure or tuberculosis (Sagrista-Sauleda, et al., 2000). Additional known frequent origins include viral and bacterial infections, rheumatic diseases, cardiovascular diseases and metabolic disorders (e.g., hypothyroidism) as well as radiotherapy (Dunne, et al., 2011; Wagner, et al., 2011).

Transudative effusions are present in 15 % of cases, and are accompanied by renal failure and status post radiotherapy. The effusion event is exudative in approximately 30 % of cases, and is caused by malignant tumors, and viral or bacterial inflammatory processes (▶ Figure 3.18d).

Literature

Agrawal V, Doelken P, Sahn SA. Pleural fluid analysis in chylous pleural effusion. Chest. 2008; 133: 1436–1441.

Clarification of Pleural Effusions

Laboratory	Total protein ratio > 0.5		Neutrophilic granulocytes > 500/μL	LDH ratio > 0.6	

Diagnosis

No   Yes ⟶ Exudate ⟵ Yes   No

Transudate

Neutrophilic granulocytes < 500/μL

Clarification of additional origins/ additional procedures	DD Transudate: Decompensated left heart failure, pulmonary embolism, liver cirrhosis, nephrotic syndrome, Appearance: clear yellowish	DD Exudate: malignant tumor, pneumonia, and tuberculosis, Appearance: turbid

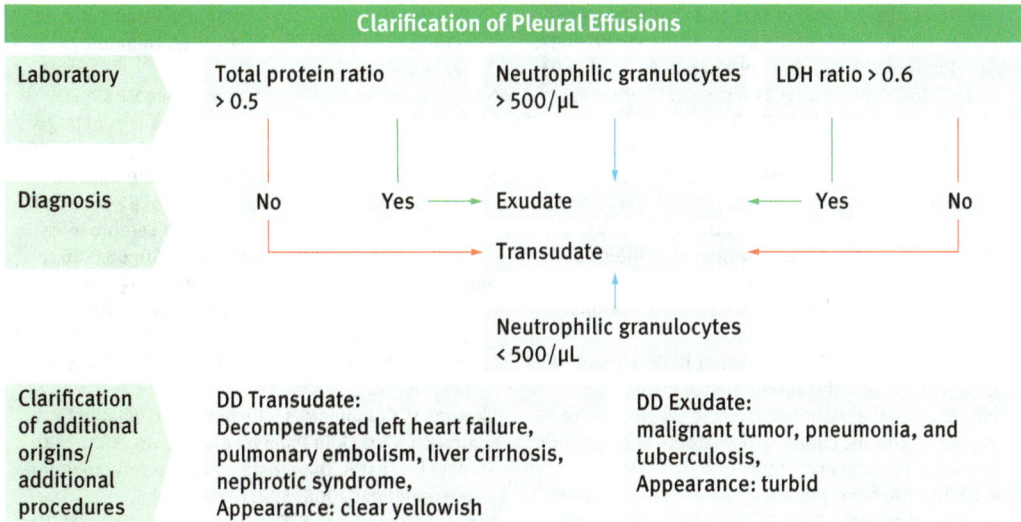

Figure 3.18c Clarification of Pleural Effusions.

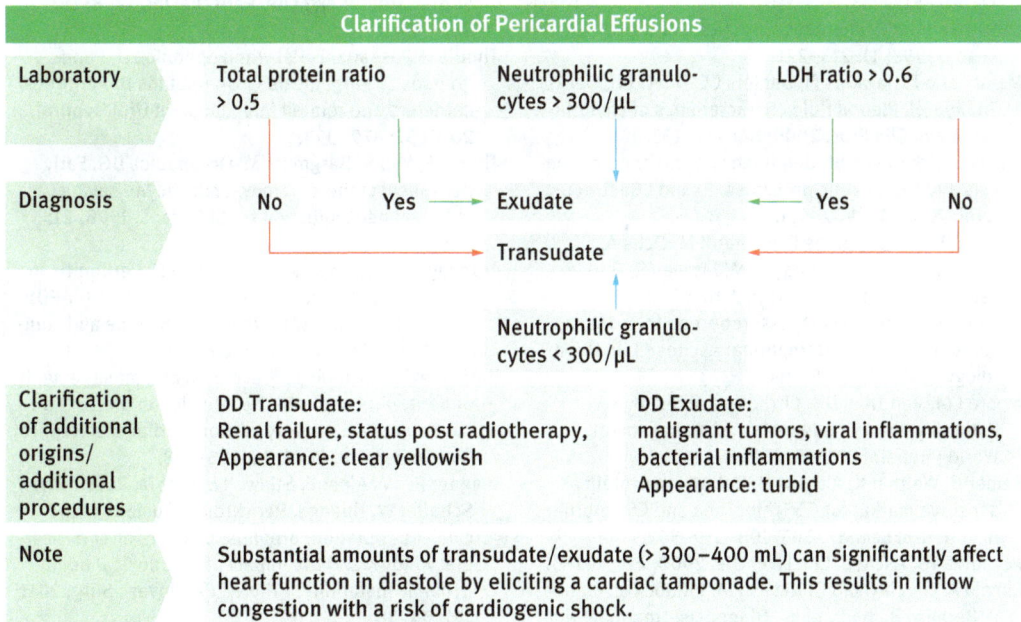

Clarification of Pericardial Effusions

Laboratory	Total protein ratio > 0.5		Neutrophilic granulo- cytes > 300/μL	LDH ratio > 0.6	

Diagnosis

No   Yes ⟶ Exudate ⟵ Yes   No

Transudate

Neutrophilic granulo- cytes < 300/μL

Clarification of additional origins/ additional procedures	DD Transudate: Renal failure, status post radiotherapy, Appearance: clear yellowish	DD Exudate: malignant tumors, viral inflammations, bacterial inflammations Appearance: turbid

Note	Substantial amounts of transudate/exudate (> 300–400 mL) can significantly affect heart function in diastole by eliciting a cardiac tamponade. This results in inflow congestion with a risk of cardiogenic shock.

Abb. 3.18d Clarification of Pericardial Effusions.

Arrer E, Meco C, Oberascher G, Piotrowski W, Albegger K, Wolfgang Patsch W. β-Trace protein as a marker for cerebrospinal fluid rhinorrhea. Clin. Chem. 2004; 50: 661–663.

Doerr CH, Allen MS, Nichols FC, Ryu JH. Etiology of chylothorax in 203 patients. Mayo Clin Proc. 2005; 80: 867–870.

Dunne JV, Chou JP, Viswanathan M, Wilcox P, Huang SH. Cardiac tamponade and large pericardial effusions in systemic sclerosis: A report of four cases and a review of the literature. Clin Rheumatol. 2011; (Epub ahead of print).

EASL clinical practice guidelines on the management of ascites, spontaneous bacterial peritonitis, and hepatorenal syndrome in cirrhosis. European Association for the Study of the Liver. 2010; 53: 397–417.

Fried L, Piraino B. Peritonitis, in: Khanna R., Krediet RT. (Hrsg.): Nolph and Gokal's textbook of peritoneal dialysis. Third edition: 2009 Springer.

Heffner JE, Brown LK, Barbieri CA. Diagnostic value of tests that discriminate between exudative and transudative pleural effusions. Chest. 1997; 111:970–980.

Ji HL, Nie HG. Electrolyte and fluid transport in mesothelial cells. J Epithel Biol Pharmacol. 2008; 1: 1–7.

Kiafar C, Gilani N. Hepatic hydrothorax: current concepts of pathophysiology and treatment options. Ann Hepatol. 2008; 7: 313–320.

Kristof RA, Grimm JM, Stoffel-Wagner B. Cerebrospinal fluid leakage into the subdural space: possible influence on the pathogenesis and recurrence frequency of chronic subdural hematoma and subdural hygroma. J Neurosurg. 2008; 108: 275–280.

Lew SQ. Hydrothorax: pleural effusion associated with peritoneal dialysis. Perit Dial Int. 2010; 30: 13–18.

Light RW, MacGregor MI, Luchsinger PC, Ball WC. Pleural effusions: the diagnostic separation of transudates and exudates. Ann Intern Med. 1972; 77: 507–513.

Loddenkemper R. Thoracoscopy: State of the art. Eur Resp J. 1998; 11: 213–221.

Maldonado F, Hawkins FJ, Daniels CE, Doerr CH, Decker PA, Ryu JH. Pleural fluid characteristics of chylothorax. Mayo Clin Proc. 2009; 84: 129–133.

Møller S, Henriksen JH, Bendtsen F. Ascites: pathogenesis and therapeutic principles. Scand J Gastroenterol. 2009; 44: 902–911.

Moore KP, Wong F, Gines P, Bernardi M, Ochs A, Salerno F, Angeli P, Porayko M, Moreau R, Garcia-Tsao G, Jimenez W, Planas R, Arroyo V. The management of ascites in cirrhosis: report on the consensus conference of the International Ascites Club. Hepatology. 2003; 38: 258–266.

Moore CM, Van Thiel DH. Cirrhotic ascites review: Pathophysiology, diagnosis and management. World J Hepatol 2013; 5: 251–263.

Reiber H, Walther K, Althaus H. Beta-trace protein as sensitive marker for CSF rhinorhea and CSF otorhea. Acta Neurol Scand. 2003; 108: 359–362.

Reynolds TB. Ascites. Clin Liver Dis. 2000; 4: 151–168.

Rimola A, Garcia-Tsao G, Navasa M, Piddock LJ, Planas R, Bernard B. Inadomi JM. Diagnosis, treatment and prophylaxis of spontaneous bacterial peritonitis: a consensus document. International Ascites Club. J Hepatol. 2000; 32: 142–153.

Runyon BA, AASLD. Introduction to the revised American Association for the Study of Liver Diseases Practice Guideline management of adult patients with ascites due to cirrhosis 2012. Hepatology 2013; 57: 1651–1653.

Sagrista-Sauleda J, Merce J, Permanyer-Miralda G, Soler-Soler J. Clinical clues to the causes of large pericardial effusions. Am J Med. 2000; 109: 95–101.

Schnabel C, DiMartino E, Gilsbach JM, Riediger D, Gressner AM, Kunz D. Comparison of β2-transferrin and β-trace protein as a marker for cerebrospinal fluid rhinorrhea. Clin Chem. 2004; 50: 661–663.

Selgas R, Paiva A, Bajo MA, Cirugede A, Aguilera A, Diaz C, Hevia C. Consequences of peritonitis episodes appearing late during peritoneal dialysis (PD) in patients able to continue PD. Adv Perit Dial. 1998; 14: 168–172.

Skouras V, Kalomenidis I. Chylothorax: diagnostic approach. Curr Opin Pulm Med. 2010; 16: 387–393.

Stanzel F, Ernst A. Diagnostik der Pleuraerkrankungen. Pneumologe. 2008; 5: 211–218.

Thodis E, Bhaskaran S, Pasadakis P, Bargman JM. Vas SI., Oreopoulos DG. Decrease in Staphylococcus Aureus Exit-Site infections and peritonitis in CAPD patients by local application of Mupirocin Ointment at the catheter exit site. Perit Dial Int. 1998; 18: 261–270.

Thodis E, Passadakis P, Lyrantzopooulos N, Panagoutsos S, Vargemezis V, Oreopoulos D. Peritoneal catheters and related infections. Int Urol Nephrol. 2005; 37: 379–393.

Thodis E, Vas S, Bargman JM, Oreopoulos DG. Early peritoneal catheter removal may be life saving in fungal peritonitis. Int J Artif Organs. 1998; 21: 489.

Tranaeus A, Heimburger O, Lindholm B. Peritonitis in continuous ambulatory peritoneal dialysis (CAPD): diagnostic findings, therapeutic outcome and complications. Perit Dial Int. 1989; 9: 179.

Vargemezis V, Thodis E. Prevention and management of peritonitis and exit-site infection in patients on continuous ambulatory peritoneal dialysis. Nephrol Dial Transplant. 2001; 16: 106–108.

Wagner PL, McAleer E, Stillwell E, Bott M, Rusch VW, Schaffer W, Huang J. Pericardial effusions in the cancer population: prognostic factors after pericardial window and the impact of paradoxical hemodynamic instability. J Thorac Cardiovasc Surg. 2011; 141: 34–38.

Wanten GJ, van Oost P, Schneeberger PM, Koolen MI. Nasal carriage and peritonitis by staphylococcus aureus in patients on continuous ambulatory peritoneal dialysis: A prospective study. Perit Dial Int. 1996; 16: 352–356.

4 Practical Examples of Targeted Stepwise Diagnosis

Matthias Imöhl, Axel Stachon

4.1 Endocrinology

Classical endocrinology deals with the endocrine glands and their hormone production. In addition, the endocrine glands, such as the pituitary, thyroid, parathyroid, the islets of Langerhans of the pancreas, adrenal glands, and gonads, communicate intensively with other organs via the nervous system, hormones, cytokines and growth factors. This endocrinological networking with physiological ramifications in other functional areas complicates the study of the significance and function of hormones. Thus, the characterization of hormone receptors (e.g., leptin or growth hormone receptors) often reveals unexpected relationships with functional areas of the organism that are not primarily endocrinological. The endocrine system is mainly studied by determining various hormone concentrations, which provide a physician in clinical practice with valuable diagnostic information. As a result, assuming a proper diagnosis, effective treatments are available for most endocrine disorders.

4.1.1 Thyroid gland

The thyroid gland makes two chemically related hormones, thyroxine (T4) and triiodothyronine (T3). Through their effects on hormone receptors in the cell nucleus, these hormones play a crucial role in growth and cell differentiation. In this way, they help to maintain the heat balance and metabolic homeostasis in humans. Thyroid function disorders occur relatively frequently. As with other regulatory systems, these can be separated into types: primary thyroid gland dysfunction, when the origin of the disorder lies in the peripheral gland; a secondary type in which the origin is in the pituitary gland; and, a tertiary type that is caused by the hypothalamus. Autoimmune processes play a special role in thyroid gland dysfunction. Thyroid gland autoimmune diseases either stimulate the gland to produce excess thyroid hormone (hyperthyroidism) or destroy the gland, which results in a hormone deficiency (hypothyroidism). Autoimmune thyroiditis (AIT) is an autoimmune disease of the thyroid gland that was first described in 1912 by Hashimoto as "lymphomatous goiter" (Hashimoto, 1912). The disease is best defined by the characteristic histological changes. Autoimmune thyroiditis is the most common origin of spontaneously occurring hypothyroidism in adults (Feldkamp, 2009). Graves' disease is responsible for 60–80 percent of hyperthyroidism cases. The prevalence varies in different populations, and is mainly dependent on the iodine supply. High iodine intake is linked with an increased prevalence of Graves' disease. The hyperthyroidism in Graves' disease is caused by thyroid-stimulating immunoglobulins (TSIs), which are formed in the thyroid gland, bone marrow and lymph nodes.

4.1.1.1 Hyperthyroidism

In pronounced cases, the clinical diagnosis of overt hyperthyroidism is a visual diagnosis. Often the medical history already points in this direction: nervousness, weight loss with strong appetite, tachycardia, restlessness, frequent urges to defecate, and heat intolerance are the most common symptoms. Goiter is observed in hyperthyroidism patients in approximately 80 percent of cases; however, a normal-sized thyroid is frequently found in immune thyroid disease cases. On the other hand, a diagnosis of Graves' disease always relatively straightforward if a noise can be auscultated above the thyroid gland or if endocrine orbitopathy is present (Allolio, 2010).

Gestational hyperthyroidism occurs in about 30 percent of pregnant women during the first trimester. Very high serum hCG concentrations can trigger overt hyperthyroidism in one percent of cases. In general, these regress in late pregnancy following thyrostatic therapy. However, it is quite possible that the thyroid metabolism status can be misinterpreted as normal when using the "classic" TSH reference values, even though a hypo-, or hyperthyroid imbalance already exists (Spielhagen, 2009).

To rule out hyperthyroidism in the presence of suspicious symptomatology, it is sufficient to determine a basal TSH value using an ultrasensitive method. A normal TSH level can rule out hyperthyroidism with very high probability. The precursor to overt hyperthyroidism is subclinical hyperthyroidism. It is characterized by serum TSH values of < 0.1 mU/L with normal fT3 and fT4 levels (Wiersinga, 1995). There are no uniform recommendations for handling of subclinical hyperthyroidism. The AACE recommends that all patients with subclinical hyperthyroidism undergo regular clinical monitoring, along with an individual approach to treatment where necessary (Baskin, 2002). Aside from this, in cases of a serious illness concomitant with hyperthyroidism, wherein the fT3 and fT4 hormone concentrations are within the normal range, evaluation of the findings can be quite difficult.

4.1.1.2 Hypothyroidism

The most common thyroid disorder is hypothyroidism. It is defined by an insufficient supply of thyroid hormone to the organs. Depending on the origin of the reduced thyroid gland secretion, a distinction is found between primary, secondary and tertiary hypothyroidism. Secondary hypothyroidism – caused by a lack of TSH – and tertiary hypothyroidism – the result of hypothalamic damage with a TRH deficiency – are rare. Hypothyroidism can be easily treated in most patients with an adequate thyroid hormone replacement therapy (Müssig, 2009). The various forms of hypothyroidism can be divided by origin into congenital and acquired. The most common origin of acquired hypothyroidism is autoimmune thyroiditis (AIT), which is characterized by a lymphocytic and plasma cellular infiltration of the thyroid gland. Throughout the world, iodine deficiency is also one of the more common origins of acquired hypothyroidism. For this reason, the AACE/AME/ETA Guideline for clarification of multinodular goiter in regions of the world with iodine deficiency recommends reliably ruling out thyroid autonomy, using scintigraphy and cytological examination of samples from fine needle aspiration from selected cold or scintigraphically indifferent areas, even in the presence of normal TSH values (Gharib, et al., 2010). Moreover, it was observed in a long-term study that even with TSH levels above about 2.5 mU/L, the thyroid gland can frequently develop overt hypothyroidism over the course of years (Vanderpump, 1995). In areas with a sufficient iodine intake, in addition to autoimmune diseases (Hashimoto's thyroiditis), iatrogenic measures (hyperthyroidism treatments) must also be taken into account in many cases as a cause of hypothyroidism (Fauci, 2009). The most common origin of congenital hypothyroidism (about 80–90 percent of cases) is an organ developmental disorder (dysgenesis).

4.1.1.3 Pre- and Post-analytical Principles

A normal TSH result rules out primary thyroid gland dysfunction with high probability. However, there are clinical situations in which the TSH determination can be misleading as a screening test, especially if the fT4 is not determined at the same time. Any serious systemic disease (non-thyroid disease) can result in abnormal levels of TSH and the peripheral thyroid hormones. Although hypothyroidism is the most common origin of an elevated TSH level, in rare cases a TSH-producing pituitary tumor or thyroid hormone resistance can be responsible. Conversely, while suppressed TSH values (< 0.1 mU/L) normally indicate hyperthyroidism, such values can also occur during the first trimester of pregnancy (due to a high hCG concentration), following hyperthyroidism treatment (since the TSH can remain low for several weeks), and under the influence of certain medications (e.g., high doses of glucocorticoids or dopamine).

4.1.1.4 Laboratory Analysis

TSH: TSH determination is the method of choice for ruling out hypothyroidism or hyperthyroidism. A normal TSH level can rule out hyperthyroidism with high probability. Assuming that the hypothalamus and anterior pituitary are functioning normally, the plasma TSH concentration reflects the supply of thyroid hormones to the tissues. The TSH concentration is inversely and exponentially correlated with the fT4. TSH is a glycoprotein, i.e., it contains sugar residues, which lead to different TSH molecule sub-fractions. This behavior can lead to problems in the biochemical quantification of TSH, compounded by the lack (to date) of a "gold standard" for TSH determination. TSH measurements are thus always based on an international standard preparation and, as an international consensus guideline requires, must be compared with the laboratory's own reference ranges for healthy subjects (Demers and Spencer, 2001). The currently available detection methods are based on the use of specific antibodies to TSH as part of an immunometric assay (Brabant, 2009). The predictive value of the TSH determination critically depends on the use of a 3rd- or 4th-generation procedure, with which valid measurements of concentrations in the range of 0.01–0.02 mU/L can be obtained. According to the quality guidelines, the "functional sensitivity" specification for a method requires that the lowest measured value can be determined with a coefficient of variation of less than 20 percent. Numerous physiological and pharmacological influences must be considered when assessing the measurement results. TSH follows a circadian rhythm, reaching a maximum at night and the lowest values in the afternoon. Moreover, the patient's sex, diet, and presence of any serious systemic diseases or depressive disorders can lead to increases or decreases in the TSH concentration. An additional consideration from the pathophysiology perspective is the absence (to date) of a uniquely assigned, age-dependent increase in TSH concentration (Biondi and Cooper, 2008; Bonomi et al, 2009; Brabant, 2006). Moreover, acute sleep deprivation significantly increases the basal TSH, whereas fasting can reduce the serum TSH concentration to about half of the initial value (Brabant, 2006). Acute administration of glucocorticoids leads to a rapid, transient suppression of TSH concentration (Brabant, 1989). Likewise, medications such as dopamine, heparin and opioids can cause changes in the TSH values.

Total T4 (tT4), free T4 (fT4), total T3 (tT3), free T3 (fT3): fT4 is formed only in the thyroid gland, and is secreted into the circulation. Protein-bound T4 arises when fT4 binds to plasma proteins, such as thyroxine-binding globulin, transthyretin, albumin, and apolipoproteins. The binding of fT4 correlates with the concentration and affinity of the binding proteins and is inversely proportional to their saturation with fT4 (Nelson and Wilcox, 1996). The tT4 and fT4 concentrations reflect the hormone secretion from the thyroid tissue as well as the tissue availability of T4 during T4 treatment (Lindstedt, 1994). Approximately 80 percent of circulating T3 is formed in the tissues through

conversion from T4, while 20 percent is directly secreted by the thyroid gland. In plasma, T3 is primarily bound to TBG, and less to transthyretin. fT3 has 5 times higher metabolic activity than fT4. For this reason, the tT3 and fT3 concentrations reflect the conversion of T4 to T3 (Klee, 1996). Also, when making thyroid hormone determinations, as likewise for TSH, it must be kept in mind that the results can vary according to the measurement method and patient's age.

Thyroid peroxidase antibodies (TPO Ab): TPO (thyroid peroxidase) is a membrane-bound heme protein. In thyroid hormone synthesis, it is involved in the iodination of the tyrosine residues and in the oxidative coupling of the two tyrosine residues in thyroglobulin. For TPO Ab always involves antibodies of class IgG1 or IgG4. The presence of TPO Ab indicates an autoimmune thyroid disease, or an increased risk of thyroid dysfunction. TPO Ab is found, usually at high titers, in almost all patients who have autoimmune hypothyroidism, and up to 80 percent of patients with Graves' disease. Some false positive results are found in TPO assays, due to cross-reaction with thyroglobulin antibodies. Moderately elevated TPO Ab concentrations are also found with non-immunogenic thyroid diseases or functional thyroid autonomy. This can likewise be the case with other immune diseases, e.g., Addison's disease, pernicious anemia, type 1 diabetes mellitus, vitiligo or in diseases that activate the immune system such as chronic active hepatitis B, primary biliary cirrhosis, or hepatitis C. The detection of autoantibodies with (still) normal thyroid function is insufficient grounds for a diagnosis of thyroid disease. Dysfunction usually occurs only after years. Nevertheless, the detection of antibodies substantiates a disposition to develop an organ-specific autoimmunity (Gartner, 2009).

Thyroglobulin antibodies (Tg Ab): TG Ab plays a smaller role in the diagnosis of immune-mediated thyroid disease than does TPO Ab. Tg Ab levels are elevated in 60–70 percent of patients with Hashimoto's thyroiditis and primary myxedema, and in 20–40 percent of patients with Graves' disease (Mann, 1997). Tg Ab levels are only significant in cases where an autoimmune thyroid disease is suspected and TPO Ab cannot be detected. In addition, the detection of Tg Ab can explain impaired thyroglobulin recovery.

TSH receptor antibody (TSHR Ab): TSH receptor antibodies bind to the TSH receptors on thyroid cells, and as TSH agonists serve to increase adenylate cyclase activity. In this way, thyroid hormone production and secretion are increased (Creutzfeldt, 1996). The antibodies that target the receptor are heterogeneous, and have stimulating and blocking properties. Their integral effect, however, is a stimulating effect on the receptor (Thomas, 1998). The TSHR Ab assay has the very high specificity of 99.1 percent for Graves' disease, and is thus an important diagnostic parameter.

The main detection methods, with their corresponding reference ranges, are summarized in ▶ Table 4.1.

Stepwise Diagnostics for Hyperthyroidism

The clinical diagnosis of hyperthyroidism is often unproblematic in patients who have the classic symptoms. Evidence for hyperthyroidism must actively be sought in oligo- or monosymptomatic patients, so that the slightest suspicion should warrant a TSH determination. Decreased TSH values should always be followed up with fT3 and fT4 determinations. With increases in one or both thyroid hormones, further clarification should be conducted by measuring the TSHR Ab, TPO Ab and Tg Ab. Positive evidence of thyroid gland antibodies indicates the presence of immunogenic hyperthyroidism. A diagnosis of non-immunogenic hyperthyroidism is made when the thyroid gland antibody determination result is unremarkable. Normal fT3 and fT4 concentrations and TSH values of < 0.1 mU/L indicate latent or subclinical hyperthyroidism (Baskin, 2006). Other origins must also be considered here, such as the administration of certain drugs (e.g., cortisol), anterior pituitary deficiency, pregnancy in the first trimester, or status post hypothyroidism. Gestational hyperthyroidism occurs in about 30 percent of pregnant women during the first trimester. Very high serum hCG concentrations can trigger overt hyperthyroidism in one percent of cases. In general, these regress in late pregnancy following thyrostatic therapy. In other unclear cases, the fT3 and fT4 concentrations should be rechecked at 6–12 weeks.

In the absence of a thyroid disease within the previous 12 months, the presence of nodular goiter in an iodine-deficient region, or hyperthyroidism under treatment, a TSH level within the normal range largely rules out hyperthyroidism. An additional fT4 determination should be considered when a patient presents with a medical history or clinical signs of the diseases listed above. Likewise, elevated TSH concentrations require a fT4 determination. Hyperthyroidism can be ruled out if the result fT4 is unremarkable. A finding of increased fT4 concentration points to

Table 4.1 Measurement methods and reference ranges in thyroid gland diagnostics.

Analyte	Material	Measurement method	Reference range
TSH	Serum or plasma	Immunoassay (4th-generation), e.g., radio-, enzyme, fluorescence, or luminescence immunoassay	0.4–(2.5) 4.12 mU/L (Hollowell, 2002; Garber, 2012)*
fT3	Serum or plasma	Immunoassay (4th-generation), e.g., radio-, enzyme, fluorescence, or luminescence immunoassay	5.4–12.3 pmol/L (Rocker, et al., 1988)
fT4	Serum or plasma	Immunoassay (4th-generation), e.g., radio-, enzyme, fluorescence, or luminescence immunoassay	10–23 pmol/L (Heinze, 1995; Engler, et al., 1992)
TPO Ab	Serum or plasma	Immunofluorescence test Passive hemagglutination Immunoassay	< 100 IU/L (Sundbeck, 1995)
Tg Ab	Serum or plasma	Immunoassay	Specified as a titer, depends on the manufacturer used
TSHR Ab	Serum or plasma	Radioligand assay	Specified as a titer, depends on the manufacturer used

* Each laboratory is recommended to determine population-based reference ranges (Garber, 2012)

Table 4.2 Origins of an acquired increase in peripheral thyroid hormone levels in euthyroid patients.

Disease	Origin	Characteristics
Acquired excess	Medications (estrogens), pregnancy, cirrhosis, hepatitis	Elevated total T4, T3; normal fT3, fT4
Excess transthyretin	Endocrine pancreatic tumor	mostly normal T3, T4
Medications: propranolol, iopanoic acid, amiodarone	Reduced T3-T4 conversion	Elevated T4, lowered T3, normal or elevated TSH
Euthyroid sick syndrome	Acute diseases, especially psychiatric disorders	Transiently elevated fT4, lowered TSH; T3, T4 can also be lowered

hyperthyroidism, e.g., due to a TSH-secreting adenoma or thyroid hormone resistance. Other origins of an acquired increase in peripheral thyroid hormone levels in euthyroid patients are shown in ▶ Table 4.2. The usual procedure for confirming the diagnosis and further clarifying hyperthyroidism is shown in ▶ Figure 4.1.

Symptoms and findings: nervousness, diarrhea, weight loss, tachycardia, systolic hypertension

Stepwise Diagnostics for Hypothyroidism

Usually, a physical examination, medical history, and basal serum TSH determination are sufficient to rule out primary hypothyroidism. An elevated TSH value requires an fT4 determination. A TPO Ab determination should follow a finding of reduced fT4 concentration to clarify the etiology, in particular to detect chronic lymphocytic thyroiditis (Boucai and Surks, 2009). A lowered fT4 with detectable TPO Ab points to autoimmune thyroiditis (AIT). However, only approximately 70–80 percent of patients with AIT test positive for TPO antibodies in the blood, so that a negative TPO antibody determination result does not rule out autoimmune thyroiditis. A finding of unremarkable fT4 concentration in the presence of elevated TSH can, if necessary, be followed up with a TRH test for further clarification regarding latent subclinical hypothyroidism. Similarly, these findings should be rechecked after 6–12 weeks. TSH levels between 2.5–4.12 mU/L in a patient who exhibits clinical hypothyroidism symptoms indicate subclinical hypothyroidism. In this case, it is useful to advise the patient in detail with regard to further monitoring and possibly trying T4 therapy. If the TSH levels lie in the normal range and

no clinical symptoms are present, hypothyroidism can be ruled out. In rare cases, patients with a clinical suspicion of hypothyroidism will exhibit a decreased TSH concentration. This raises the question of further clarification to consider, e.g., euthyroid sick syndrome or anterior pituitary insufficiency. The use of certain medications (e.g., amiodarone, steroids, dopamine agonists) can also elicit such a constellation of findings. In this case, a determination of the fT4 concentration is useful for further clarification. The diagnostic procedure for suspected hypothyroidism is summarized in ▶ Figure 4.2.

Literature

Allolio B, Schule HM, Hsg. (2010). Praktische Endokrinologie. Urban und Fischer.

Baskin J (2002). Thyroid guidelines. AACE American Association of Clinical Endocrinologists and Associazione Medici Endocrinologi medical guidelines for clinical practise for the diagnosis and management od thyroid nodules, 8: 457–469.

Biondi B, Cooper D (2008). The clinical significance of subclinical thyrois dysfunction. Endocr Rev, 29: 76–131.

Bonomi M, Busnelli M, Beck-Peccoz P, Constanzo D, Antonica F, Dolci C, Pilotta A, Buzi F, Persani L, (2009). A family with complete resistance to thyrotropin-releasing hormone. N Engl J Med, 360: 731–734.

Boucai L, Surks MI (2009). Reference limits for serum TSH and free T4 are significantly influenced by race and age in an urban outpatient medical practice. Clin Endocrinol (Oxf), 70: 788–793.

Brabant A, Brabant G, Schurmeyer T, Ranft U, Schmidt FW, Hesch RD, von zur Muhlen A (1989). The role of glucocorticoids in the regulation of thyrotropin. Acta Endocrinol (Copenh), 121: 95–100.

Brabant G, Beck-Peccoz P (2006: 154). Is there a need to redefine the upper normal limit of TSH? Eur J Endocrinol, 5: 633–637.

Ruling In/out Hyperthyroidism

Initial examination/incidental findings

TSH

Lowered —— No ——→ Within reference range —— No → Elevated

Yes

Yes

Yes

Laboratory

Determination of fT4 and fT3

Thyroid disease within previous 12 months (esp. hyperthyroidism under treatment, T4 therapy), elderly patients, hyperthyroid symptoms, nodular goiter in aniodine-deficient region

Yes

fT4 and/or fT3 elevated —— No

No

Determination of fT4

Yes

Detection of TSHR Ab, TPO Ab, Tg Ab

fT4 elevated

Yes   No

No   Yes

Diagnosis

Immunogenic Hyperthyroidism

Non-immunogenic Hyperthyroidism

Latent/subclinical Hyperthyroidism (Assuming other causes are ruled out: *inter alia*, cortisol administration, anterior pituitary deficiency, 1st trimester pregnancy, status post hypothyroidism)

Hyperthyroidism Ruled Out

TSH-secreting Adenoma, Thyroid Hormone Resistance, Hyperthyroidism

Clarification of additional origins/additional procedures

Recheck every 6–12 weeks

If necessary, further clarification acc. Table 4.2

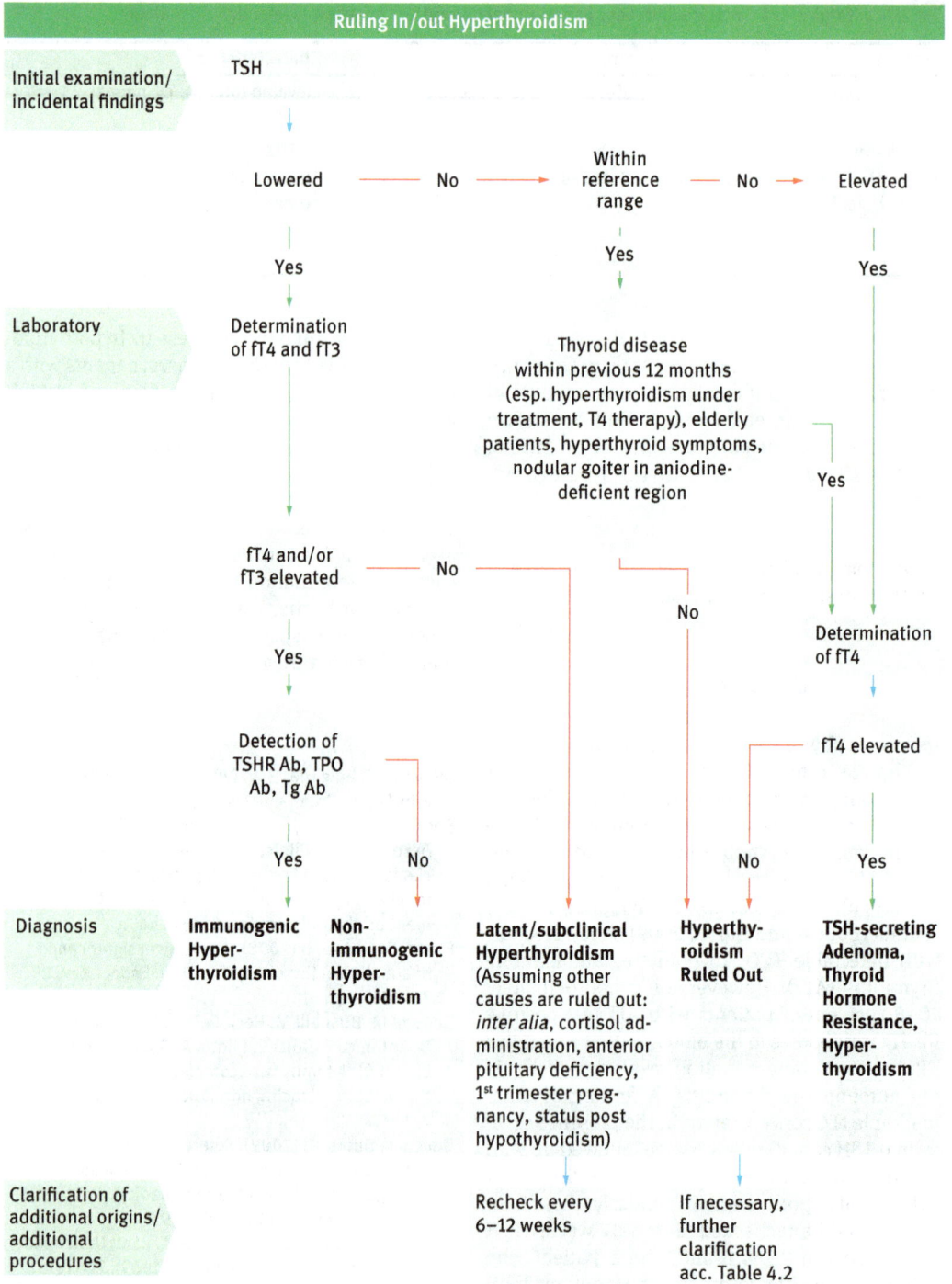

Figure 4.1 Diagnostic procedure for clarifying hyperthyroidism.

Brabant G, Kahaly J, Schicha H, Reiners C, (7. August 2006). Milde Formen der Schilddrüsenfehlfunktion. Deutsches Arzteblatt Jg, 103: 2110–2114.

Brabant G (2009). Neue TSH-Normalbereiche – ab wann therapieren? Dtsch Med Wochenschr, 134: 2510–2513.

Demers LM, Spencer C (2001). Laboratory support for the diagnosis and monitoring of thyroid disease NACB guidelines. Price Clin Chem, 47: 2067.

Engler H, Staub JJ, Kunz M, Althaus B, Ryff A, Viollier E, Girard J (1992). Ist eine isolierte TSH-Erhöhung behandlungsbedürftig? Schweiz Med Wschr 122: 66–69.

Fauci, BK (2009). Harrisons Innere Medizin Band 2. ABW Wissenschaftsverlag.

Feldkamp J (2009). Autoimmunthyreoiditis: Diagnostik und Therapie. Dtsch Med Wochenschr 134: 2504–2509.

Feldt R (1996). Analytical and clinical performance goals for testing autoantibodies to Thyroperoxidase, thyreoglobulin, and thyrotropin receptor. Clin Chem 42: 160–163.

Garber JR, Cobin RH, Gharib H, Hennessey JV, Klein I, Mechanick JI, Pessah-Pollack R, Singer PA, Woeber KA (2012). Clinical Practice Guidelines for Hypothyroidism in Adults: Cosponsored by the Am. Ass. of Clin. Endocrin. and the Am. Thyroid Ass. Thyroid 22: 1200–1235

Gartner R (2009). Diagnostik und Therapie von Schilddrüsenerkrankungen: effizient und evidenzbasiert. Dtsch Med Wochenschr, 134: 2497.

Gharib H, Papini E, Pasche R, Duick DS, Valcavi R, Hegedus L et al. (2010). American Association of Clinical Endocrinologists, Italien Association of Clinical Endocrinologists and European Thyroid Association Medical Guidelines For Clinical Practice For the Diagnosis and Management of Thyroid Nodules. Endocr Pract, Hot Thyroidology, J Endocrin Invest.

Hashimoto H (1912). Zur Kenntnis der lymphomatosen Veränderung der Schilddruse (Struma lymphomatosa). Arch Klin Chir, 97: 219.

Heinze HG (1995). Diskrepanz zwisachen peripheren Schilddrüsenhormonwerten und TSH-Spiegeln. Dtsch Med Wschr 120: 1639–1640.

Hollowell JG, Staehling NW, Flanders WD, Hannon WH, Gunter EW, Spencer CA, Brawermann LE (2002). Serum TSH, T4, and thyroid antibodies in the United States population (1988 to 1994): NHANES III. J. Clin Endocrinol Metab 87: 488–499.

Klee GG (1996). Clinical usage recommendations and analytic performance goals for total and free triiodothyronine measurements. Clin Chem 42: 155–159.

Lindstedt G, Berg G, Janssons S, Torring O, Valdemarsson S, Warin B, Nystrom E, (1994). Clinical use of laboratory hyroid tests and investigations. JIFCC 6: 136–141.

Mann K 1997. Sekretion der Deutschen Gesellschaft für Endokrinologie. Diagnostik und Therapie von Schilddrüsenkrankheiten. Empfehlung zur Qualitätssicherung. Internist 38: 177–185.

Müssig K, MK (2009). Hyperthyreose infolge einer Pseudomalabsorbtion von L-Thyroxin – Fall 12/2009. Dtsch Med Wochenschr, 134: 2514.

Nelson JC, Wilcox R 1996. Analytical performance of free and total thyroxine assays. Clin Chem 42: 146–154.

Rocker L, Janiszewski CH, Hopfenmuller W 1988. Referenzwerteermittlung von Schilddrüsenparametern im mSerum für den Raum Berlin (West) unter besonderer Beruksichtigung von Alters- und Geschlechtsabhängigkeit. Lab Med, 12: 213–222.

Spielhagen C, BK 2009. Schilddrüsendiagnostik in der Schwangerschaft. Referenzwerte und klinische Anwendung. J lab Med 33: 7–10.

Sundbeck G, Eden S, Jagenburg S, Lundberg P-A, Lindstedt G 1995. Prevalence of serum antithyroid peroxidase antibodies in 85-year old woman. Clin Chem 41: 707–712.

Thomas, L 1998. Labor und Diagnose. TH-Books Verlagsgesellschaft mbH.

Vanderpump MP, TW 1995. The incidence of thyroid disorders in the community: a twenty-year follow-up of the Whickham Survey. Clin Endocrinol (Oxf), 43: 55–68.

Wiersinga WM 1995. Subclinical hypothyrism and hyperthyroidism. Prevalence and clinical relevance. Neth J Med; 46: 197–204.

4.1.2 Adrenal glands

4.1.2.1 Cushing syndrome

Medical history and clinical picture: The term Cushing syndrome now encompasses all clinical pictures of hypercortisolism, i.e., central, adrenal, ectopic, and other forms. The disorder was first described in 1932 by Harvey W. Cushing, from whom the modern disease name derives (Cushing, 1932). The clinical symptoms of Cushing syndrome are summarized in ▶ Table 4.3 in order of frequency.

Cushing syndrome is rare. The various forms of the disease (▶ Table 4.4) can occur at all ages, but show a peak between 25 and 50 years (Boscaro, et al., 2001). Interestingly, a significant increase in the incidence of Cushing syndrome has been described in recent years in some monitoring studies (Boscaro and Arnaldi, 2009). Pituitary Cushing disease, which is responsible for about 70 % of Cushing syndrome cases, has an incidence of 1–10 per million per year. Women are affected three to ten times more often than men (Boscaro

Diagnostics for Suspected Hypothyroidism			
Initial examination/ incidental findings	TSH		
	Elevated ——————— No ———→		Within reference range
	Yes		Yes
Laboratory	Determination of fT4 and TPO Ab		TSH 2.5–4.2 mU/L and clinical symptoms
	fT4 lowered		
	Yes	No	Yes
	TPO Ab positive		
	Yes	No	
Diagnosis	**Autoimmune Hypothyroidism**	**Primary Hypothyroidism**	**Latent Subclinical Hypothyroidism, Suspected Immunothyroiditis** / **Subclinical Hypothyroidism?**
Clarification of additional origins/additional procedures	T4 therapy	Clarification of origins	TRH test? Recheck in 6–12 months / Counseling patient, TSH, fT4 recheck, TRH test? Try T4 therapy if necessary

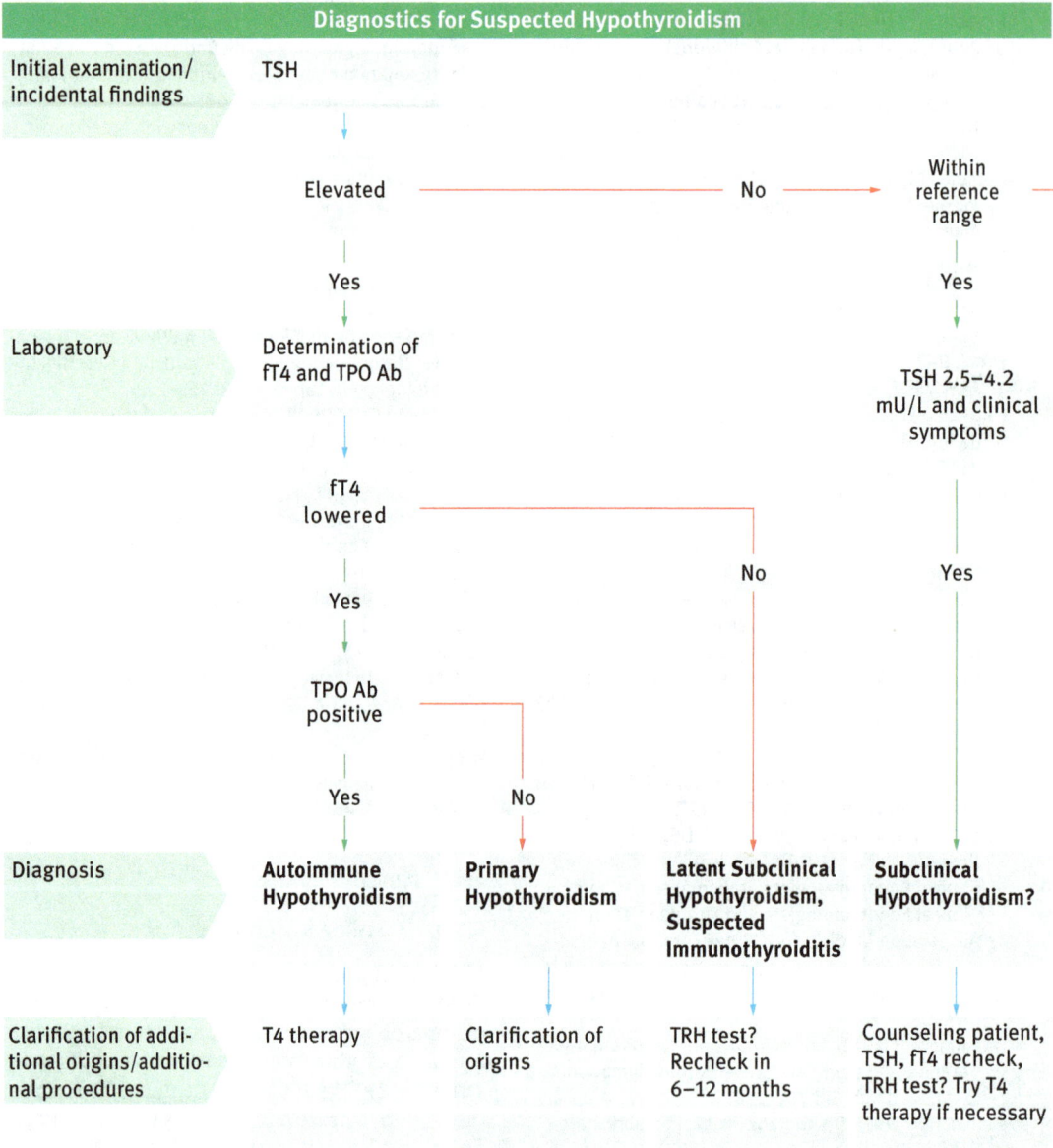

Figure 4.2 Diagnostic procedure for clarifying hypothyroidism.

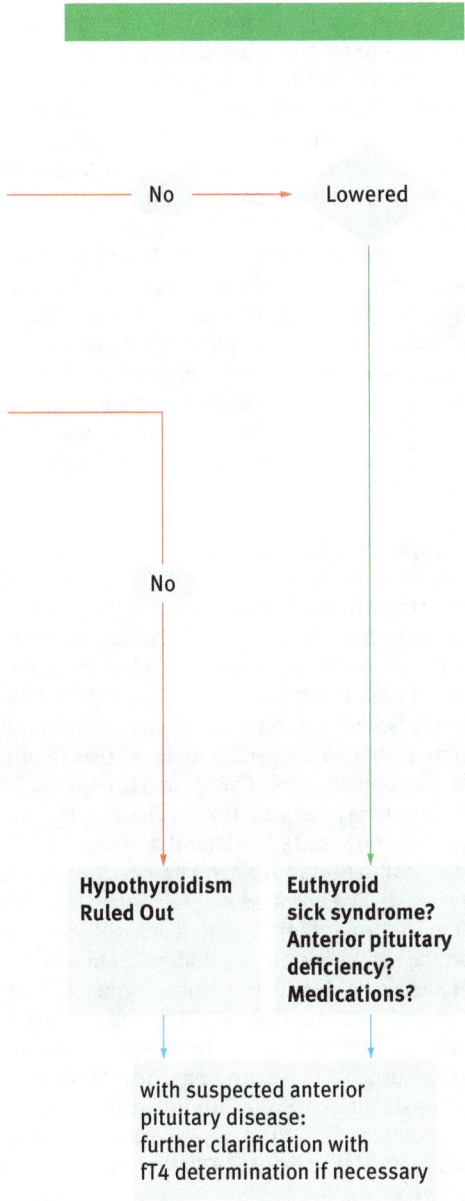

and Arnaldi, 2009; Boscaro, et al., 2001). Cushing Syndrome cases attributable to other causes are correspondingly rare (Findling, et al., 1991; Oldfield, et al., 1991; Orth, 1995).

Pre- and Post-analytical Principles: Corticotropin-releasing hormone (CRH) is synthesized in

No ——→ Lowered

No

Hypothyroidism Ruled Out

Euthyroid sick syndrome? Anterior pituitary deficiency? Medications?

with suspected anterior pituitary disease: further clarification with fT4 determination if necessary

Table 4.3 Symptoms of Cushing syndrome and their relative frequency.

Symptoms	Frequency (in %)
Red, rounded face (full moon, plethora)	90
Abdominal obesity	65
Diabetic metabolism	85
Hypertension	80
Hypogonadism (amenorrhea, loss of libido and potency)	75
Psychological changes	70
Osteoporosis	65
Striae rubrae, hemorrhagic diathesis	60
Muscle weakness	65
Hirsutism (women)	70
Ankle edema	55
Bull neck/buffalo hump	55
Acne	55
Back and other bone pains	50
Poor wound healing	35
Kidney stones	20
Polycythemia	20

Table 4.4 Origins of Cushing syndrome and their relative prevalence.

Origins	Prevalence (in %)
ACTH-dependent Cushing syndrome	
ACTH-secreting pituitary adenoma (Cushing disease)	70
Ectopic ACTH syndrome	12
Ectopic CRH syndrome	< 1
Pseudo-Cushing syndrome	< 2
ACTH-independent Cushing syndrome	
Adrenocortical adenoma	10
Adrenocortical carcinoma	8
Bilateral micronodular dysplasia (PPNAD)	1
Bilateral macronodular hyperplasia (AIMAH)	< 1

hypothalamus, where its secretion is regulated by a variety of neurotransmitters, and is the most powerful regulator of adrenocorticotropic hormone (ACTH) secretion. As a glandotropic hormone, ACTH governs the production and release of glucocorticoids in the adrenal cortex. CRH and ACTH secretion are primarily inhibited by cortisol (negative feed-back), whereby the steeper the cortisol increase, the more severe the inhibitory effect (differential effect) and the greater the amount of cortisol in circulation over a given period of time (integral effect) (Eberwine, et al., 1987; Herman, et al., 1992; Vale, et al., 1983).

Cushing syndrome can be divided into ACTH-dependent forms, in which inadequately high ACTH levels stimulate adrenal cortisol production, and ACTH-independent forms, in which pathological processes in the adrenal cortex cause excessive cortisol production that involves suppressing CRH and ACTH secretion (▶ Table 4.4).

ACTH-dependent Cushing Syndrome

Cushing Disease: Cushing disease refers only to those cases of hypercortisolism that have an ACTH-forming pituitary tumor as the underlying cause. These are responsible for 70 % of all Cushing Syndrome cases. Most are microadenomas (< 1 cm diameter), rarer are macroadenomas or hyperplasia of the corticotropic cells, and extremely rarely carcinomas. Adenomas arise from a single progenitor cell. While chronically increased CRH secretion can lead to a hyperplasia of corticotropic cells of the anterior pituitary, it does not lead to an adenoma. Adenoma-induced overproduction of ACTH leads to a bilateral adrenocortical hyperplasia with increased cortisol production. This in turn inhibits endogenous CRH and ACTH secretion.

The normal circadian ACTH rhythm is lost with Cushing disease (Boyar, et al., 1979; Hellman, et al., 1970; Liu, et al., 1987; Sederberg-Olsen, et al., 1973), so that cortisol secretion does not follow the normal circadian rhythm. The morning ACTH and cortisol levels can be normal, but the evening concentrations are increased. The increased cortisol secretion is reflected in increased cortisol elimination. Chronically elevated cortisol levels inhibit CRH secretion and lead to atrophy of the non-adenomatous modified corticotropic cells of the anterior pituitary. Essentially, there is resistance between ACTH secretion and the negative feedback

by glucocorticoids, with a shift of the threshold to a higher reference point (Liddle, 1960).

Patients with Cushing disease exhibit excessive ACTH and cortisol responses following stimulation with CRH, and incomplete inhibition of cortisol and ACTH secretion in the dexamethasone suppression test (Fukata, et al., 1988; Grossman, et al., 1988; Oldfield, et al., 1991; Orth, et al., 1982; Pieters, et al., 1983). Apparently, the adenoma cells are relatively resistant to glucocorticoids, while being relatively sensitive to CRH. A significant increase in blood ACTH following CRH administration is absent in approximately 10 % of patients with microadenomas, which is attributed to a lack of the necessary receptor or post receptor mechanisms (Hermus, et al., 1986; Nieman, et al., 1986; Orth, 1992).

Ectopic ACTH syndrome: In ectopic ACTH syndrome, there is inadequate ACTH secretion due to a tumor located outside the pituitary. The most frequent cause is small-cell lung cancer. However, a variety of other tumors can also lead to ectopic ACTH production (Becker and Aron, 1994; Liddle, et al., 1969; Wigg, et al., 1999), *inter alia* carcinoid tumors that are often difficult to localize (Findling and Doppman, 1994; Trainer and Grossman, 1991; Wajchenberg, et al., 1994). The ectopic ACTH production causes a bilateral adrenocortical hyperplasia with an inadequate cortisol secretion increase. The elevated serum cortisol concentrations in turn inhibit hypothalamic CRH secretion, which results in pituitary undersecretion of ACTH. However, with a few exceptions (particularly in bronchial carcinoids), ACTH secretion by the tumor will not be affected by the increased blood glucocorticoid concentrations. Accordingly, high-dose dexamethasone administration likewise does not lead to a drop in serum cortisol (Clark, et al., 1990; Mason, et al., 1972; Nieman, et al., 1986; Strott, et al., 1968).

Ectopic CRH syndrome: Ectopic CRH syndrome is a very rare variant of Cushing syndrome. It differs from ectopic ACTH syndrome in that the inadequate CRH production from a tumor located outside the hypothalamus leads to hypertrophy of the anterior pituitary corticotropic cells, which is accompanied by an inadequate increase in ACTH secretion (Orth, 1992). This latter in turn leads to bilateral adrenocortical hyperplasia with an excess in blood cortisol, which presumably suppresses hypothalamic CRH secretion (Belsky, et al., 1985).

Plasma CRH concentrations should increase in ectopic CRH syndrome (Fjellestad-Paulsen, et al., 1988; Jessop, et al., 1987; Schteingart, et al., 1986), and CRH-stimulated ACTH secretion should be suppressible following high-dose dexamethasone administration (DeBold, et al., 1989; Hohnloser, et al., 1989; O'Brien, et al., 1992). However, the suppressibility of ACTH is absent in many cases, because in addition to CRH these tumors frequently also secrete inadequate ACTH. Ectopic CRH syndrome predominantly involves bronchial carcinoids (Schteingart, et al., 1986; Zarate, et al., 1986).

Pseudo-Cushing Syndrome: Patients with severe depression can exhibit laboratory diagnostic aspects of Cushing syndrome (Plotsky, et al., 1998). Approximately 80 % of patients with severe depression can have a pathological dexamethasone suppression test result that reflects a disruption of cortisol secretion (Gold, et al., 1986; Halbreich, et al., 1985; Pfohl, et al., 1985), wherein the basal cortisol levels are slightly increased at best (Orth, 1995).

Chronic alcoholism is also a very rare cause of pseudo-Cushing syndrome. Longtime excessive use of alcohol can produce Cushing symptomatology and lead to a suppression of the circadian cortisol secretion cycle or a pathological dexamethasone suppression test result (Groote and Meinders, 1996). The underlying pathobiochemistry is still unclear. The patient's medical history and alcohol withdrawal will help with the differential diagnosis, so that the clinical and laboratory medical findings will normalize within a few weeks of abstinence (Boscaro, et al., 2001).

Pseudo-Cushing syndrome can also occur in HIV patients, as described under antiviral therapy, in which cases the normal basal cortisol levels are only inadequately inhibitable in the dexamethasone suppression test (Miller, et al., 1998).

Medicines, in particular anti-epileptic drugs (phenytoin), but also spironolactone and estrogens (oral contraceptives), likewise clearly elicit increased basal cortisol levels and pathological results in the dexamethasone suppression test, without further evidence of Cushing syndrome or Cushing disease being found. This underlines the importance of taking a careful medication history. The phrase "hypercortisolism in the absence of (true) Cushing syndrome" is being increasingly used instead of the phrase "pseudo-Cushing syndrome" (Guignat and Bertherat, 2010).

ACTH-independent Cushing syndrome

Cushing syndrome due to a primary disease of the adrenal cortex. The elevated cortisol levels lead to suppression of CRH and ACTH secretion in the sense of negative feedback coupling.

Adrenocortical tumors: benign and malignant adrenocortical tumors are the most common origins of ACTH-independent Cushing syndrome (Carpenter, 1986). In correlation to their size, adrenocortical carcinomas produce large quantities of various steroids. Thus, based on the tissue mass, cortisol biosynthesis is relatively insufficient and the amount of cortisol precursors is disproportionately high. By contrast, adrenocortical adenomas are characterized by efficient, usually excessive cortisol biosynthesis.

Since a unilateral, cortisol-producing adrenocortical tumor suppresses ACTH secretion, the contralateral adrenal cortex and the remaining ipsilateral adrenocortical tissue are usually atrophied. Indications of hypertrophy mean that the possibility of asymmetric macronodular hyperplasia must be considered (Doppman, et al., 1988).

Bilateral Micronodular Dysplasia: Bilateral micronodular dysplasia (PPNAD) is one of the rare causes of Cushing syndrome (Shenoy, et al., 1984). About half of all cases affect children and adults under 30 years of age, and the rest are based on a genetic, autosomal dominant disease referred to as the "Carney complex" (Carney, et al., 1985; Stratakis, 2001).

Bilateral Macronodular Hyperplasia: ACTH-independent bilateral macronodular adrenocortical hyperplasia (AIMAH) is considered to be an extremely rare cause of primary adrenal-related Cushing syndrome (Zeiger, et al., 1991). It is even rarer than the likewise comparatively rare bilateral micronodular dysplasia (PPNAD). In laboratory terms, both AIMAH and PPNAD are characterized by ACTH-independent endogenous hypercortisolism due to bilateral nodular changes in the adrenal cortex. The etiology of AIMAH is still unclear, but it is probably a primary adrenocortical disease (Wada, et al., 1996). Overall, the pathophysiology of AIMAH has been shown to be heterogeneous.

Sample Stability and Analytical Peculiarities

Cortisol: Cortisol can be stored before carrying out the analysis at 22 °C or 4 °C for 4 days (2013; Kern and Fehm, 2008; Schneider, et al., 2007.). Cortisol in saliva appears to be stable for a longer time: stability for several weeks at both room and refrigerator temperatures has been described (Nieman, et al., 2008).

Depending on the immunoassay used, cross-reactivity with other corticosteroids will be present in the cortisol determination (about 1–5 % for 11-desoxycortisol and corticosterone, more than 20 % for prednisolone) (2013).

ACTH: ACTH is rapidly degraded in the blood. The sampling should be done in cooled, plastic tubes containing EDTA or heparin because ACTH is strongly adsorbed on glass surfaces. After sample collection, the tube should be cooled in an ice-water mixture during transport to the laboratory, and the sample should be centrifuged within 4 h of collection. A decrease of > 10 % in the ACTH concentration occurs during storage of the plasma after > 24 h at 4 °C, and after > 19 h at 22 °C. Hemolysis and high bilirubin levels do not interfere with the usual test systems, while strongly lipemic specimens must be clarified by ultracentrifugation (2000; 2013; Kern and Fehm, 2008; Reisch, et al., 2007).

Basic diagnostic approach

General: The diagnosis and differential diagnosis of Cushing syndrome is often difficult, complex and costly, especially since many of the clinical symptoms also occur with other, much more common diseases. On the other hand, especially in mild cases, frequently only a few symptoms of Cushing syndrome are found (Boscaro and Arnaldi, 2009). As a further confound, the obesity that is spreading in epidemic proportions can also lead to a Cushingoid appearance in many cases (Findling and Raff, 2006).

The low-dose dexamethasone suppression test can rule out Cushing syndrome with high reliability. In case of insufficient suppression, the free cortisol determination in a 24-hour urine sample is used to confirm a diagnosis. In doubtful cases, a daily cortisol profile can also be carried out, for example, with blood sampling at 8, 18 and 24 hours, where the 24-hour value has particular significance for the diagnosis of Cushing syndrome. As an alternative to the nighttime serum cortisol determination, the saliva determination is finding increasing use. The diagnosis of Cushing syndrome should primarily be based on two or more of the first-line pathological tests (e.g., low-dose dexamethasone suppression test, free cortisol in the 24-hour urine, increased nighttime cortisol levels). While the low-dose dexamethasone suppression test and free cortisol determination in the 24-hour urine are generally considered the most effective methods (Boscaro and Arnaldi, 2009; Elamin, et al., 2008), some authors have discussed a higher sensitivity and specificity of the nighttime cortisol determination in saliva for the diagnosis of Cushing syndrome (Findling and Raff, 2006). However, there are also other tests that can be used to confirm the diagnosis or to rule out Cushing syndrome (Findling and Raff, 2006; Nieman, et al., 2008; Pecori Giraldi, 2009; Vilar, et al., 2007).

Only after confirmation of the underlying disease through hormone analysis is localization diagnostics indicated (Newell-Price and Grossman, 2007; Vilar, et al., 2007). The diagnostic procedure for clarifying Cushing syndrome is shown in ▶ Figure 4.3a.

> **Symptoms and findings:** Full-moon face, abdominal obesity, diabetes mellitus, hypertension, osteoporosis, striae rubrae, hirsutism, amenorrhea

Free cortisol in the 24-hour urine: Free cortisol measurement in the 24-hour urine has the advantage of being an integrated measurement of the serum cortisol concentrations that fluctuate widely throughout the day (Newell-Price and Grossman, 1999). The diagnostic sensitivity for free cortisol is 95–100 %, and the specificity is 94–98 % (Crapo, 1979; Mengden, et al., 1992). The collection period begins after the first morning urine and ends with the morning urine of the next day. Due to the possibility of cumulative errors, even when the patients are well instructed, and the possibility even in Cushing syndrome patients of day-to-day variations in cortisol secretion, the determination should be repeated if borderline findings are ob-

Confirming a Cushing Syndrome Diagnosis

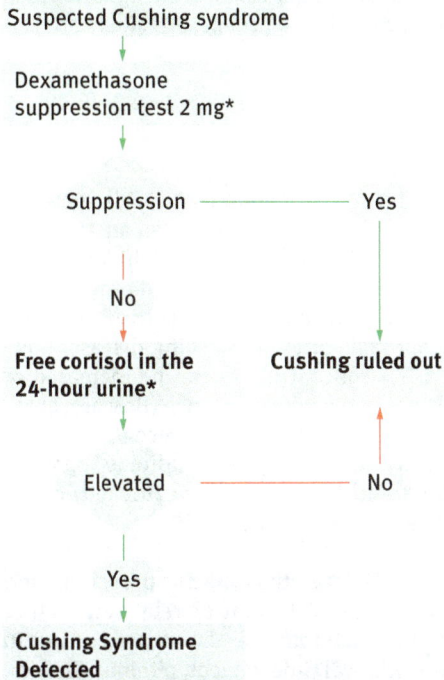

Suspected Cushing syndrome

↓

Dexamethasone
suppression test 2 mg*

↓

Suppression ——————— Yes

|

No

↓

Free cortisol in the   Cushing ruled out
24-hour urine*

↓   ↑

Elevated ——————— No

|

Yes

↓

**Cushing Syndrome
Detected**

* Increased nighttime cortisol levels in serum or saliva
that are obtained in isolation or as part of a daily
cortisol profile can be likewise used to confirm a
diagnosis of Cushing syndrome. The diagnosis is
confirmed when two of the three tests (low-dose
dexamethasone suppression test, free cortisol in
24 hour urine, increased nighttime cortisol levels)
show pathological results.

Figure 4.3a Confirming a Cushing syndrome diagnosis.

tained, especially if the measurements are being done on an outpatient basis (Nieman and Iliad, 2005).

To ensure a proper 24-hour collection period, the determination of creatinine concentration in the urine can be used, as the day-to-day variation is less than 10 % (Boscaro, et al., 2001). If an improperly conducted urine collection is suspected during the collection period, the urine cortisol concentration must not be based on the urine creatinine concentration because while the creatinine elimination rate remains relatively constant over 24 hours, the cortisol elimination rate varies episodically (Orth, 1995). Urine cortisol determination is of limited suitability in patients with impaired renal function (Boscaro, et al., 2001; Nieman and Ilias, 2005). Many experts recommend that the determination of free cortisol in the 24-hour urine should be performed at least twice (Guignat and Bertherat, 2010; Lila, et al., 2013; Nieman, et al., 2008; Nieman and Ilias, 2005). If no elevated values are found from repeated determinations, Cushing syndrome is very unlikely (Newell-Price, et al., 1998. Vilar, et al., 2007).

Low-dose Dexamethasone Suppression Test: Since the low-dose dexamethasone suppression test was first described by Liddle in 1960 (eight-fold administration of 0.5 mg dexamethasone every six hours), it has been the most important functional test for ruling out Cushing syndrome (Liddle, 1960). Currently it usually involves the oral administration of 1–2 mg dexamethasone by 11:00 pm or midnight, with a cortisol determination performed at 8:00 am or 9:00 am the following morning (Bertagna, et al., 2009; Chase, 2008; Gilbert and Lim, 2008; Lila, et al., 2013; Nugent, et al., 1965). Some authors also recommend the administration of 0.5 mg dexamethasone (Kageyama, et al., 2012; Oki, et al., 2009). A suppression less than 30 µg/L (< 80 nmol/L) is normal; higher levels following dexamethasone administration indicate an autonomous hypercortisolism. Ideally, the cortisol level should also be determined in the morning before the oral dexamethasone dose is administered, not the least on plausibility grounds. In the context of clarifying Cushing syndrome, the diagnostic sensitivity of the test is about 97–100 % (Crapo, 1979; Hankin, et al., 1977; Kennedy, et al., 1984; Newell-Price, et al., 1998; Newell-Price, et al., 1995; Yanovsky, et al., 1993). Its diagnostic specificity varies depending on the test population and implementation. If a cut-off value of < 18.5 µg/L (< 50 nmol/L) is chosen, the specificity is 97–100 % (Boscaro, et al., 2001; Newell-Price, et al., 1998). The predictive value of all variants of the dexamethasone-inhibition test depend on individual factors, including different absorption and the rates of metabolism of dexamethasone, medications taken, any hormonal contraception used, pregnancy, psychiatric diseases, alcoholism, stress, lack of compliance, chronic renal failure, and hypothyroidism.

Circadian Rhythm and Night Sleep: In healthy individuals with a normal circadian rhythm, the serum cortisol levels begin to rise 3:00 am–4:00

am, reach a maximum at 7:00 am–9:00 am, then decrease continuously over the further course of the day, and achieve the lowest values during the first half of the night (Nieman, et al., 2008). While asleep at night, cortisol secretion is largely unaffected by exogenous factors. During this phase, if the serum cortisol value does not drop below 50 μg/L, there is a high probability of Cushing syndrome. In addition, a single nighttime blood draw at midnight can confirm (John, et al., 2010; Newell-Price, et al., 1998) or rule out (Vilar, et al., 2007) Cushing syndrome. Moreover, the determination of free cortisol in saliva is increasingly being used to determine the nighttime cortisol levels (2008; Alexandraki and Grossman, 2010; Carrozza, et al., 2010; Findling and Raff, 2006; Manetti, et al., 2012; Nunes, et al., 2009), and there appears to be no difference between determinations done at 11:00 pm or midnight (Findling and Raff, 2006). It is possible that the nighttime cortisol determination in saliva has even higher sensitivity and specificity for the diagnosis of Cushing syndrome than the low-dose dexamethasone suppression test and the free cortisol in 24-hour urine (Findling and Raff, 2006). Many publications recommend a minimum of two determinations (Carrasco, et al., 2012; Findling and Raff, 2006; Guignat and Bertherat, 2010; Liu, et al., 2005; Nieman, et al., 2008; Viardot, et al., 2005).

Free Cortisol in the Saliva: The cortisol concentration in saliva substantially corresponds to the free, biologically active cortisol in the serum, and is independent of saliva flow. Unlike the serum cortisol, the concentration is not affected by changes in the transcortin concentration. The saliva cortisol analysis is suitable for both functional tests (Boscaro, et al., 2000; Laudat, et al., 1988) and nighttime cortisol determination (Beko, et al., 2010; Carrozza, et al., 2010; Sakihara, et al., 2010). An increase in the serum cortisol reflected within minutes in the salivary cortisol (Read, et al., 1990). The great advantage of the free cortisol determination from saliva is the possibility of simple sample collection, e.g., in the independent sample collection by the patient in the home environment or with pediatric patients (Boscaro and Arnaldi, 2009).

After a long time during which the saliva analysis did not find broad implementation (Tunn, et al., 1992), it has now made its way into routine diagnostics and guidelines (AWMF, 2010; Find-

ling and Raff, 2006; Guignat and Bertherat, 2010; Manetti, et al., 2012; Nieman, et al., 2008; Nieman and Ilias, 2005; Nunes, et al., 2009; Raff, 2012).

4.1.2.2 Clarification of Cushing Syndrome

Differential diagnosis

ACTH: The determination of ACTH is the most suitable for distinguishing between an ACTH-dependent or ACTH-independent origin for a Cushing syndrome case. Undetectable morning ACTH levels indicate an autonomous cortisol secretion of the adrenal cortex. In Cushing disease, however, ACTH concentrations can be increased or can also be in the reference range (Boscaro, et al., 2001). The higher the ACTH concentration, the more likely an ectopic ACTH syndrome is present (Findling and Doppman, 1994; Howlett, et al., 1986; Trainer and Grossman, 1991).

High-dose Dexamethasone Suppression Test: Following administration of relatively higher doses of dexamethasone, the serum cortisol in patients with ACTH-dependent, pituitary Cushing syndrome drops below 50 % of the initial value in most cases. However, in ACTH-independent, i.e., adrenal Cushing syndrome, there is no cortisol suppression. In turn, patients with ectopic ACTH syndrome can occasionally exhibit cortisol suppression to below 50 % of the initial value.

The test runs with either a single dose of 8 mg dexamethasone *per os* at 11:00 pm (Tyrrell, et al., 1986) or over 48 hours with the administration of 2 mg of dexamethasone every six hours (total of 16 mg) (Liddle, 1960). The sensitivities and specificities described in the literature vary between 60 % and 100 %, depending on the selected cutoff value, application period, and the time of blood sampling (Bruno, et al., 1985; Crapo, 1979; Dichek, et al., 1994; Flack, et al., 1992; Grossman, et al., 1988; Hermus, et al., 1986; Howlett, et al., 1986; Kaye and Crapo, 1990; Nieman and Ilias, 2005; Tyrrell, et al., 1986), and the 8 mg quick test generally seems to have a higher sensitivity (Dichek, et al., 1994; Tyrrell, et al., 1986). Also described are inhibition tests with the administration of dexamethasone *per infusionem*, which can circumvent the malabsorption in question, an increased clearance rate, or even poor compliance. Finally, the suppression following administration of much higher dexamethasone doses (32 mg over

24 hours) seems to be more effective than the usual 8 mg dose. Such a test variant thus offers an option for further clarification of a pituitary Cushing syndrome not suppressible by an 8 mg dose (al-Saadi, et al., 1998).

CRH Test: After emplacing a venous access, the test should be preceded by a rest period of 2 hours. This is followed by the first sample collection to determine the basal ACTH and cortisol levels, followed by the slow intravenous administration of 100 µg CRH. More samples are taken, for example, at 15, 30, 45, and 60 minutes following CRH administration.

In contrast to tumors with ectopic ACTH secretion, most ACTH-secreting pituitary adenomas have CRH receptors and generally show exceptionally high ACTH and cortisol responses following CRH administration. Thus, for an ACTH increase of more than 35 % of the initial value, the diagnostic sensitivity and specificity for the presence of pituitary Cushing syndrome is 93 % or 100 %, respectively (Nieman, et al., 1993). Occasionally, cases with ectopic ACTH secretion can also exhibit an ACTH increase following CRH stimulation.

CRH tests can be performed either in the morning (Grossman, et al., 1988) or the evening (Nieman, et al., 1986), but conducting the test in the morning is usually favored (Newell-Price and Grossman, 2001; Nieman, et al., 1993; Orth, et al., 1982). A CRH test will not yield the expected response in 7–14 % of patients with confirmed Cushing disease (Newell-Price and Grossman, 2001). However, most of these nonresponders will exhibit suppression in the high-dose dexamethasone suppression test (Grossman, et al., 1988; Hermus, et al., 1986). Very rarely, suppression in the high-dose dexamethasone suppression test together with a response following CRH administration could also be caused by an ACTH-secreting bronchial carcinoma (Malchoff, et al., 1988).

Petrosal Sinus Catheter: In this procedure, two catheters are inserted into the distal ends of the inferior petrosal sinuses and for each side separately ACTH in the sinus blood is measured before and after CRH administration, including simultaneous ACTH measurement in the cubital venous blood. The result facilitates a distinction between pituitary Cushing syndrome and ectopic ACTH syndrome. If the ratio of the "central" and "peripheral" ACTH levels following CRH stimulation is > 2.0, this corresponds to a sensitivity of 95–97 % and a specificity of 100 % for the presence of Cushing disease (Kaltsas, et al., 1999). In other publications, a ratio of > 2.0 before or > 3.0 after CRH administration was taken as proof of the presence of Cushing disease (Findling and Raff, 2006; Nieman and Ilias, 2005; Oldfield, et al., 1991).

With an ACTH concentration gradient between left- and right-side of > 1.4, it is possible to achieve the side localization of a pituitary microadenoma with a diagnostic sensitivity of 83 % (Boscaro, et al., 2000; Kaltsas, et al., 1999). However, the large number of possible anatomic variations can significantly complicate the test interpretation in individual cases. Overall, this test should be reserved for patients for whom the high-dose dexamethasone-inhibition test, CRH tests and complementary imaging techniques are unsuccessful in confidently distinguishing between pituitary Cushing syndrome and ectopic ACTH syndrome (Boscaro, et al., 2001; Findling and Raff, 2006; Utz and Biller, 2007).

The usual procedure to confirm a diagnosis of Cushing syndrome is shown in ▶ Figure 4.3a, and the further clarification and localization diagnosis is shown in ▶ Figure 4.3b.

4.1.2.3 Hypocortisolism

Medical History and Clinical Picture

Hypocortisolism refers to a cortisol deficiency. It can occur in a primary adrenocortical insufficiency (Addison's disease), or be the result of secondary adrenocortical insufficiency. The clinical symptoms of adrenocortical insufficiency can be due either to a deficiency of glucocorticoids or of mineralocorticoids (▶ Table 4.5), wherein a mineralocorticoid deficiency occurs only in primary adrenocortical insufficiency, while by contrast the renin-angiotensin-aldosterone system is not affected by a secondary adrenocortical insufficiency (Hahner, 2010; Kern and Fehm, 2008; Stewart, 2008; Ten, et al., 2001; Williams and Dluhy, 2008). Due to partial homology between ACTH and melanocyte-stimulating hormone (MSH), primary adrenocortical insufficiency with elevated ACTH values results in classical skin and mucosal hyperpigmentation (Leelarathna, et al., 2009; Nieman and Chanco Turner, 2006). Correspondingly, in secondary adrenocortical insufficiency with

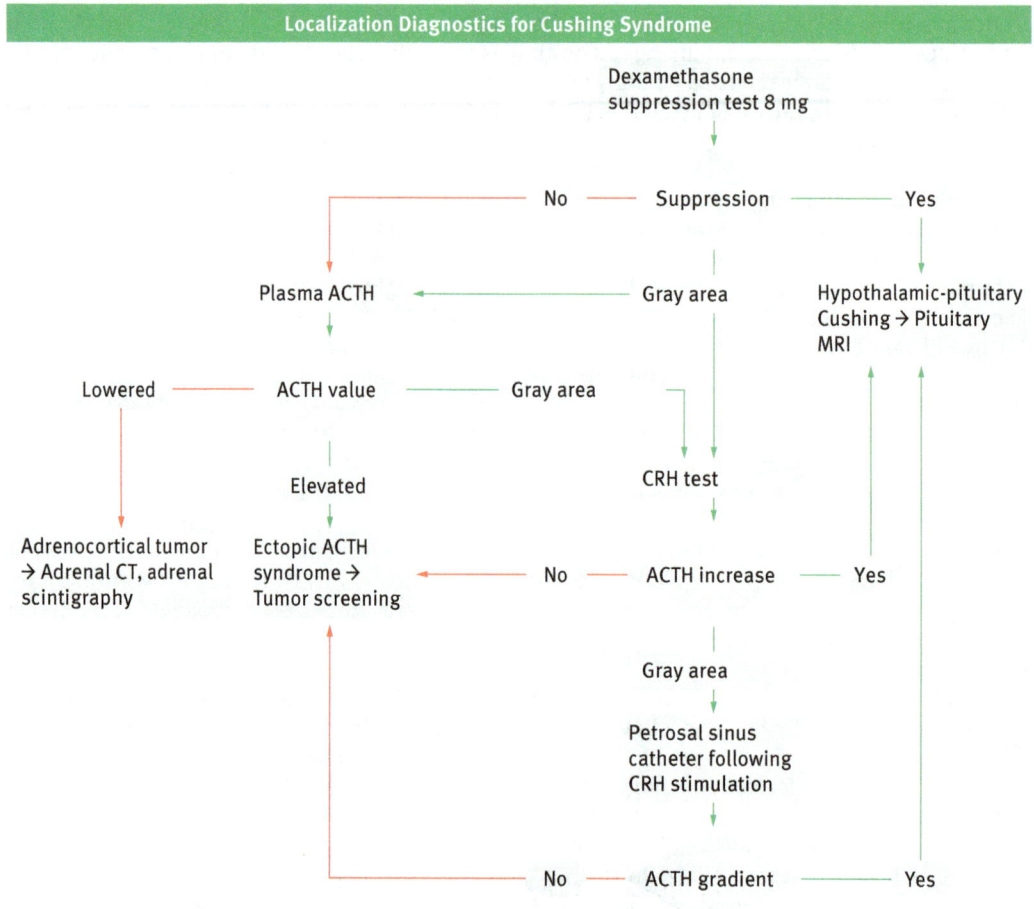

Figure 4.3b Diagnostic procedure for localization diagnostics for confirmed Cushing Syndrome.

decreased or low normal ACTH values, this hyperpigmentation is absent. The hyperpigmentation is usually absent by the time the diagnosis is made, if the adrenal glands undergo very rapid destruction in primary adrenocortical insufficiency (Williams and Dluhy, 2008). Women are more often affected by adrenocortical insufficiency than men, and the mean age at diagnosis is between 30 and 40 years.

The following basically applies: with suspected presence of a clinically-threatening, acute adrenocortical insufficiency (adrenal crisis), endocrine function tests must not delay initiation of treatment. In these cases, the pretreatment diagnostic measures should be limited to blood draws, which will facilitate the determinations of cortisol and ACTH, and possibly complementary parameters such as electrolytes, renin, aldosterone, and DHEAS. The function tests should then be rescheduled for a later date.

Pre- and Post-analytical Principles

Primary adrenocortical insufficiency is rare. The incidence in Western populations is approximately 4.7–6.2 per million/year, with an upward trend (Arlt and Allolio, 2003; Vaidya, et al., 2009). The most common origin of primary adrenocortical insufficiency in developing countries is tuber-

Table 4.5 Symptoms of adrenocortical insufficiency and their relative frequency. The symptoms caused by a mineralocorticoid deficiency are found only in primary adrenocortical insufficiency (Kern and Fehm, 2008; Williams and Dluhy, 2008; Stewart, 2008; Hahner, 2010; Ten, et al., 2001).

Symptoms	Frequency (in %)
Weakness	99–100
Weight loss	97–100
Skin pigmentation	94–98
Anorexia, nausea, vomiting	75–100
Hypotension (< 110/70 mmHg)	87–94
Pigmentation of mucous membranes	82–94
Hyponatremia (mineralocorticoid deficiency, primary adrenocortical insufficiency)	88
Hyperkalemia (mineralocorticoid deficiency, primary adrenocortical insufficiency)	64
Anemia	40
Stomach pains	34
Salt craving (mineralocorticoid deficiency, primary adrenocortical insufficiency)	16–22
Diarrhea	16–20
Constipation	19
Eosinophilia	17
Syncope	16
Vitiligo	9–20
Hypercalcemia	6

culous adrenalitis. In the industrialized nations, however, 80–90 % of all patients with primary adrenocortical insufficiency are found to have autoimmune adrenalitis (Betterle, et al., 2001).

Secondary adrenocortical insufficiency is most commonly caused by mass lesions in the area of the hypothalamus or pituitary gland. The rarer causes include, for example, autoimmune hypophysitis or pituitary apoplexy (Arlt and Allolio, 2003; Ten, et al., 2001).

An overview of possible origins of adrenocortical insufficiency is contained in ▶ Table 4.6.

Basic diagnostic approach

General: In the early phase of slow destruction of the adrenal cortex, the routine laboratory parameters are not necessarily altered, and basal steroid secretion can also be normal. However, there is a reduction in adrenal reserve, as a result of which only insufficient cortisol will be released under conditions of stress.

Since cortisol secretion is at its highest in the early morning hours, determinations of the basal cortisol and ACTH levels at this time are most likely to differentiate between adrenocortical insufficiency and proper adrenal function. In this way, morning cortisol levels of < 30 μg/L (< 80 nmol/L) between 8:00 am and 9:00 am indicate adrenal insufficiency (Kern and Fehm, 2008), while values > 145 μg/L (> 400 nmol/L) (Hagg,

Table 4.6 Causes of adrenocortical insufficiency (Williams and Dluhy, 2008; Stewart, 2008; Hahner, 2010; Ten, et al., 2001).

Causes of primary adrenocortical insufficiency	Causes of secondary adrenocortical insufficiency
Autoimmune adrenalitis (80–90 % of cases in Western industrialized nations)	Pituitary tumors, other tumors of the hypothalamus-pituitary region (craniopharyngioma, meningioma, metastases)
Infectious adrenalitis (tuberculous, fungal, CMV, HIV)	
Bilateral adrenalectomy	Operation or radiation in the hypothalamus-pituitary region
Tumor infiltration	lymphocytic hypophysitis
Bilateral adrenal hemorrhage	Pituitary infiltration (tuberculosis, sarcoidosis, Wegener's granulomatosis)
Medication-induced adrenocortical insufficiency (mitotane, metyrapone, ketoconazole, aminoglutethimide, etomidate, suramin)	Pituitary apoplexy
	Postpartum hypopituitarism (Sheehan syndrome)
Congenital origins (adrenoleukodystrophy, AGS, Triple-A syndrome, familial glucocorticoid deficiency syndrome, congenital adrenal hypoplasia)	Skull-brain trauma
Infiltrations (amyloidosis, hemochromatosis)	Congenital (e.g., mutations of TPIT, POMC)
	Suppression of the hypothalamus-pituitary axis by steroids (exogenous following glucocorticoid therapy, endogenous via tumor-related production)

et al,. 1987) or > 190 μg/L (> 525 nmol/L) (Kern and Fehm, 2008) would rule this out.

Cortisol physiologically inhibits TSH secretion (Hahner, 2010; Hangaard, et al., 1996), which is why slight TSH elevations of up to 10 mIU/L are often found with untreated adrenocortical insufficiency (Arlt, 2009; Leelarathna, et al., 2009; Topliss, et al., 1980).

The renin concentration or activity is increased in primary adrenocortical insufficiency, and its determination can be useful in distinguishing between primary and secondary adrenocortical insufficiency (Chakera and Vaidya, 2010; Vaidya, et al., 2009). Serum aldosterone also should be determined in patients with primary adrenocortical insufficiency (Hahner, et al., 2003).

An adrenal androgen deficiency can occur in both primary and secondary adrenocortical insufficiency. Levels of dehydroepiandrosterone (DHEA) and dehydroepiandrosterone sulfate (DHEAS) are reduced or below the detection limit in this case (Hahner, et al., 2003). ACTH stimulates androgen secretion (Leelarathna, et al., 2009; Stewart, 2008). Due to the age dependency, DHEA and DHEAS determinations only make sense in patients up to an age of approximately 40 years (Arlt, 2009).

Clarification of Hypocortisolism

ACTH-Test: The gold standard for suspected adrenocortical insufficiency is the ACTH stimulation test (Leelarathna, et al., 2009; Vaidya, et al., 2009). In practice, an ACTH test should be performed directly in patients with suspected hypocortisolism, without doing any intensive monitoring of cortisol basal levels (Stewart, 2008). The ACTH test is independent of the time of day, and can be performed at any time.

In general, the ACTH test is carried out as a quick test with a blood sample previously obtained for ACTH determination. At 30 and/or 60 minutes following iv administration of synthetic ACTH (250 μg 1–24 ACTH), another blood sample is drawn to determine the stimulated serum cortisol value. In the presence of normal adrenocortical function, stimulation leads to an increase in the serum cortisol value to at least 180–200 μg/L (500–550 nmol/L) (Arlt, 2009; Clark, et al., 1998; Hahner, et al., 2003; Oelkers, et al., 1992; Stewart, et al., 1988; Vaidya, et al., 2009; Wood, et al., 1965). In primary adrenal insufficiency, the

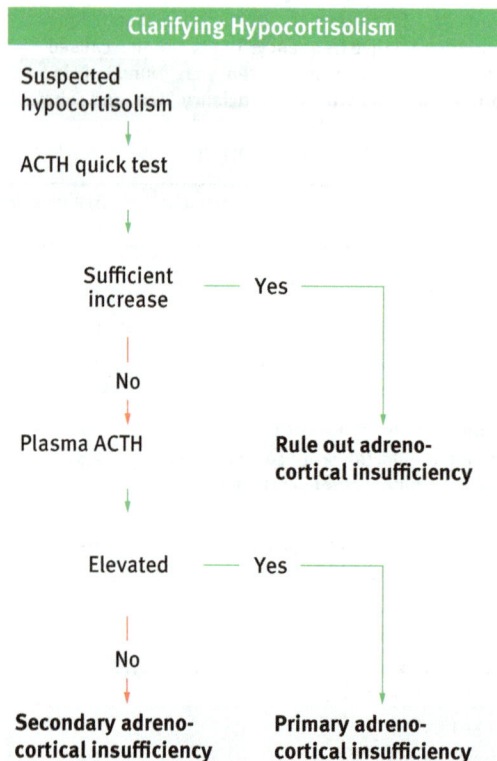

Figure 4.4 Diagnostic procedure for clarifying hypocortisolism.

cortisol increase is almost completely absent at elevated basal plasma ACTH levels. In secondary adrenocortical insufficiency, a slight but insufficient increase is usually observed (Allolio, 2010).

Since the decreased response is based on the relative degree of atrophy of the adrenal cortex, which occurs only after a long-standing ACTH deficiency, the ACTH test can be normal with a secondary adrenal insufficiency case of recent onset. Thus, the ACTH test should not be done within the first two to six weeks following pituitary surgery or an insult, and cannot be used to assess the pituitary-adrenocortical axis due to the lack of diagnostic sensitivity (Allolio, 2010; Arlt, 2009; Kern and Fehm, 2008).

With an ACTH deficiency of longer standing, the insulin hypoglycemia test (insulin tolerance test) (Arlt, 2009; Hahner, et al., 2003) or the metopirone test (Kern and Fehm, 2008) offers a possible complementary or alternative for confirming a secondary adrenocortical insufficiency.

ACTH: Following an insufficient cortisol increase in the ACTH test, a primary adrenocortical insufficiency (Addison's disease) can be distinguished from a secondary adrenocortical insufficiency using the ACTH value (Vaidya et al., 2009).

The ACTH concentration increases in primary adrenocortical insufficiency, and is generally well above 22 pmol/L (Hahner, 2010). By contrast, on secondary adrenocortical insufficiency, the ACTH concentration is lowered or lies in the bottom of the reference range (Hahner, et al., 2003).

The usual diagnostic procedure for clarifying hypocortisolism is shown in ▶ Figure 4.4.

> **Symptoms and findings:** Weakness, hypotension, weight loss, possibly hyperpigmentation

Literature

2000. Die Qualität diagnostischer Proben – Empfehlung der Arbeitsgruppe Präanalytik der Deutschen Gesellschaft für Klinische Chemie und der Deutschen Gesellschaft für Laboratoriumsmedizin.

2008. Syndrome de Cushing – Protocole national de diagnostic et de soins. Haute Autorite de Sante.

2013. Lab Tests Online, www.labtestsonline.de, accessed 25. 03. 2013.

al-Saadi N, Diederich S, Oelkers W. 1998. A very high dose dexamethasone suppression test for differential diagnosis of Cushing syndrome. Clin Endocrinol (Oxf) 48(1): 45–51.

Alexandraki KI, Grossman AB. 2010. Novel insights in the diagnosis of Cushing's syndrome. Neuroendocrinology 92 Suppl 1: 35–43.

Allolio B. 2010. Diagnostische Methoden bei Nebennierenerkrankungen. In: Allolio B, Schulte HM, editors. Praktische Endokrinologie. Munchen: Urban & Fischer. p 209–215.

Arlt W. 2009. The approach to the adult with newly diagnosed adrenal insufficiency. J Clin Endocrinol Metab 94(4): 1059–67.

Arlt W, Allolio B. 2003. Adrenal insufficiency. Lancet 361(9372): 1881–93.

AWMF. 2010. Leitlinien der Gesellschaft für Kinderheilkunde und Jugendmedizin (DGKJ): Cushing-Syndrom. Nr. 027/033.

Becker M, Aron DC. 1994. Ectopic ACTH syndrome and CRH-mediated Cushing syndrome. Endocrinol Metab Clin North Am 23(3): 585–606.

Beko G, Varga I, Glaz E, Sereg M, Feldman K, Toth M, Racz K, Patocs A. 2010. Cutoff values of midnight salivary cortisol for the diagnosis of overt hypercortisolism are highly influenced by methods. Clin Chim Acta 411(5–6): 364–7.

Belsky JL, Cuello B, Swanson LW, Simmons DM, Jarrett RM, Braza F. 1985. Cushing syndrome due to ectopic production of corticotropin-releasing factor. J Clin Endocrinol Metab 60(3): 496–500.

Bertagna X, Guignat L, Groussin L, Bertherat J. 2009. Cushing disease. Best Pract Res Clin Endocrinol Metab 23(5): 607–23.

Betterle C, Dalpra C, Greggio N, Volpato M, Zanchetta R. 2001. Autoimmunity in isolated Addison's disease and in polyglandular autoimmune diseases type 1, 2 and 4. Ann Endocrinol (Paris) 62(2): 193–201.

Boscaro M, Arnaldi G. 2009. Approach to the patient with possible Cushing syndrome. J Clin Endocrinol Metab 94(9): 3121–31.

Boscaro M, Barzon L, Fallo F, Sonino N. 2001. Cushing syndrome. Lancet 357(9258): 783–91.

Boscaro M, Barzon L, Sonino N. 2000. The diagnosis of Cushing syndrome: atypical presentations and laboratory shortcomings. Arch Intern Med 160(20): 3045–53.

Boyar RM, Witkin M, Carruth A, Ramsey J. 1979. Circadian cortisol secretory rhythms in Cushing disease. J Clin Endocrinol Metab 48(5): 760–5.

Bruno OD, Rossi MA, Contreras LN, Gomez RM, Galparsoro G, Cazado E, Kral M, Leber B, Arias D. 1985. Nocturnal high-dose dexamethasone suppression test in the aetiological diagnosis of Cushing syndrome. Acta Endocrinol (Copenh) 109(2): 158–62.

Carney JA, Gordon H, Carpenter PC, Shenoy BV, Go VL. 1985. The complex of myxomas, spotty pigmentation, and endocrine overactivity. Medicine (Baltimore) 64(4): 270–83.

Carpenter PC. 1986. Cushing syndrome: update of diagnosis and management. Mayo Clin Proc 61(1): 49–58.

Carrasco CA, Garcia M, Goycoolea M, Cerda J, Bertherat J, Padilla O, Meza D, Wohllk N, Quiroga T. 2012. Reproducibility and performance of one or two samples of salivary cortisol in the diagnosis of Cushing's syndrome using an automated immunoassay system. Endocrine 41(3): 487–93.

Carrozza C, Corsello SM, Paragliola RM, Ingraudo F, Palumbo S, Locantore P, Sferrazza A, Pontecorvi A, Zuppi C. 2010. Clinical accuracy of midnight salivary cortisol measured by automated electrochemiluminescence immunoassay method in Cushing syndrome. Ann Clin Biochem 47(Pt 3): 228–32.

Chakera AJ, Vaidya B. Addison disease in adults: diagnosis and management. Am J Med 123(5): 409–13.

Chase C. 2008. The diagnosis of Cushing's syndrome: an Endocrine Society clinical practice guideline. The Endocrine Society.

Clark AJ, Stewart MF, Lavender PM, Farrell W, Crosby SR, Rees LH, White A. 1990. Defective glucocorticoid regulation of proopiomelanocortin gene expression and peptide secretion in a small cell lung cancer cell line. J Clin Endocrinol Metab 70(2): 485–90.

Clark PM, Neylon I, Raggatt PR, Sheppard MC, Stewart PM. 1998. Defining the normal cortisol response to the short Synacthen test: implications for the investigation of hypothalamic-pituitary disorders. Clin Endocrinol (Oxf) 49(3): 287–92.

Crapo L. 1979. Cushing syndrome: a review of diagnostic tests. Metabolism 28(9): 955–77.

Cushing HW. 1932. The basophil adenomas of the pituitary body and their clinical manifestations (pituitary basophilism). Bull Johns Hopkins Hosp 50: 137–195.

DeBold CR, Jackson RV, Kamilaris TC, Sheldon WR, Jr., Decherney GS, Island DP, Orth DN. 1989. Effects of ovine corticotropin-releasing hormone on adrenocorticotropin secretion in the absence of glucocorticoid feedback inhibition in man. J Clin Endocrinol Metab 68(2): 431–7.

Dichek HL, Nieman LK, Oldfield EH, Pass HI, Malley JD, Cutler GB, Jr. 1994. A comparison of the standard high dose dexamethasone suppression test and the overnight 8-mg dexamethasone suppression test for the differential diagnosis of adrenocorticotropindependent Cushing syndrome. J Clin Endocrinol Metab 78(2): 418–22.

Doppman JL, Miller DL, Dwyer AJ, Loughlin T, Nieman L, Cutler GB, Chrousos GP, Oldfield E, Loriaux DL. 1988. Macronodulär adrenal hyperplasia in Cushing disease. Radiology 166(2): 347–52.

Eberwine JH, Jonassen JA, Evinger MJ, Roberts JL. 1987. Complex transcriptional regulation by glucocorticoids and corticotropin-releasing hormone of proopiomelanocortin gene expression in rat pituitary cultures. DNA 6(5): 483–92.

Elamin MB, Murad MH, Mullan R, Erickson D, Harris K, Nadeem S, Ennis R, Erwin PJ, Montori VM. 2008. Accuracy of diagnostic tests for Cushing syndrome: a systematic review and metaanalyses. J Clin Endocrinol Metab 93(5): 1553–62.

Findling JW, Doppman JL. 1994. Biochemical and radiologic diagnosis of Cushing syndrome. Endocrinol Metab Clin North Am 23(3): 511–37.

Findling JW, Kehoe ME, Shaker JL, Raff H. 1991. Routine inferior petrosal sinus sampling in the differential diagnosis of adrenocorticotropin (ACTH)-dependent Cushing syndrome: early recognition of the occult ectopic ACTH syndrome. J Clin Endocrinol Metab 73(2): 408–13.

Findling JW, Raff H. 2006. Cushing syndrome: important issues in diagnosis and management. J Clin Endocrinol Metab 91(10): 3746–53.

Fjellestad-Paulsen A, Abrahamsson PA, Bjartell A, Grino M, Grimelius L, Hedeland H, Falkmer S. 1988. Carcinoma of the prostate with Cushing syndrome. A case report with histochemical and chemical demonstration of immunoreactive corticotropin-releasing hormone in plasma and tumoral tissue. Acta Endocrinol (Copenh) 119(4): 506–16.

Flack MR, Oldfield EH, Cutler GB, Jr., Zweig MH, Malley JD, Chrousos GP, Loriaux DL, Nieman LK. 1992. Urine free cortisol in the high-dose dexamethasone suppression test for the differential diagnosis of the Cushing syndrome. Ann Intern Med 116(3): 211–7.

Fukata J, Nakai Y, Imura H, Abe K, Aono T, Demura H, Fujita T, Hibi I, Ibayashi H, Igarashi M and others. 1988. Human corticotropin-releasing hormone test in normal subjects and patients with hypothalamic, pituitary or adrenocortical disorders. Endocrinol Jpn 35(3): 491–502.

Gilbert R, Lim EM. 2008. The diagnosis of Cushing's syndrome: an endocrine society clinical practice guideline. Clin Biochem Rev 29(3): 103-6.

Gold PW, Loriaux DL, Roy A, Kling MA, Calabrese JR, Kellner CH, Nieman LK, Post RM, Pickar D, Gallucci W and others. 1986. Responses to corticotropin-releasing hormone in the hypercortisolism of depression and Cushing disease. Pathophysiologic and diagnostic implications. N Engl J Med 314(21): 1329–35.

Groote VR, Meinders AE. 1996. On the mechanism of alcohol-induced pseudo-Cushing syndrome. Endocr Rev 17(3): 262–8.

Grossman AB, Howlett TA, Perry L, Coy DH, Savage MO, Lavender P, Rees LH, Besser GM. 1988. CRF in the differential diagnosis of Cushing syndrome: a comparison with the dexamethasone suppression test. Clin Endocrinol (Oxf) 29(2): 167–78.

Guignat L, Bertherat J. 2010. The Diagnosis of Cushing syndrome: An Endocrine Society Clinical Practice Guideline – Commentary from a European Perspective. Eur J Endocrinol.

Hagg E, Asplund K, Lithner F. 1987. Value of basal plasma cortisol assays in the assessment of pituitaryadrenal insufficiency. Clin Endocrinol (Oxf) 26(2): 221–6.

Hahner S. 2010. Nebennierenrindeninsuffizienz In: Allolio B, Schulte HM, editors. Praktische Endokrinologie. Munchen: Urban & Fischer. p 238–245.

Hahner S, Arlt W, Allolio B. 2003. (Adrenal crisis. Diagnostic and therapeutic management of acute adrenal cortex insufficiency). Internist (Berl) 44(10): 1243–52.

Halbreich U, Asnis GM, Shindledecker R, Zumoff B, Nathan RS. 1985. Cortisol secretion in endogenous depression. II. Time-related functions. Arch Gen Psychiatry 42(9): 909–14.

Hangaard J, Andersen M, Grodum E, Koldkjaer O, Hagen C. 1996. Pulsatile thyrotropin secretion in patients with Addison's disease during variable glucocorticoid therapy. J Clin Endocrinol Metab 81(7): 2502–7.

Hankin ME, Theile HM, Steinbeck AW. 1977. An evaluation of laboratory tests for the detection and differential diagnosis of Cushing syndrome. Clin Endocrinol (Oxf) 6(3): 185–96.

Hellman L, Weitzman ED, Roffwarg H, Fukushima DK, Yoshida K. 1970. Cortisol is secreted episodically in Cushing syndrome. J Clin Endocrinol Metab 30(5): 686–9.

Herman JP, Schafer MK, Thompson RC, Watson SJ. 1992. Rapid regulation of corticotropin-releasing hormone gene transcription in vivo. Mol Endocrinol 6(7): 1061–9.

Hermus AR, Pieters GF, Pesman GJ, Smals AG, Benraad TJ, Kloppenborg PW. 1986. The corticotropin-releasing hormone test versus the high-dose dexamethasone test in the differential diagnosis of Cushing syndrome. Lancet 2(8506): 540–4.

Hohnloser J, Von Werder K, Muller OA. 1989. Acute dexamethasone suppression of ACTH secretion stimulated by human corticotrophin releasing hormone, AVP and hypoglycaemia. Clin Endocrinol (Oxf) 31(2): 175–84.

Howlett TA, Drury PL, Perry L, Doniach I, Rees LH, Besser GM. 1986. Diagnosis and management of ACTH-dependent Cushing syndrome: comparison of the features in ectopic and pituitary ACTH production. Clin Endocrinol (Oxf) 24(6): 699–713.

Jessop DS, Cunnah D, Millar JG, Neville E, Coates P, Doniach I, Besser GM, Rees LH. 1987. A phaeochromocytoma presenting with Cushing syndrome associated with increased concentrations of circulating corticotrophin-releasing factor. J Endocrinol 113(1): 133–8.

John M, Lila AR, Bandgar T, Menon PS, Shah NS. 2010. Diagnostic efficacy of midnight cortisol and midnight ACTH in the diagnosis and localisation of Cushing syndrome. Pituitary 13(1): 48–53.

Kageyama K, Oki Y, Sakihara S, Nigawara T, Terui K, Suda T. 2012. Evaluation of the diagnostic cri-teria for Cushing's disease in Japan [Review]. Endocr J.

Kaltsas GA, Giannulis MG, Newell-Price JD, Dacie JE, Thakkar C, Afshar F, Monson JP, Grossman AB, Besser GM, Trainer PJ. 1999. A critical analysis of the value of simultaneous inferior petrosal sinus sampling in Cushing disease and the occult ectopic adrenocorticotropin syndrome. J Clin Endocrinol Metab 84(2): 487–92.

Kaye TB, Crapo L. 1990. The Cushing syndrome: an update on diagnostic tests. Ann Intern Med 112(6): 434–44.

Kennedy L, Atkinson AB, Johnston H, Sheridan B, Hadden DR. 1984. Serum cortisol concentrations during low dose dexamethasone suppression test to screen for Cushing syndrome. Br Med J (Clin Res Ed) 289(6453): 1188–91.

Kern W, Fehm HL. 2008. Hypothalamus-Hypophysen-Nebennierenrinden-System. In: Thomas L, editor. Labor und Diagnose. Frankfurt/Main: TH-Books Verlagsgesellschaft mbH. p 1441–1460.

Laudat MH, Cerdas S, Fournier C, Guiban D, Guilhaume B, Luton JP. 1988. Salivary cortisol measurement: a practical approach to assess pituitary-adrenal function. J Clin Endocrinol Metab 66(2): 343–8.

Leelarathna L, Powrie JK, Carroll PV. 2009. Thomas Addison's disease after 154 years: modern diagnostic perspectives on an old condition. QJM 102(8): 569–73.

Liddle GW. 1960. Tests of pituitary-adrenal suppressibility in the diagnosis of Cushing syndrome. J Clin Endocrinol Metab 20: 1539–60.

Liddle GW, Nicholson WE, Island DP, Orth DN, Abe K, Lowder SC. 1969. Clinical and laboratory studies of ectopic humoral syndromes. Recent Prog Horm Res 25: 283–314.

Lila AR, Sarathi V, Jagtap VS, Bandgar T, Menon P, Shah NS. 2013. Cushing's syndrome: Stepwise approach to diagnosis. Indian J Endocrinol Metab 15 Suppl 4: 317–21.

Liu H, Bravata DM, Cabaccan J, Raff H, Ryzen E. 2005. Elevated late-night salivary cortisol levels in elderly male type 2 diabetic veterans. Clin Endocrinol (Oxf) 63(6): 642–9.

Liu JH, Kazer RR, Rasmüssen DD. 1987. Characterization of the twenty-four hour secretion patterns of adrenocorticotropin and cortisol in normal women and patients with Cushing disease. J Clin Endocrinol Metab 64(5): 1027–35.

Malchoff CD, Orth DN, Abboud C, Carney JA, Pairolero PC, Carey RM. 1988. Ectopic ACTH syndrome caused by a bronchial carcinoid tumor responsive to dexamethasone, metyrapone, and corticotropin-releasing factor. Am J Med 84(4): 760–4.

Manetti L, Rossi G, Grasso L, Raffaelli V, Scattina I, Del Sarto S, Cosottini M, Iannelli A, Gasperi M, Bogazzi F and others. 2012. Usefulness of salivary cortisol in the diagnosis of hypercortisolism: comparison with serum and urinary cortisol. Eur J Endocrinol 168(3): 315–21.

Mason AM, Ratcliffe JG, Buckle RM, Mason AS. 1972. ACTH secretion by bronchial carcinoid tumours. Clin Endocrinol (Oxf) 1(1): 3–25.

Mengden T, Hubmann P, Muller J, Greminger P, Vetter W. 1992. Urinary free cortisol versus 17-hydroxycorticosteroids: a comparative study of their diagnostic value in Cushing syndrome. Clin Investig 70(7): 545–8.

Miller KK, Daly PA, Sentochnik D, Doweiko J, Samore M, Basgoz NO, Grinspoon SK. 1998. Pseudo-Cushing syndrome in human immuno-deficiency virus-infected patients. Clin Infect Dis 27(1): 68–72.

Newell-Price J, Grossman A. 1999. Diagnosis and management of Cushing syndrome. Lancet 353(9170): 2087–8.

Newell-Price J, Grossman AB. 2001. The differential diagnosis of Cushing syndrome. Ann Endocrinol (Paris) 62(2): 173–9.

Newell-Price J, Grossman AB. 2007. Differential diagnosis of Cushing syndrome. Arq Bras Endocrinol Metabol 51(8): 1199–206.

Newell-Price J, Trainer P, Besser M, Grossman A. 1998. The diagnosis and differential diagnosis of Cushing syndrome and pseudo-Cushing's states. Endocr Rev 19(5): 647–72.

Newell-Price J, Trainer P, Perry L, Wass J, Grossman A, Besser M. 1995. A single sleeping midnight cortisol has 100 % sensitivity for the diagnosis of Cushing syndrome. Clin Endocrinol (Oxf) 43(5): 545–50.

Nieman LK, Biller BM, Findling JW, Newell-Price J, Savage MO, Stewart PM, Montori VM. 2008. The diagnosis of Cushing syndrome: an Endocrine Society Clinical Practice Guideline. J Clin Endocrinol Metab 93(5): 1526–40.

Nieman LK, Chanco Turner ML. 2006. Addison's disease. Clin Dermatol 24(4): 276–80.

Nieman LK, Chrousos GP, Oldfield EH, Avgerinos PC, Cutler GB, Jr., Loriaux DL. 1986. The ovine corticotropin-releasing hormone stimulation test and the dexamethasone suppression test in the differential diagnosis of Cushing syndrome. Ann Intern Med 105(6): 862–7.

Nieman LK, Ilias I. 2005. Evaluation and treatment of Cushing syndrome. Am J Med 118(12):1340–6.

Nieman LK, Oldfield EH, Wesley R, Chrousos GP, Loriaux DL, Cutler GB, Jr. 1993. A simplified morning ovine corticotropin-releasing hormone stimulation test for the differential diagnosis of adrenocorticotropin-dependent Cushing syndrome. J Clin Endocrinol Metab 77(5): 1308–12.

Nugent CA, Nichols T, Tyler FH. 1965. Diagnosis of Cushing syndrome; Single Dose Dexamethasone Suppression Test. Arch Intern Med 116: 172–6.

Nunes ML, Vattaut S, Corcuff JB, Rault A, Loiseau H, Gatta B, Valli N, Letenneur L, Tabarin A. 2009. Late-night salivary cortisol for diagnosis of overt and subclinical Cushing syndrome in hospitalized and ambulatory patients. J Clin Endocrinol Metab 94(2): 456–62.

O'Brien T, Young WF, Jr., Davila DG, Scheithauer BW, Kovacs K, Horvath E, Vale W, van Heerden JA. 1992. Cushing syndrome associated with ectopic production of corticotrophin-releasing hormone, corticotrophin and vasopressin by a phaeochromocytoma. Clin Endocrinol (Oxf) 37(5): 460–7.

Oelkers W, Diederich S, Bahr V. 1992. Diagnosis and therapy surveillance in Addison's disease: rapid adrenocorticotropin (ACTH) test and measurement of plasma ACTH, renin activity, and aldosterone. J Clin Endocrinol Metab 75(1): 259–64.

Oki Y, Hashimoto K, Hirata Y, Iwasaki Y, Nigawara T, Doi M, Sakihara S, Kageyama K, Suda T. 2009. Development and validation of a 0.5 mg dexamethasone suppression test as an initial screening test for the diagnosis of ACTH-dependent Cushing's syndrome. Endocr J 56(7): 897–904.

Oldfield EH, Doppman JL, Nieman LK, Chrousos GP, Miller DL, Katz DA, Cutler GB, Jr., Loriaux DL. 1991. Petrosal sinus sampling with and without corticotropin-releasing hormone for the differential diagnosis of Cushing syndrome. N Engl J Med 325(13): 897–905.

Orth DN. 1992. Corticotropin-releasing hormone in humans. Endocr Rev 13(2): 164–91.

Orth DN. 1995. Cushing syndrome. N Engl J Med 332(12): 791–803.

Orth DN, DeBold CR, DeCherney GS, Jackson RV, Alexander AN, Rivier J, Rivier C, Spiess J, Vale W. 1982. Pituitary microadenomas causing Cushing disease respond to corticotropin-releasing factor. J Clin Endocrinol Metab 55(5): 1017–9.

Pecori Giraldi F. 2009. Recent challenges in the diagnosis of Cushing syndrome. Horm Res 71 Suppl 1: 123–7.

Pfohl B, Sherman B, Schlechte J, Winokur G. 1985. Differences in plasma ACTH and cortisol between depressed patients and normal controls. Biol Psychiatry 20(10): 1055–72.

Pieters GF, Hermus AR, Smals AG, Bartelink AK, Benraad TJ, Kloppenborg PW. 1983. Responsiveness of the hypophyseal-adrenocortical axis to corticotropin-releasing factor in pituitary-dependent Cushing disease. J Clin Endocrinol Metab 57(3): 513–6.

Plotsky PM, Owens MJ, Nemeroff CB. 1998. Psychoneuroendocrinology of depression. Hypothalamicpituitary-adrenal axis. Psychiatr Clin North Am 21(2): 293–307.

Raff H. 2012. Cushing's syndrome: diagnosis and surveillance using salivary cortisol. Pituitary 15(1): 64–70.

Read GF, Walker RF, Wilson DW, Griffiths K. 1990. Steroid analysis in saliva for the assessment of endocrine function. Ann N Y Acad Sci 595: 260–74.

Reisch N, Reincke M, Bidlingmaier M. 2007. Preanalytical stability of adrenocorticotropic hormone depends on time to centrifugation rather than temperature. Clin Chem 53(2): 358–9.

Sakihara S, Kageyama K, Oki Y, Doi M, Iwasaki Y, Takayasu S, Moriyama T, Terui K, Nigawara T, Hirata Y and others. 2010. Evaluation of plasma, salivary, and urinary cortisol levels for diagnosis of Cushing syndrome. Endocr J 57(4): 331–7.

Schneider S, Brummer V, Carnahan H, Dubrowski A, Askew CD, Struder HK. 2007. Stress hormone stability: processing of blood samples collected during parabolic flight. A pre-flight comparison of different protocols. Clin Biochem 40(16–17): 1332–5.

Schteingart DE, Lloyd RV, Akil H, Chandler WF, Ibarra-Perez G, Rosen SG, Ogletree R. 1986. Cushing syndrome secondary to ectopic corticotropin-releasing hormone-adrenocorticotropin secretion. J Clin Endocrinol Metab 63(3): 770–5.

Sederberg-Olsen P, Binder C, Kehlet H, Neville AM, Nielsen LM. 1973. Episodic variation in plasma corticosteroids in subjects with Cushing syndrome of differing etiology. J Clin Endocrinol Metab 36(5): 906–10.

Shenoy BV, Carpenter PC, Carney JA. 1984. Bilateral primary pigmented nodulär adrenocortical disease. Rare cause of the Cushing syndrome. Am J Surg Pathol 8(5): 335–44.

Stewart PM. 2008. The Adrenal Cortex. In: Kronenberg HM, Melmed S, Polonsky KS, Larsen PR, editors. Williams Textbook of Endocrinology. Philadelphia: Saunders Elsevier. p 445–503.

Stewart PM, Corrie J, Seckl JR, Edwards CR, Padfield PL. 1988. A rational approach for assessing the hypothalamo-pituitary-adrenal axis. Lancet 1(8596): 1208–10.

Stratakis CA. 2001. Genetics of adrenocortical tumors: Carney complex. Ann Endocrinol (Paris) 62(2):180–4.

Strott CA, Nugent CA, Tyler FH. 1968. Cushing syndrome caused by bronchial adenomas. Am J Med 44(1): 97–104.

Ten S, New M, Maclaren N. 2001. Clinical review 130: Addison's disease 2001. J Clin Endocrinol Metab 86(7): 2909–22.

Topliss DJ, White EL, Stockigt JR. 1980. Significance of thyrotropin excess in untreated primary adrenal insufficiency. J Clin Endocrinol Metab 50(1): 52–6.

Trainer PJ, Grossman A. 1991. The diagnosis and differential diagnosis of Cushing syndrome. Clin Endocrinol (Oxf) 34(4): 317–30.

Tunn S, Mollmann H, Barth J, Derendorf H, Krieg M. 1992. Simultaneous measurement of cortisol in serum and saliva after different forms of cortisol administration. Clin Chem 38(8 Pt 1): 1491–4.

Tyrrell JB, Findling JW, Aron DC, Fitzgerald PA, Forsham PH. 1986. An overnight high-dose dexamethasone suppression test for rapid differential diagnosis of Cushing syndrome. Ann Intern Med 104(2):180–6.

Utz A, Biller BM. 2007. The role of bilateral inferior petrosal sinus sampling in the diagnosis of Cushing syndrome. Arq Bras Endocrinol Metabol 51(8): 1329–38.

Vaidya B, Chakera AJ, Dick C. 2009. Addison's disease. BMJ 339: b2385.

Vale W, Vaughan J, Smith M, Yamamoto G, Rivier J, Rivier C. 1983. Effects of synthetic ovine corticotropin-releasing factor, glucocorticoids, catecholamines, neurohypophysial peptides, and other substances on cultured corticotropic cells. Endocrinology 113(3): 1121–31.

Viardot A, Huber P, Puder JJ, Zulewski H, Keller U, Muller B. 2005. Reproducibility of nighttime salivary cortisol and its use in the diagnosis of hypercortisolism compared with urinary free cortisol and overnight dexamethasone suppression test. J Clin Endocrinol Metab 90(10): 5730–6.

Vilar L, Freitas Mda C, Faria M, Montenegro R, Casulari LA, Naves L, Bruno OD. 2007. Pitfalls in the diagnosis of Cushing syndrome. Arq Bras Endocrinol Metabol 51(8): 1207–16.

Wada N, Kubo M, Kijima H, Ishizuka T, Saeki T, Koike T, Sasano H. 1996. Adrenocorticotropin-independent bilateral macronodulär adrenocortical hyperplasia: immunohistochemical studies of steroidogenic enzymes and post-operative course in two men. Eur J Endocrinol 134(5): 583–7.

Wajchenberg BL, Mendonca BB, Liberman B, Pereira MA, Carneiro PC, Wakamatsu A, Kirschner MA. 1994. Ectopic adrenocorticotropic hormone syndrome. Endocr Rev 15(6): 752–87.

Wigg SJ, Ehrlich AR, Fuller PJ. 1999. Cushing syndrome secondary to ectopic ACTH secretion from metastatic breast carcinoma. Clin Endocrinol (Oxf) 50(5): 675–8.

Williams GH, Dluhy RG. 2008. Disorders of the Adrenal Cortex. In: Fauci AS, Braunwald E, Kasper DL, Hauser SL, Longo DL, Jameson JL, Loscalzo J, editors. Harrison's Principles of Internal Medicine: McGraw-Hill. p 2247–2268.

Wood JB, Frankland AW, James VH, Landon J. 1965. A Rapid Test of Adrenocortical Function. Lancet 1 (7379): 243–5.

Yanovski JA, Cutler GB, Jr., Chrousos GP, Nieman LK. 1993. Corticotropin-releasing hormone stimulation following low-dose dexamethasone administration. A new test to distinguish Cushing syndrome from pseudo-Cushing's states. JAMA 269(17): 2232–8.

Zarate A, Kovacs K, Flores M, Moran C, Felix I. 1986. ACTH and CRF-producing bronchial carcinoid associated with Cushing syndrome. Clin Endocrinol (Oxf) 24(5): 523–9.

Zeiger MA, Nieman LK, Cutler GB, Chrousos GP, Doppman JL, Travis WD, Norton JA. 1991. Primary bilateral adrenocortical origins of Cushing syndrome. Surgery 110(6): 1106–15.

Arnold von Eckardstein, Elisabeth Minder

4.2 Diabetes and Metabolism

4.2.1 Diabetes mellitus

4.2.1.1 Diagnosis and Risk Assessment

In 1979/1980, the National Diabetes Data Group and the World Health Organization (WHO) first established the diagnostic criteria for diabetes mellitus based in epidemiological data, namely: 1. The presence of classic symptoms associated with evidence of hyperglycemia; 2. Glucose concentrations >7.8 mmol/L (>140 mg/dL) in fasting plasma (fasting plasma glucose = FPG); 3. Glucose concentrations >11.1 mmol/L (>200 mg/dL) 2 hours after oral glucose loading (2h PG after OGTT) (National Diabetes Group 1979). The 2h PG in OGTT was the reference parameter because this cut-off value best correlated in the then current cross-sectional analyzes of epidemiological data with the occurrence of retinopathy. These definitions were revised in the late 1990s due to a number of new prospective epidemiological study results from the American Diabetes Association (ADA) and WHO (American Diabetes Association, 1997; World Health Organization 1999). The diagnostic FPG cut-off value was lowered to 7.0 mmol/L (126 mg/dL), because exceeding of this limit value gave the most sensitive prediction of exceeding the 2h PG value of 11.1 mmol/L (200 mg/dL) in the OGTT. In addition, the ADA adopted the detection of > 11.1 mmol/L increased random glucose plasma concentration as a diagnostic criterion, i.e., independent of prandial status, while the WHO maintained the OGTT criteria. Moreover, the ADA adopted the impaired fasting glucose (IFG: 6.1–7.0 mmol/L = 110–126 mg/dL, later revised to 5.6–7.0 mmol/L = 100–126 mg/dL) as a prognostic criterion for establishing an increased risk for the later development of diabetes mellitus (American Diabetes Association in 1997, 2010), while WHO retained the definition of impaired glucose tolerance (IGT) as a 2h PG value of 7.8–11.1 mmol/L (140–200 mg/dL) in the OGTT (World Health Organization 1999).

In early 2010, the ADA published another revision of the criteria for the diagnosis and classification of diabetes mellitus (American Diabetes Association in 2010, 2012). These new recommendations, reconfirmed in 2012, summarized the previous ADA and WHO definitions for the diagnosis of diabetes mellitus, and adopted the cut-off value for glycated hemoglobin A1 (HbA1c) in the diagnosis of overt diabetes mellitus, as proposed one year earlier by an international group of experts (International Expert Committee 2009). The definitions are summarized in ▶ Table 4.7. The term "pre-diabetes" was replaced by a "category of increased risk for diabetes mellitus" (▶ Table 4.8).

The main arguments for including the HbA1c concentration among the diabetes mellitus diagnostic criteria relate to the unreliability of the plasma glucose concentration due to diurnal and prandial fluctuations (and also acute stress!), the instability of glucose in collected blood samples due to glycolysis, and the analytical interference by medications (International Expert Committee, 2009). The HbA1c value is an intra-individually stable biomarker in which the concentration reflects glycemia over the past 8–12 weeks, and the pre-analytical factors are easier to control than those for glucose. The HbA1c value correlates over the entire concentration range with the risk of microvascular complications. Through worldwide standardization by the NGSP/DCCT and IFCC, the current method independence of HbA1c measurements is sufficiently optimized so that the parameter can be used diagnostically across wide populations. Significant known disadvantages of the HbA1c parameter are greater imprecision compared to glucose measurements, especially when using point-of-care testing (POCT) devices (Lenters-Westra and Slingerland, 2010), and possible misjudgments in patients who have altered

Table 4.7 Definition of diabetes mellitus according to the criteria of the American Diabetes Association (2010).

Criteria	
1.	HbA1c ≥ 6.5 % according to the NGSP (> 48 mmol/mol according to IFCC) *
or	
2.	Fasting plasma glucose (FPG) ≥ 126 mg/dL (7.0 mmol/L). Fasting is defined as no caloric intake for at least 8 h. *
or	
3.	2-hour plasma glucose ≥ 11.1 mmol/L (> 200 mg/dL) during an OGTT. The test should be conducted according the WHO protocol, namely drinking a water solution with 75 g unhydrated glucose.*
or	
4.	A patient with classic symptoms of hyperglycemia or in hyperglycemic crisis with a plasma glucose ≥ 11.1 mmol/L (> 200 mg/dL) independent of prandial status.

* In the absence of pronounced hyperglycemia, criteria 1–3 should be confirmed through repeat testing.
FPG = fasting plasma glucose, NGSP = National Glycohemoglobin Standardization Program, IFCC = International Federation of Clinical Chemistry

Table 4.8 Definition of pre-diabetes mellitus "category of increased risk for diabetes mellitus" according to the criteria of the American Diabetes Association (2010).

Criteria*

- FPG 5.6–6.9 mmol/L (100–125 mg/dL) (IFG)
- 2h PG following 75 g OGTT of 7.8–11.0 mmol/L (140–199 mg/dL) (IGT)
- HbA1c of 5.7–6.4 % according to NGSP (39–48 mmol/mol according to IFCC)

* The risk is continuous for all 3 tests, i.e., the risk begins below the lower limit and increases disproportionately starting from the top of the range. FPG = fasting plasma glucose, IFG = impaired fasting glucose = increased glucose concentration in the fasting plasma; 2h PG: 2-hour plasma glucose, IGT = impaired glucose tolerance

red blood cell survival times, chronic renal failure, heavy alcohol consumption, or genetic hemoglobin or hyperglycation variants. In addition, the HbA1c test is considerably more expensive than glucose measurement.

Results from population-wide evaluation studies in America, Europe and Asia show a lower sensitivity of the HbA1c criterion for diagnosing overt diabetes mellitus, as compared to the glucose criterion. A validation of the HbA1c criterion conducted in Germany among 2660 participants in the KORA study, 31–75 years old and without known diabetes mellitus, showed that the HbA1c and glucose criteria (i.e., FPG and OGTT) diagnose people with diabetes mellitus differently (Rathmann, et al., 2011): only 20 % of all participants who fulfilled at least one of the two diagnostic criteria for diabetes mellitus had both an elevated HbA1c and a pathological OGTT. Among the newly diagnosed diabetics, an HbA1c value of > 6.5 % (> 48 mmol/mol) was observed in only 0.7 % of 31–60 year-olds and in 2.9 % of 61–75-year-olds, while at 2.3 % or 7.9 % (resp.) had pathologic OGTT results. Therefore, it appears that overall in Germany, the American HbA1c criterion is less sensitive than the glucose criterion for diagnosing both overt and latent diabetes mellitus. For these reasons, experts from the German Diabetes Association (DDG) have proposed to adopt the ADA recommendations in modified form (▶ Figure 4.5) (Kerner, et al., 2010) (http://www.deutsche-diabetes-gesellschaft.de/redaktion/news/Stellungnahme_HbA1c_final.pdf).

1. The main difference is the differentiation of different cut-off values for ruling in (HbA1c ≥ 6.5 % or ≥ 48 mmol/mol) and ruling out (HbA1c < 5.7 % and < 39 mmol/mol) diabetes mellitus.
2. In the gray area corresponding to the "ADA-category with an increased risk for diabetes mellitus" (5.7 % < HbA1c < 6.5 %, or 39 mmol/mol < HbA1c < 48 mmol/mol), further clarification is needed with measurements of FPG and 2h PG following OGTT.
3. The use of the HbA1c criteria requires the use of standard methods according to NGSP/DCCT and/or IFCC
4. HbA1c measurements should be performed for all persons who are at an increased risk of diabetes according to the German Diabetes Risk Test (▶ Table 4.9) (Schulze, et al., 2007) (http://www.dife.de/de/presse/Diabetes_Test_Fragebogen.pdf)
5. In the presence of diabetes symptoms (weight loss, polyuria, polydipsia), primary diabetes should be diagnosed based on glucose measurements.
6. The following conditions that affect the HbA1c concentration independent of glycemia likewise require primary glucose measurements:
   a) Globin variants (HbS, HbE, HbF, HbD, etc.);
   b) Altered red blood cell survival time (hemolytic anemia, iron deficiency anemia, kidney disease, liver disease, enhanced erythropoiesis under the anemia treatment);
   c) Chemical modifications of hemoglobin (carbamylated Hb from uremia, acetylated Hb at high-dose, long-term vitamin C treatment);
   d) Inhibition of glycation from continuous vitamin C or vitamin E treatment;
   e) Pregnancy (although contrary to the international recommendations) (for the differentiation between gestational diabetes and diabetes in pregnancy, see Table 4.13).

The ADA recommends an examination for the presence of diabetes mellitus in all persons older than 45 years of age, and all persons with a BMI > 25 kg/m^2 regardless of age, who have one or more of the risk factors shown in ▶ Table 4.10. The DDG also recommends the examination of persons who score more than 40 points in the German Diabetes Risk Test (Schulze, et al., 2007) (http://www.dife.de/de/presse/Diabetes_Test_Fragebogen.pdf).

Recommendations of the German Diabetes Association for Diabetes Mellitus Diagnostics			
Initial examination/ incidental findings	Diabetes symptoms Weight loss, polyuria, polydipsia) and/or elevated diabetes risk (Tables 4.9 and 4.10)		
	HbA1c		
Laboratory	≥ 6.4% ≥ 47 mmol/mol	5.7–6.5% 39–48 mmol/mol	< 5,7% < 39 mmol/mol
Expanded laboratory	Fasting plasma glucose and OGTT		
	FPG ≥ 7.0 mmol/L (≥ 126 mg/dL) and/or 2h PG ≥ 11.1 mmol/L (≥ 200 mg/dL)	FPG ≥ 5.6–6.9 mmol/L (100–125 mg/dL) and/or 2h PG 7.8–11.0 mmol/L (140–199 mg/dL)	FPG ≥ 5.6–7.0 mmol/L (< 100 mg/dL) and/or 2h PG < 7.8 mmol/L (< 140 mg/dL)
Diagnosis	Diabetes	Pre-diabetes "Condition with increased risk for diabetes mellitus"	No diabetes
Further procedures	Therapy according to guidelines. Recognition of additional risk factors (see Figures 4.7, 4.8, 4.9)	Explanation of diabetes risk, lifestyle intervention, treatment of risk factors. Reevaluation of risk and HbA1c retest after 1 year. If necessary, recognition of additional risk factors (see Figures 4.7, 4.8, 4.9)	

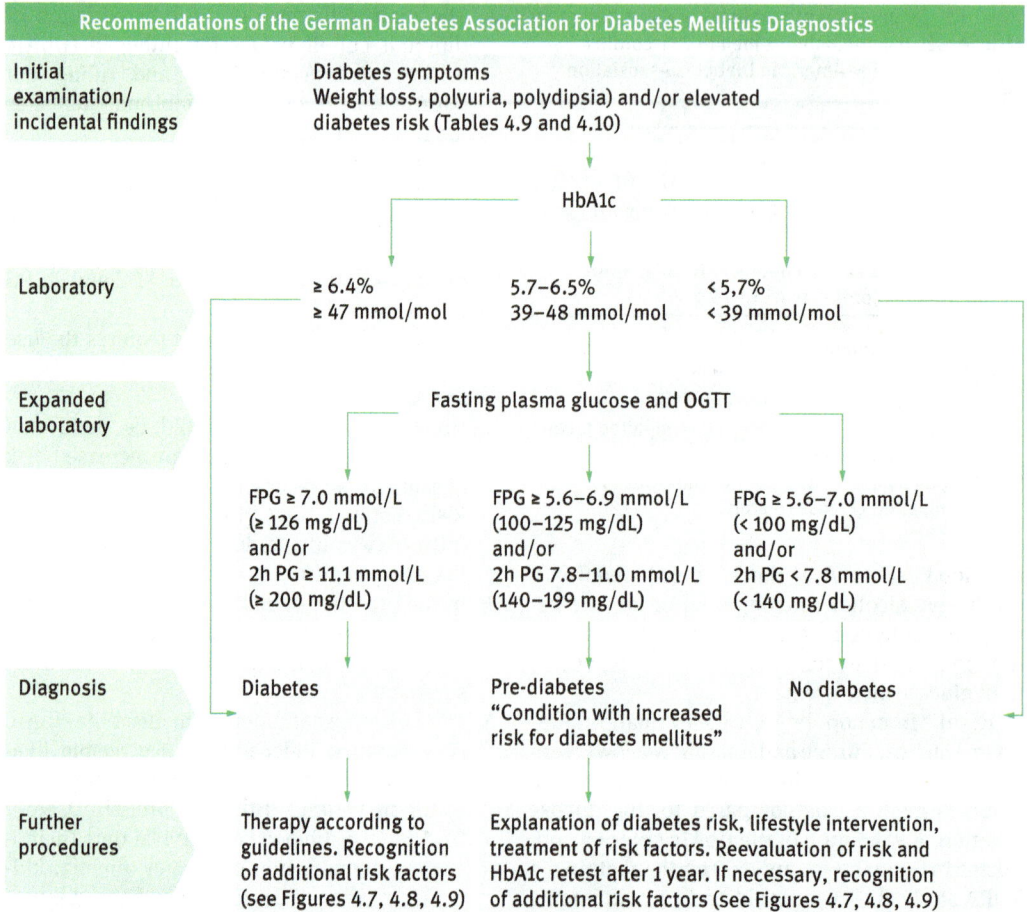

Figure 4.5 Flow diagram for diagnosing diabetes mellitus (modified from Kerner, et al., 2010, and http://www.deutsche-diabetes-gesellschaft.de/redaktion/ news/Stellungnahme_HbA1c_final.pdf); FPG = fasting plasma glucose, OGTT = oral glucose tolerance test, 2h PG = 2-hour plasma glucose following OGTT.

Type 2 diabetes mellitus mostly occurs in the adult years, but late manifestation of type 1 diabetes mellitus (LADA = latent insulin diabetes in adulthood) is also possible. ▶ Table 4.11 contrasts the differential diagnostic criteria for these two principal diagnoses. With suspected type 1 diabetes mellitus, testing for anti-glutamic acid decarboxylase antibodies (anti-GAD65) is recommended, since these occur in 90–95 % of type 1 diabetics cases (Kerner, et al., 2010).

4.2.1.2 Gestational Diabetes Mellitus (GDM)

The early diagnosis of gestational diabetes mellitus (GDM) together with proper and optimal treatment improves the prognosis for both mother and child. The optimal control of diabetes during pregnancy means achieving euglycemia in all stages of pregnancy, as well before conception (with pre-existing diabetes) and after birth. New international guidelines for achieving this goal

Table 4.9 Identification of persons at increased risk for diabetes
(http://www.dife.de/de/presse/Diabetes_Test_Fragebogen.pdf).

Parameter: Question	Selection criteria	Points
Age:	< 35	0 points
What is your age in years?	35–39	1 point
	40–44	3 points
	45–49	5 points
	50–54	7 points
Physical activity:	No	1 point
Do you get exercise at least 5 hours per week? (e.g., sports, garden work, bicycling)	Yes	0 points
High blood pressure	No	0 points
Have you been diagnosed even once with high blood pressure?	Yes	5 points
Whole-grain bread consumption:	0	5 points
How many slices of whole-grain bread do you eat per day?	1	4 points
	2	3 points
	3	2 points
	4	1 point
	> 4	0 points
Meat consumption:	None or quite seldom	0 points
How often do you eat beef, pork, or lamb?	1–2 times per week	1 point
(not sausages)	3–4 times per week	2 points
	5–6 times per week	4 points
	Every day	5 points
	Several times per day	8 points
Coffee:	0–1	2 points
How many cups of coffee do you drink per day?	2–5	1 point
	> 5	0 points
Smoking:	I have never smoked	0 points
How would you describe your tobacco use?	I once smoked fewer than 20 cigarettes per day	0 points
	I once smoked 20 or more cigarettes per day	3 points
	I smoke fewer than 20 cigarettes per day	0 points
	I smoke 20 or more cigarettes per day	6 points
Alcohol: How many alcoholic drinks do you consume per day?	I seldom or never drink alcohol	2 points
	1–4	0 points
	>4	2 points
Body height:	< 152	11 points
What is your body height in centimeters?	152–159	9 points
	160–167	7 points
	168–175	5 points
	176–183	3 points
	184–191	1 point
	≥ 192	0 points

Table 4.9 (cont.).

Parameter: Question	Selection criteria	Points
Waist circumference:	< 75	0 points
What is your waist circumference in centimeters?	75–79	4 points
	80–84	8 points
	85–89	12 points
	90–94	16 points
	95–99	20 points
	100–104	24 points
	105–109	28 points
	110–114	32 points
	115–119	36 points
	≥ 120	40 points

Evaluation:
0–29 points: low diabetes risk (< 1 % in 5 years)
30–39 points: still low diabetes risk (1–2 % in 5 years)
40–49 points: increased diabetes risk (2–5 % in 5 years)
50–59 points: high diabetes risk (5–10 % in 5 years)
> 59 points: very high diabetes risk (> 10 % in 5 years)

Table 4.10 Groups of people recommended for diabetes mellitus screening according to the recommendations of the American Diabetes Association (2010).

1. Adults who are overweight or obese (BMI ≥ 25 kg/m²*), who have one or more of the following risk factors:
   • Minimal physical activity;
   • Close relative with diabetes;
   • Ancestors from high-risk ethnic groups: (e.g., African, American Indian, Latin American, Asian, Pacific Islander);
   • Women who have born a child with a birth weight > 4.5 kg, or who developed gestational diabetes;
   • High blood pressure (≥ 140/90 mmHg, or under anti-hypertensive treatment);
   • HDL cholesterol < 0.90 mmol/L (< 35 mg/dL);
   • Triglycerides > 2.8 mmol/L (> 250 mg/dL);
   • Women with polycystic ovary syndrome;
   • HbA1c ≥ 5.7 % (> 39 mmol/mol), IGT, or IFG at an earlier examination;
   • Other clinical conditions associated with insulin resistance (e.g., pronounced obesity, acanthosis nigricans);
   • History of cardiovascular disease.
2. In the absence of the above criteria, diabetes testing should begin from 45 years
3. With a normal result, the test should be repeated every 3 years. More frequent examinations, if necessary, and depending on the risk status (see point 1) or test results (see Table 4.8).

were published by the International Association of Diabetes and Pregnancy Study Groups (IADPSG), which is composed of obstetricians, pediatricians, diabetologists and epidemiologists, (International Association of Diabetes and Pregnancy Study Groups Consensus Panel 2010; Castorino, et al., 2011). ▶ Tables 4.12 and 4.13 summarize the threshold values for diagnosing GDM or overt diabetes mellitus during pregnancy, as well as strategies for their detection (▶ Figure 4.6.) (International Association of Diabetes and Pregnancy Study Groups Consensus Panel, 2010; http://www.deutsche-diabetes-gesellschaft.de/redaktion/news/EbLL_GDM_ENDFASSUNG_2011_01_28_E1.pdf).

Table 4.11 Differential diagnostic criteria for type 1 and type 2 diabetes mellitus (Kerner, et al., 2010).

	Type 1 diabetes mellitus	Type 2 diabetes mellitus
Age of onset	Mostly in children, adolescents, and young adults	Mostly in middle-aged and older adults
Appearance, onset	subacute to acute	usually insidious
Symptoms	Frequently polyuria, polydipsia, weight loss, fatigue	Frequently no complaints
Body weight	Usually normal weight	Usually overweight (abdominal obesity)
Ketosis predisposition	Pronounced	Absent or low
Insulin secretion	Decreased or absent	initially subnormal to high
Insulin resistance	None	Often pronounced
familial predisposition	Low (concordance in monozygotic twins <50 %)	Typical (concordance in monozygotic twins > 50 %)
Diabetes associated antibodies (ICA, GAD65, IA-2, IAA)*	ca. 90–95 % at onset	Absent
Lipoprotein metabolism	Unremarkable	Common low HDL cholesterol and elevated triglycerides
Response to betacytotropic antidiabetics	Usually absent	Quite good at first
Insulin therapy	Necessary	Usually required only after years of disease progression due to reduced insulin secretion

ICA = islet cell antibodies, GAD65 = antibodies against glutamate decarboxylase, IA-2 = antibodies against tyrosine phosphatase 2, IAA = insulin autoantibodies

Table 4.12 Threshold values for diagnosing gestational diabetes mellitus (International Association of Diabetes and Pregnancy Study Groups, 2010: Castorino, et al., 2011).

Parameter	Threshold glucose concentration value *	
	mmol/L	mg/dL
Fasting plasma glucose	5.1	92
1h plasma glucose (75 g OGTT)	10.0	180
2h plasma glucose	8.5	153

* For a diagnosis of gestational diabetes, one or more of these threshold values must be exceeded.

In contrast to previous recommendations, results from the Hyperglycemia and Adverse Pregnancy Outcome (HAPO) study have prompted a new recommendation for diabetes screening in all pregnant women through direct application of the 75g OGTT procedure in the 24th–28th week of pregnancy. The previously used 50g OGTT procedure was defined as obsolete, especially because the implied 2-step approach delayed the diagnosis and thus also treatment of GDM until the 30h–34th week of pregnancy, by which time the hyperglycemia and macrosomia effects were already present. Also new is the differentiation between GDM and overt diabetes. These recommendations were adopted by the ADA in 2012.

A broad application appears necessary to minimize any complications during pregnancy (e.g., deformities, miscarriages), but also the increased risk of macrosomal children for obesity, diabetes and cardiovascular diseases during the childhood and/or adult years.

Women with GDM are at increased risk of about 30 % for developing overt diabetes within 5 years postpartum (Ekelund, et al., 2010). Positive HbA1c and FPG tests during pregnancy, the number of previous pregnancies, and a family history of diabetes mellitus are independent risk factors for the later occurrence of postpartum diabetes mellitus. An HbA1c value of > 5.7 % (> 39 mmol/mol) and an FPG value of > 5.2 mmol/L increase diabetes

Table 4.13 Threshold values for diagnosing diabetes mellitus of pregnancy (International Association of Diabetes and Pregnancy Study Groups, 2010: Castorino, et al., 2011).

Parameter	Consensus threshold value
FPG[1]	≥ 7.0 mmol/L (> 126 mg/dL)
HbA1c[2]	≥ 6.5 % according to NGSP, > 48 mmol/mol according to IFCC
Random plasma glucose concentration	≥ 11.1 mmol/L (≥ 200 mg/dL) + Confirmation[2]

[1] One of the two criteria must be fulfilled to diagnose overt diabetes in pregnancy.

[2] If a plasma glucose concentration determined through random (postprandial) testing exceeds this threshold value, the presumptive diagnosis must be confirmed using FPG or HbA1c.

risk by factors of 4 or 6, resp. Correspondingly, these women must be regularly examined in view of their increased risk of diabetes and regarding their glycemia. 10 % of women with GDM have islet cell antibodies and an increased risk for the development of type 1 diabetes mellitus.

4.2.1.3 Monitoring Diabetes Mellitus

Glycemia control

Cardiovascular complications are the leading cause of morbidity and mortality in patients with diabetes mellitus. The Diabetes Control and Complications Trial (DCCT) and the United Kingdom Prospective Diabetes Study (UKPDS) consistently showed that intensive glycemic control favorably influenced the development and progression of microvascular complications in patients with type 1 or type 2 diabetes. It is controversial, however, whether intensive glucose lowering also prevents macrovascular events. Extended follow-up in the two abovementioned studies showed that intensive glycemic control reduces the incidence of heart attack and death due to cardiovascular causes. In contrast, the ACCORD, ADVANCE and VADT studies found that intensive glycemic control had either no or even a harmful effect on cardiovascular events (Brown, et al., 2010). The results of a British registration study of almost 48,000 patients with diabetes suggest

that glycemic control that is too strict increases overall mortality and the rate of cardiovascular events (Curie, et al., 2010). The adjusted HbA1c levels showed a U-shaped relationship with overall mortality. The lowest mortality was associated with the deciles that comprise the HbA1c interval of 7.5–7.6 % (55– 56 mmol/mol). Despite these alarming study results, the DDG currently maintains its treatment target for HbA1c of < 6.5 % (< 48 mmol/mol) (▶ Figure 4.7) (Matthaei, et al., 2010), instead of the value of < 7 % (52 mmol/mol) used in other countries. However, it accepts that avoidance of side effects (hypoglycemia, significant weight gain) plays a high priority, so that the target HbA1c value should be left at 7.0 (52 mmol/mol) if achieving the goal of < 6.5 % (< 48 mmol/mol) elicits the abovementioned side effects.

Microalbuminuria and eGFR

Diabetes mellitus is the most common cause of chronic renal failure. 20–40 % of diabetes patients develop chronic kidney disease. Although the term "diabetic nephropathy" combines various clinical pictures with respect to etiology and pathogenesis, left untreated these usually lead to end-stage renal failure, which makes dialysis treatment necessary. Early forms of diabetic nephropathy can manifest as selective glomerular proteinuria, which is referred to as microalbuminuria. Depending on the examination method (albumin +/– creatinine) and material (spot or total urine) and possibly the collection period (one-time or 24 hour), various diagnostic cut-off values have been defined (▶ Table 4.14). Microalbuminuria is not only a risk factor for the progression of diabetic nephropathy, but also indicates an increased risk (by a factor of 2) of developing cardiovascular disease or dying. The degree of albuminuria and the progression of diabetic nephropathy are modulated by multiple risk factors (▶ Table 4.15), which can be partly influenced by therapy, especially the optimization of glycemia, blood pressure, body weight; plasma concentrations of LDL cholesterol, HDL cholesterol and triglycerides;, as well as non-smoking. The international and national guidelines recommend annual testing for microalbuminuria in diabetes patients (▶ Figure 4.8) (http://www.versorgungs-leitlinien.de/ themen/diabetes2/dm 2_nephro/pdf/ nvl_t2dnephro_lang.pdf).

Clarification of Gestational Diabetes

Initial examination

Pregnancy

First presentation before 24 weeks

First presentation after 24 weeks

Laboratory

Increased risk?
(see Tables 4.12 and 4.13)

All

Yes

Expanded laboratory

Random plasma glucose

≥ 11.1 mmol/L
(≥ 200 mg/dL) — Yes

No

Fasting plasma glucose

≥ 7.0 mmol/L
(≥ 126 mg/dL)

5.1–6.9 mmol/L
(92–125 mg/dL)

< 5.1 mmol/L
(< 92 mg/dL)

24–28 week of pregnancy
75 g OGTT

FPG ≥ 7.0 mmol/L
(≥ 126 mg/dL)
No OGTT!

2h PG ≥ 11.1 mmol/L
(≥ 200 mg/dL)

FPG ≥ 5.1 mmol/L
(≥ 92 mg/dL)

1h PG ≥ 10.0 mmol/L
(≥ 180 mg/dL)

2h PG ≥ 8.5 mmol/L
(≥ 150 mg/dL)

Fasting plasma glucose ≥ 7.0 mmol/L and/or HbA1c 6.5%

Yes

Yes (at least 1 value)

No

Diagnosis

Overt diabetes

No →

Gestational diabetes

No Gestational diabetes

Further procedures

HbA1c
Type 1/Type 2? → GAD65
Secondary

Counseling as in known diabetes before conception

Training and treatment according to guidelines

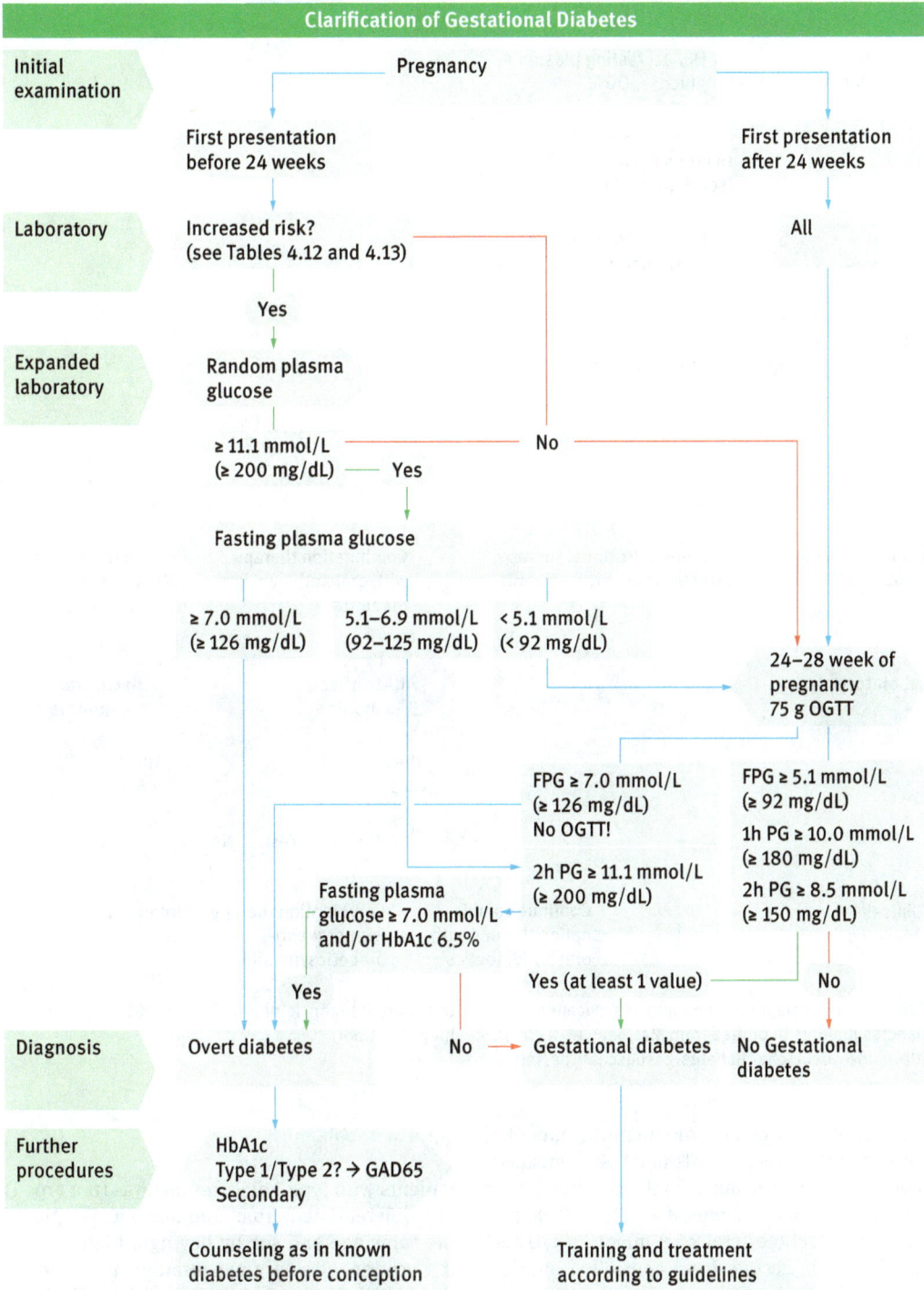

Figure 4.6 Flow diagram for the diagnosis of gestational diabetes or diabetes of pregnancy (modified from http://www.deutsche-diabetes-gesellschaft.de/redaktion/news/EbLL_GDM_ENDFAS-SUNG_2011_01_28_E1.pdf);

1:Persons at risk are described in Tables 3 and 4; SSW = weeks of pregnancy, FPG = fasting plasma glucose, OGTT = oral glucose tolerance test, 2h PG = 2-hour plasma glucose following OGTT, GAD65 = antibodies to glutamate decarboxylase 65.

Monitoring Glycemia during Diabetes Mellitus

Initial examination/incidental findings — HbA1c, fasting plasma glucose, OGTT

↓

Diagnosis: type 2 diabetes (see Figure 4.5)

↓

Clinical measures — Training, nutritional therapy, exercise therapy, metformin

↓

Laboratory — HbA1c after 3–6 months

HbA1c ≥ 6.5% — Yes → HbA1c ≥ 7.5%

No ↓ | No ↓ | Yes ↓

Clinical measures — Training, nutritional therapy, exercise therapy, metformin | Combination therapy with oral anti-diabetics | Combination therapy with oral anti-diabetics/insulin

Laboratory — HbA1c after 3–6 months | HbA1c after 3–6 months

HbA1c ≥ 6.5% | HbA1c ≥ 6.5%

No | Yes | No | Yes

Clinical measures — Continue combination therapy with oral antidiabetics | Combination therapy with oral anti-diabetics/insulin | Intensification of insulin therapy

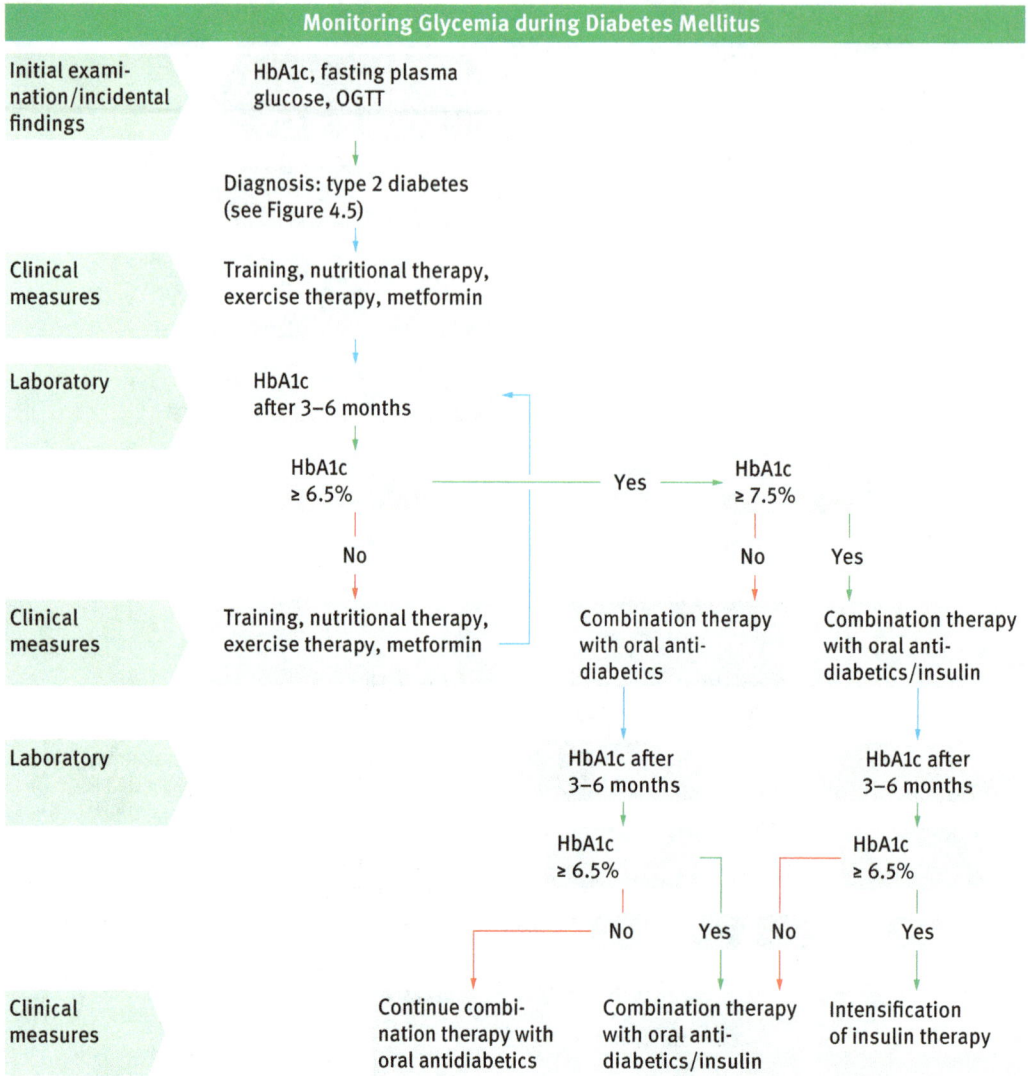

Figure 4.7 Flow diagram for monitoring glycemia in diabetes mellitus (modified from Matthaei, et al., 2010: http://www.deutsche-diabetes-gesellschaft.de/redak-tion/mitteilungen/leitlinien/PL_DDG2010_Behand-lung_Typ2.pdf).

In the presence of microalbuminuria, pursuit of the extant therapeutic goals must be intensified: HbA1c < 6.5 % or < 48 mmol/mol (possibly < 7 % or < 52 mmol/mol), blood pressure < 135–140/80 mm Hg, and LDL cholesterol < 1.8 mmol/L (< 70 mg/dL). Based on results from controlled studies, the use of angiotensin converting enzyme inhibitors or angiotensin II receptor blockers is recommended for antihypertensive therapy in diabetic patients with microalbuminuria.

Lipid metabolism

Patients with type 2 diabetes mellitus (not type 1) are differentiated from non-diabetic people of the same age and sex by having a higher mean triglyceride plasma concentration and a lower mean HDL cholesterol concentration. The low-HDL cholesterol/hypertriglyceridemia syndrome often emerges before the onset of diabetes mellitus, which is why patients with this dyslipidemia

Table 4.14 Diagnostic cut-off values* for albuminuria according to sample material.

	Total urine		Spot urine		
	(mg/24h)	µg/min	mg/L	mg/mmol creatinine	mg/g creatinine
Normal	< 30	< 20	< 20	< 2	< 30
Microalbuminuria	30–300	20–200	20–200	2–20	30–300
Macroalbuminuria	> 300	> 200	> 200	> 20	> 300

* The cut-off values used for women are approximately 1/3 lower

Table 4.15 Risk factors for diabetic nephropathy.

Controllable risk factors	Uncontrollable risk factors
Hyperglycemia	Advanced age
High blood pressure	Male sex
Albumin excretion rate	Duration of diabetes
Smoking	Onset of diabetes before age 20 years
Elevated LDL cholesterol	Simultaneous presence of retinopathy
Hypertriglyceridemia	Positive family history of hypotension and/or nephropathy
Low HDL cholesterol	Ethnic origin: African, Latin American, Native American
elevated body-mass index	

should be examined in detail for the presence of diabetes mellitus, including administration of an OGTT (▶ Table 4.10).

The plasma concentrations of LDL and HDL cholesterol as well as triglycerides affect the diabetes risk for both macro- and microvascular diseases. Accordingly, the correction of lipid metabolism disorders is an important measure to take in reducing the cardiovascular risk in diabetes patients. In fact, several studies have shown that lowering LDL cholesterol reduces the coronary risk of diabetes patients (Cholesterol Treatment Trialists Collaborators, et al., 2008), so that the LDL cholesterol target values for people with diabetes are just as low as those defined for patients with manifest atherosclerosis, namely < 2.6 mmol/L (< 100 mg/dL) or even < 1.8 mmol/L (< 70 mg/dL) (www.chd-taskforce.de/guide.htm; The Task Force for the Management of Dyslipidaemias of 2011).

The clinical benefits from treatment of hypertriglyceridemia and low HDL cholesterol appear complex: Treatment with fibrates, alone or in combination with statins, showed no benefit in terms of the reduction of cardiovascular risk (Jun, et al., 2010), but rather in relation to a reduction in the risks for nephropathy and retinopathy (Fioretto,

et al., 2010). In addition, the results of a post hoc analysis suggest that diabetic patients with HDL cholesterol levels < 1 mmol/L (< 39 mg/dL) and triglyceride plasma concentrations > 2.3 mmol/L (> 200 mg/dL) less frequently experience heart attacks while under treatment with fibrates (24). Consequently, these data should be collected from diabetic patients at least once a year to assess the lipid status (▶ Figure 4.9).

4.2.2 Lipid and Lipoprotein Metabolism

4.2.2.1 Assessment of Cardiovascular Risk

In a number of epidemiological studies and a meta-analysis of original data from these studies (Emerging Risk Factors Collaboration, et al., 2009), the incidence of coronary events was positively associated with the plasma concentrations of total cholesterol, LDL cholesterol, non-HDL cholesterol and triglycerides, and inversely associated with the plasma concentration of HDL cholesterol. The lipid risk factors interact with each other and with other risk factors, so that the cardiovascular risk increases disproportionately in the presence of multiple risk factors. In

Microalbuminuria and Estimated Glomerular Filtration Rate (eGFR) in Diabetes Mellitus

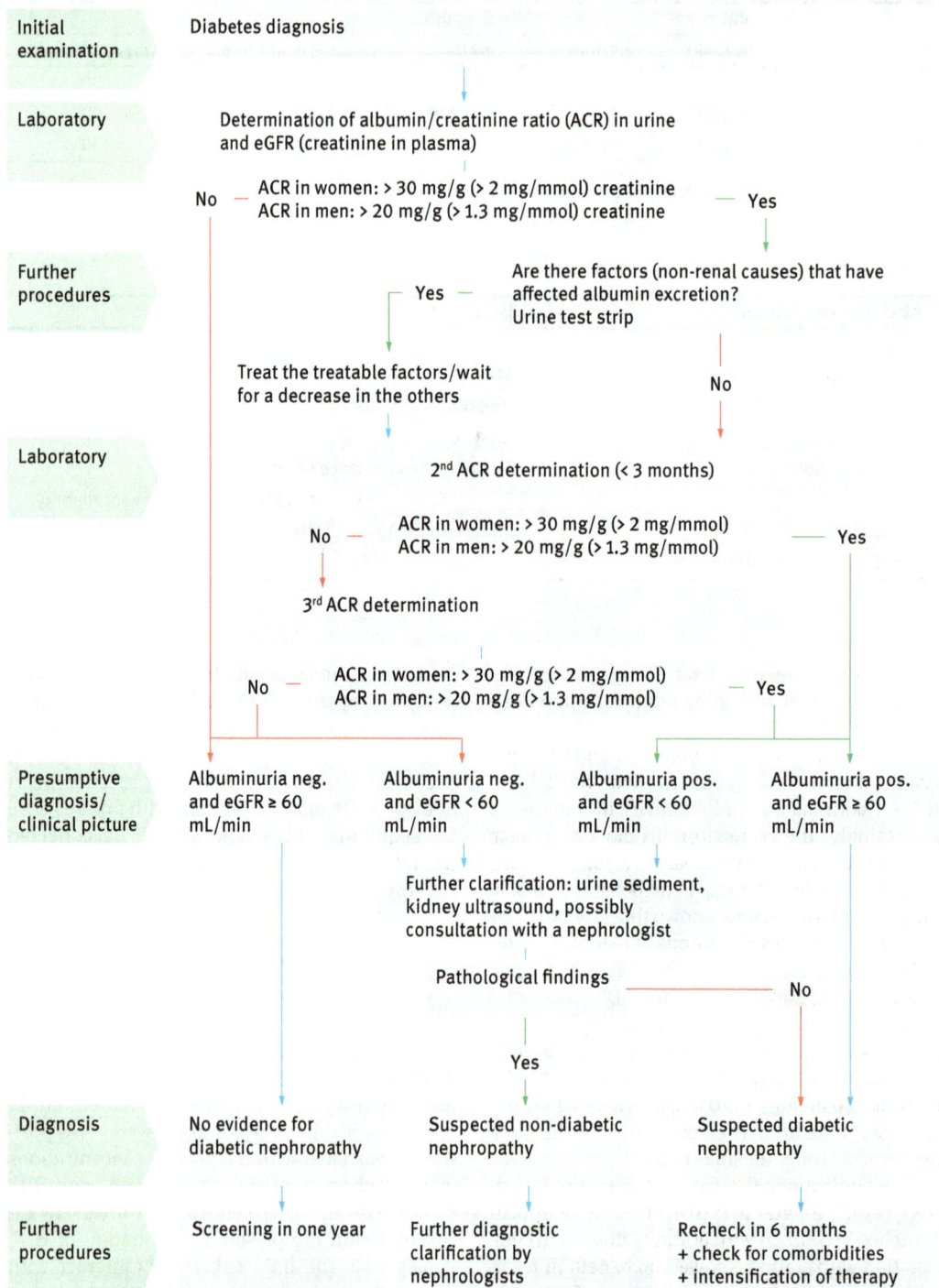

Initial examination

Diabetes diagnosis

Laboratory

Determination of albumin/creatinine ratio (ACR) in urine and eGFR (creatinine in plasma)

No — ACR in women: > 30 mg/g (> 2 mg/mmol) creatinine
ACR in men: > 20 mg/g (> 1.3 mg/mmol) creatinine — Yes

Further procedures

Yes — Are there factors (non-renal causes) that have affected albumin excretion?
Urine test strip

Treat the treatable factors/wait for a decrease in the others

No

Laboratory

2nd ACR determination (< 3 months)

No — ACR in women: > 30 mg/g (> 2 mg/mmol)
ACR in men: > 20 mg/g (> 1.3 mg/mmol) — Yes

3rd ACR determination

No — ACR in women: > 30 mg/g (> 2 mg/mmol)
ACR in men: > 20 mg/g (> 1.3 mg/mmol) — Yes

Presumptive diagnosis/ clinical picture

| Albuminuria neg. and eGFR ≥ 60 mL/min | Albuminuria neg. and eGFR < 60 mL/min | Albuminuria pos. and eGFR < 60 mL/min | Albuminuria pos. and eGFR ≥ 60 mL/min |

Further clarification: urine sediment, kidney ultrasound, possibly consultation with a nephrologist

Pathological findings —— No

Yes

Diagnosis

No evidence for diabetic nephropathy

Suspected non-diabetic nephropathy

Suspected diabetic nephropathy

Further procedures

Screening in one year

Further diagnostic clarification by nephrologists

Recheck in 6 months
+ check for comorbidities
+ intensification of therapy

Figure 4.8 Flow diagram for diagnosis of diabetic nephropathy (modified from http://www.versorgungs-sleitlinien.de/themen/diabetes2/dm 2_nephro/pdf/ nvl_t2dnephro_lang.pdf); ACR = albumin/creatinine ratio in urine, eGFR = estimated glomerular filtration rate.

Assessing Lipid Status

Initial examination/ clinical findings

Patient and family medical history
Physical examination

Symptomatic arteriosclerosis: CHD, CVD, PAOD?
Known diabetes mellitus
Known renal failure

Yes   No

Age > 45 years, BMI > 25 kg/m² or waist circumference > 94 cm (m), 80 cm (f)
Positive family medical history of diabetes mellitus or premature arteriosclerosis
Known or measured hypotension, smoker

Yes   No

Laboratory

Lipid status: Total, LDL, HDL cholesterol; triglycerides
Fasting glucose or HbA1c

Risk estimate according to Figures 4.10 and 4.11

High risk   Low risk

Yes   No   Yes

Diagnosis

| Patient with high cardiovascular risk | Intermediate or unknown risk | Patient with low cardiovascular risk | Unremarkable finding |

Expanded laboratory

Additional risk factors
• Lp(a) • (hs troponin)
• hs CRP • (NT-ProBNP) • (Albumin in urine)

Lp(a) > 500 mg/L   hs CRP > 2 mg/L
(hs troponin > 99th Percentile)
(NT-proBNP > 300 ng/L), (BNP > 100 ng/L)
(Microalbuminuria)

Yes   No

Further procedures

• Control risk factors
• Lipid-lowering therapy:
  LDL-C < 2.6 mmol/L (< 100 mg/dL)*
• Blood pressure lowering RR
  < 135/85 mm Hg
• Diabetes treatment

LDL-C
> 3.4 mmol/L
(> 130 mg/dL)

LDL-C
> 4.1 mmol/L
(> 160 mg/dL)

No   Yes   Yes   No

| Medical check-ups, frequent at first (LDL-C, CK, ALT), annually after achieving the therapeutic targets | Lifestyle recommendations Check-up after 1 year | Consider lipid-lowering therapy, lifestyle recommendations Check-up after 1 year | Lifestyle recommendations Check-up after 5 years |

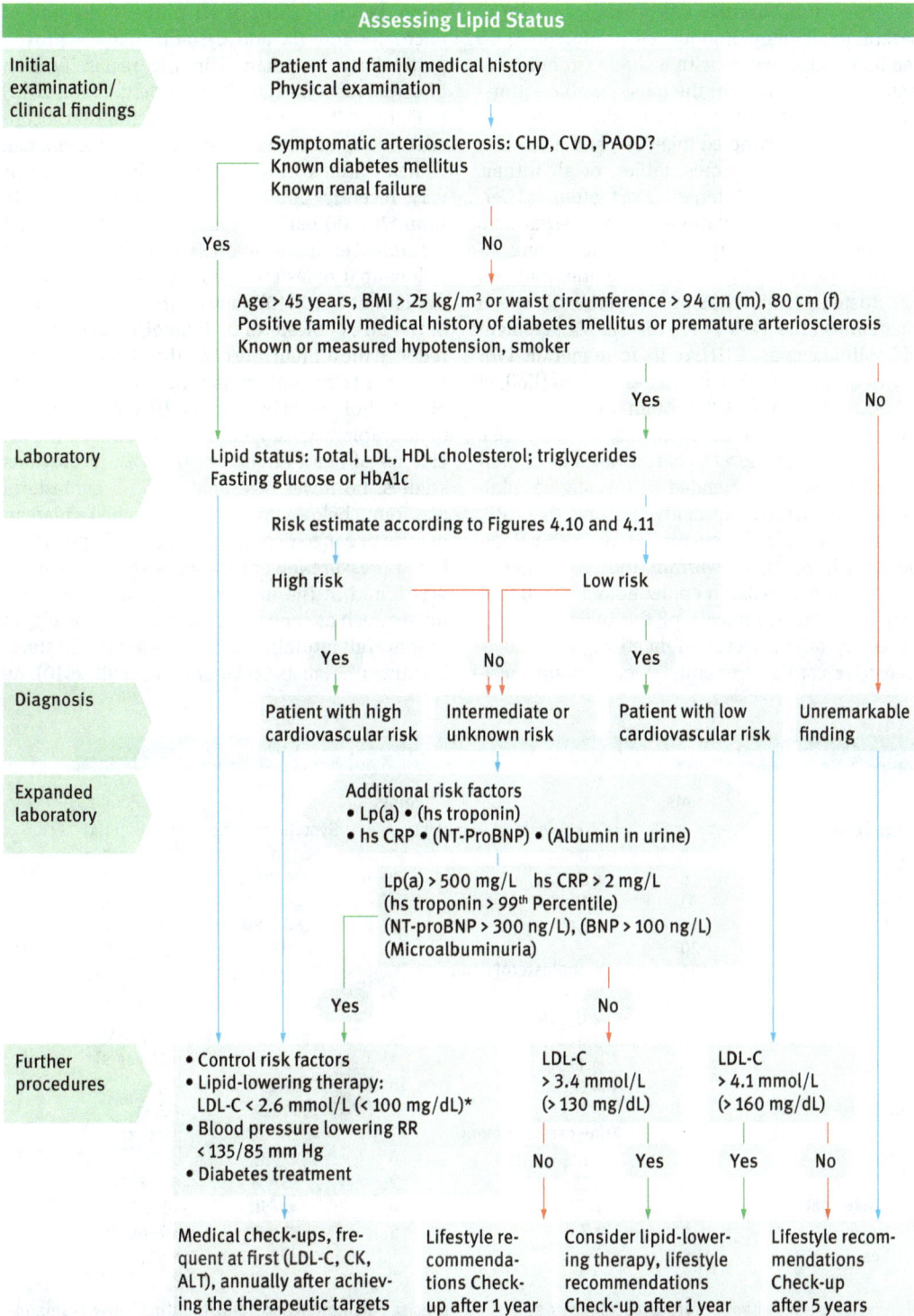

Figure 4.9 Flow diagram for assessing cardiovascular risk; CHD = coronary heart disease, CVD = cerebrovascular disease, PAOD = peripheral artery occlusive disease, BMI = body-mass index, m = male, f = female, LDL-C = LDL cholesterol, Lp(a) = lipoprotein (a), hsCRP = high sensitivity C-reactive protein, hs troponin = high sensitivity troponin, BNP = B-type natriuretic peptide, CK = creatine kinase, ALT = alanine-aminotransferase.

fact, the cardiovascular risk in the presence of several moderately pronounced risk factors is often higher than a case with a single strongly pronounced one. Thus, for the most reliable estimation possible of cardiovascular risk, the classical risk factors are gathered together, and a calculation is made using scores, tables, or algorithms accessible via the Internet. Most often in Germany, the recommendations of the International Atherosclerosis Society (PROCAM score and algorithm) (www.chd-taskforce.de/guide.htm; von Eckardstein, et al., 2005), or the Joint European Guidelines (The Task Force for the Management of Dyslipidaemias, 2011), or its form modified for use in Germany (D-SCORE) are employed (Keil, et al., 2005). (▶ Figures 4.9 through 4.11).

In patients with intermediate risk (10–20 % risk for coronary events, >1 % cardiovascular mortality risk) it is recommended to investigate additional risk factors, especially the sensitive CRP, but also the Lp(a) (Assmann, et al., 2005; Noordestgaard, 2010), to warrant the most aggressive treatment goals. In epidemiological studies, moreover, measurements of the biomarkers induced by atherosclerosis-related organ damage (sensitive cardiac troponins T or I, brain natri-uretic peptides (BNP or NT-proBNP)) as well of microalbuminuria and cystatin C, have proven particularly informative in the reclassification of cardiovascular risk (Blankenberg, et al., 2010) (▶ Figure 4.9). Lowering the LDL cholesterol concentration, mainly using statins, reduces the risk of heart attack in a dose-dependent manner. A very recently published meta-analysis of data from 170,000 participants in 26 randomized and controlled endpoint studies with at least 2 years of follow-up (Cholesterol Treatment Trialists Collaboration, et al., 2010) showed that each lowering of the LDL cholesterol by 1 mmol/L (38.4 mg/dL) reduced the annual rate of fatal and nonfatal coronary events by approximately 20 %. The lowering of LDL cholesterol by 2–3 mmol/L (77–115 mg/dL) (achievable with modern statins) reduced the incidence of heart attack by 40–50 %. In previous studies, no lower threshold for LDL cholesterol was found below which the risk reached a plateau or even began to rise again (unlike with glucose or blood pressure lowering). Moreover, no increase was found in the incidence of other serious illnesses such as cancer or other causes of death, so that overall mortality had decreased (Cholesterol Treatment Trialists Collaboration, et al., 2010). As

Estimating the Cardiovascular Risk according to the PROCAM Score

Age (years)	Points	HDL cholesterol (mmol/L)	Points	Systolic blood pressure (mmHg)	Points
35–39	0	< 0.9	10	< 120	0
40–45	6	0.9–1.15	7	120–139	2
46–50	11	1.15–1.4	4	140–159	4
51–55	16	> 1.4	0	160–189	7
56–60	20			> 189	10
61–65	23	LDL cholesterol (mmol/L)			
		< 2.6	0		
Positive family history		2.6–3.4	5		
No	0	3.4–4.2	9	Points	Coronary risk (% in 10 years)
Yes	4	4.2–5.0	13		
		> 5.0	18	0–13	< 0.5
Cigarette smoker				14–19	0.5–1
No	0	Triglycerides (mmol/L)		20–26	1–2
Yes	8	< 1.15	0	27–35	2–5
		1.15–1.72	2	36–41	5–10
Diabetes patient		1.73–2.3	3	42–50	10–20
No	0	> 2.3	4	51–58	20–40
Yes	5			> 58	> 40

Figure 4.10 Assessment of cardiovascular risk according to recommendations of the International Atherosclerosis Society (von Eckardstein, et al., 2005): precise calculation according to http://www.assmann-stiftung.de/stiftungsinstitut/procam-tests/procam-gesundheitstest/

Cholesterol chart

Cholesterol/HDL cholesterol ratio

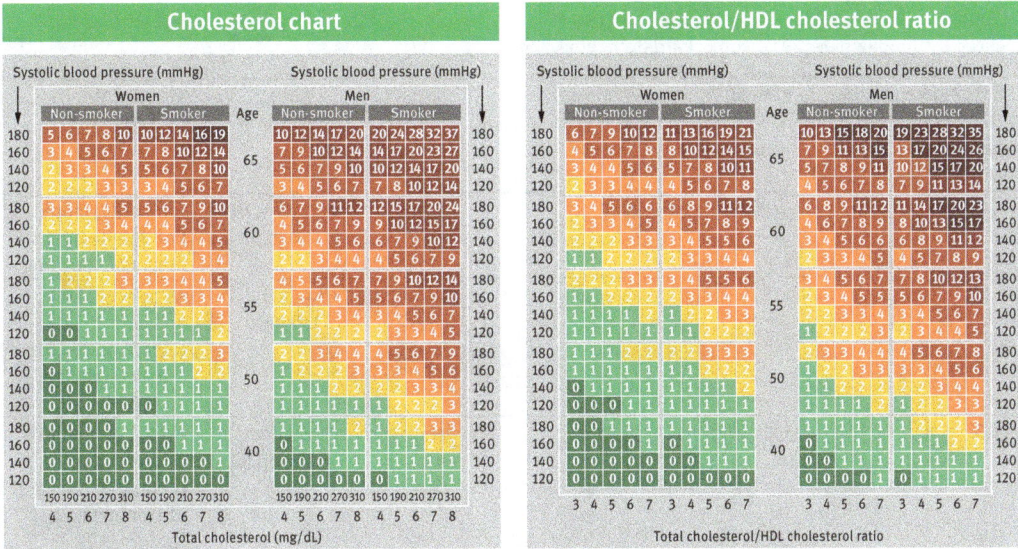

Figure 4.11 Estimating cardiovascular risk according to the General European Recommendations (modified for Germany, Keil, et al., 2005).

a result of these studies, the lowering of LDL-cholesterol below 2.6 mmol/L (100 mg/dL), or even to below <1.8 mmol/L (<70 mg/dL) is currently recommended for patients with manifest atherosclerosis, or high risk for diabetes mellitus, or in the presence of multiple risk factors (▶ Table 4.16, ▶ Figs. 4.10, 4.11) (The Task Force for the Management of Dyslipidaemias, 2011). For asymptomatic patients with moderate or low risk, higher LDL cholesterol targets are applicable (▶ Table 4.16).

The causal relationships between HDL cholesterol/triglycerides and atherosclerosis are less clear than that of LDL cholesterol, and in addition low HDL cholesterol and moderate hypertriglyceridemia often occur together and with other components of metabolic syndrome (overweight or obesity, impaired glucose tolerance or overt type 2 diabetes mellitus, high blood pressure). The statistically independent association of, mainly, HDL cholesterol and the less robust one for triglycerides (Emerging Risk Factors Collaboration, 2009), are not yet conclusive. Previous intervention studies have brought no clarity to this issue, not least because the fibrates used therein gave only slight increases/decreases in the HDL cholesterol and triglycerides concentrations, respectively. Overall, fibrates (alone or in combination with statins) confer no significant risk reduction. In *post hoc* analyses, however, it was found that fibrate treatment in patients with simultaneously low HDL cholesterol (<1 mmol/L or <38.4 mg/dL) and elevated triglycerides (>2.3 mmol/L or >200 mg/dL) conferred the benefit of lower incidence of heart attack (Jun, et al., 2010). Accordingly, there are no therapeutic target values for triglycerides and HDL cholesterol, but cut-off values for the diagnosis of metabolic syndrome and increased cardiovascular risk (▶ Table 4.17) (Alberti, et al., 2009).

4.2.2.2 Differential Diagnosis of Lipid Metabolism Disorders

Lipid metabolism disorders are often multifactorial, i.e., due to a coincidence of genetic predisposition and environmental or lifestyle factors. In particular, moderately pronounced dyslipidemia, caused by an excess (LDL cholesterol, triglycerides) or deficiency (HDL cholesterol) compared to the ideal and target values defined by the consensus recommendations for the prevention of cardiovascular disease and diabetes (▶ Table 4.16 and 4.17), cannot always be assigned to an unambiguous etiology in individual cases.

Only pronounced dyslipidemia, for example, a case that exceeds the 90th percentile or falls below the 10th percentile in the lipid metabolism

Table 4.16 Cardiovascular risk categories and target values for LDL cholesterol (The Task Force for the Management of Dyslipidaemias, 2011; von Eckardstein, et al., 2005).

IAS recommendation: risk for a cardiovascular event (fatal or nonfatal) within the next 10 years	Joint European Guidelines: risk for a fatal cardiovascular event within the next 10 years	Category	Target LDL cholesterol value	Treatment
< 10 %	< 1 %	Low	< 4.1 mmol/L (< 160 mg/dL)	Generally, motivation for lifestyle and behavior changes
10–20 %	1–5 %	Moderate	< 3.4 mmol/L (< 130 mg/dL)	As above, and if possible, drug therapy to reduce the increased risk factors
> 20 % or: known atherosclerosis	5 %–10 % or: Cholesterol > 8 mmol/L/> 320 mg/dL or: LDL-C > 6 mmol/L/> 240 mg/dL or: blood pressure > 180/110 mm Hg	High	< 2.6 mmol/L (< 100 mg/dL)	As above, and usually intensive drug therapy to reduce the increased risk factors
	> 10 % or: known atherosclerosis or: Diabetes mellitus or: chronic renal failure with GFR < 60 mL/min	Very high	< 1.8 mmol/L (< 70 mg/dL)	As above, and usually intensive drug therapy to reduce the increased risk factors

Table 4.17 Definition of metabolic syndrome (Alberti, et al., 2009).

Parameter	Categorical cut-off values	
	Men	Women
• Waist circumference (valid for Caucasians; there are other cut-off values for other ethnic groups	102 cm	88 cm
	(increased risk at 94 cm)	(increased risk at 80 cm)
• Triglyceride (or drug treatment for hypertriglyceridemia)	> 1.7 mmol/L (> 150 mg/dL)	> 1.7 mmol/L (> 150 mg/dL)
• HDL cholesterol (or drug treatment for lowered HDL cholesterol)	< 1.0 mmol/L (< 40 mg/dL)	< 1.3 mmol/L (< 50 mg/dL)
• Blood pressure (or anti-hypertensive drug therapy)	Systolic: > 130 mm Hg Diastolic: > 85 mm Hg	Systolic: > 130 mm Hg Diastolic: > 85 mm Hg
• Glucose (or treatment for hyperglycemia)	> 5.5 mmol/L (> 100 mg/dL)	> 5.5 mmol/L (> 100 mg/dL)
Metabolic syndrome is present when three of the five criteria are fulfilled		

parameter range (▶ Table 4.18), warrants the expense of an exhaustive differential diagnosis and search for a cause.

In particular, the search for monogenic causes should be strongly indicated because of their increased cost and frequently minimal therapeutic consequences. Several monogenic dyslipidemias are passed via codominant autosomal inheritance, so that family studies should be used to demonstrate vertical transmission of the lipid phenotype before expensive and time-consuming genetic or functional studies are conducted in specialized laboratories. ▶ Table 4.18 summarizes the typical primary and secondary hyperlipidemias.

▶ Figures 4.12 and 4.13 provide diagnostic pathways for the clarification of hypercholesterolemia, hypertriglyceridemia, and low HDL-cholesterol dyslipidemia (Hersberger, et al., 2008).

4.2.3 Porphyrias

Porphyrias are a group of metabolic disorders affecting heme biosynthesis. With the exception of sporadic porphyria cutanea tarda (*vide infra*), these are genetic diseases. Most porphyrias are passed along through autosomal dominant inheritance, i.e., the presence of heterozygosity and a functionally relevant mutation are sufficient for the disease to occur. As the penetrance of the disease is often low, frequently only one individual in a family is symptomatic.

Porphyrias are characterized by two main symptoms, which also affect the clarification strategies: neurovisceral attacks and photodermatosis. The test methods mentioned below are described in detail in Minder and Schneider-Yin (2008). The proposed clarification strategies are formulated from consensus-based recommendations and our experience (http://porphyria.eu; Anderson, et al., 2005; Schneider-Yin, et al., 2009) (▶ 4.14 and 4.15).

4.2.3.1 Neurovisceral Attacks

The most common symptom by far is acute abdominal symptomatology. This usually co-occurs with other typical symptoms such as nausea, vomiting, constipation, tachycardia, hypertension, and hyponatremia. Signs of peritonitis are absent, and signs of inflammation such as fever or leukocytosis are rare. Progression of the disease can lead to peripheral neuropathy with paralysis, including the respiratory muscles; paresthesia, epileptic seizures, and coma with possible death.

Porphyrias associated with this symptomatology are currently referred to as acute porphyrias. Rapid diagnosis during an acute phase by measuring the quantitative porphobilinogen in a spot urine sample standardized to creatinine facilitates giving specific treatment, with administration of heme arginate (Normosang® or panhematin®) and avoidance of porphyria-triggering drugs. With the exception of trace tests, the qualitative porphobilinogen detection methods are non-specific, and therefore result in many false positive results. During an acute porphyria attack up to at least one week after the onset of symptoms, the porphobilinogen value increases at least 5-fold. Later, and also in a latent phase, porphobilinogen can be significantly increased in some patients, while it returns to normal in others.

A normal porphobilinogen concentration value measured during a typical attack of pain rules out acute porphyria as the cause of that pain.

Three different diseases can underlie acute porphyria: acute intermittent porphyria due to a porphobilinogen (PBG) deaminase mutation, porphyria variegata caused by a protoporphyrinogen oxidase mutation, and hereditary coproporphyria caused by a coproporphyrinogen oxidase mutation. Also worth mentioning is the recessive defect in aminolevulinic acid dehydratase, which due to its extreme rarity was not included in the clarification scheme. The three acute porphyrias can be differentiated through further biochemical investigations, PBG deaminase activity, plasma fluorescence scan, and stool porphyrins. A lowered value for PBG deaminase activity together with a negative plasma fluorescence scan result and normal stool porphyrins is typical for acute intermittent porphyria. A normal value for PBG deaminase activity, a peak in the plasma fluorescence scan at 626 nm, together with elevated levels of coproporphyrin (CP) and protoporphyrin IX (PPIX) in the stool are typical for porphyria variegata. Hereditary coproporphyria exhibits a normal value for PBG deaminase activity, normally increased CP in the stool, and often shows a peak at 620 nm in the plasma fluorescence scan. These diagnoses are then to be verified by investigating the corresponding genes: hydroxymethylbilane synthase (HMBS) for the acute intermittent porphyria, protoporphyrinogen oxidase (PPOX) for variegate porphyria, and coproporphyrinogen oxidase (CPOX) for hereditary coproporphyria.

Assessment in the latent phase: Should it be necessary to clarify the presence of porphyria in a patient in whom symptoms have vanished for longer than one week, or if the porphobilinogen value increases by less than 5-fold, in addition to determining porphobilinogen we recommend the

Table 4.18 Differential diagnosis to determine the origin of pronounced lipid metabolism disorders; ABC = ATP binding cassette transporter, apo = apolipoprotein, ARH = autosomal recessive hypercholesterolemia, LCAT = lecithin-cholesterol acyltransferase, MTP = microsomal transfer protein, PCSK9 = proprotein convertase subtilisin kexin 9.

	Cholesterol	Triglycerides	LDL cholesterol	HDL cholesterol
Hyperlipidemia				
90th percentile (m/f)	7.5/7.5 mmol/L (290/290 mg/dL)	3.8/2.8 mmol/L (330/240 mg/dL)	5.0/5.0 mmol/L (190/190 mg/dL)	1.80/2.25 mmol/L (70/85 mg/dL)
Typical primary causes	Mutations in genes for LDL receptor, apoB, PCSK9, ARH, ABCG5/8 (sitosterolemia) Type III hyperlipidemia (apoE2 homozygosity, other mutations in the apoE gene) Cholesteryl ester storage disease	Chylomicronemia: Mutations in genes for lipoprotein lipase, apoC II, apoA-V, GPIHBP	Mutations in genes for LDL receptor, apoB, PCSK9, ARH, ABCG5/8 (sitosterolemia)	Mutations in genes for CETP, hepatic lipase
Typical secondary causes	Hypothyroidism Cholestasis Anorexia nervosa Nephrotic syndrome Cushing syndrome	Diabetes mellitus Renal failure Hepatitis Inflammations Pregnancy	Hypothyroidism Cholestasis Anorexia nervosa	
Typical medication or nutrient effects	Gestagens HIV protease inhibitors Immunosuppressants	Estrogens Diuretics Neuroleptics Glucocorticoids Retinoids Alcohol	Gestagens HIV protease inhibitors Immunosuppressants	Estrogens Anticonvulsants
Hypolipidemia				
10th percentile (m/f)	4.7/4.7 mmol/L 180/180 mg/dL	0.7/0.9 mmol/L 80/60 mg/dL	2.3/2.3 mmol/L 90/90 mg/dL	0.90/1.15 mmol/L 35/45 mg/dL
Typical primary causes	A/hypobetalipoproteinemia (mutations in apoB, MTP)		A/hypobetalipoproteinemia (mutations in apoB, MTP)	Mutations in genes for apoA-I, LCAT, ABCA1 (Tangier disease)
Typical secondary causes	Liver failure, sepsis, catabolic states	Liver failure	Liver failure, sepsis, catabolic states	Diabetes (metabolic syndrome), liver failure, right heart failure, acute inflammation, malignant tumors (hemato-oncological disease)
Typical medication or nutrient effects				Androgens, anabolic steroids, some beta blockers

Clarifying Hypercholesterolemia

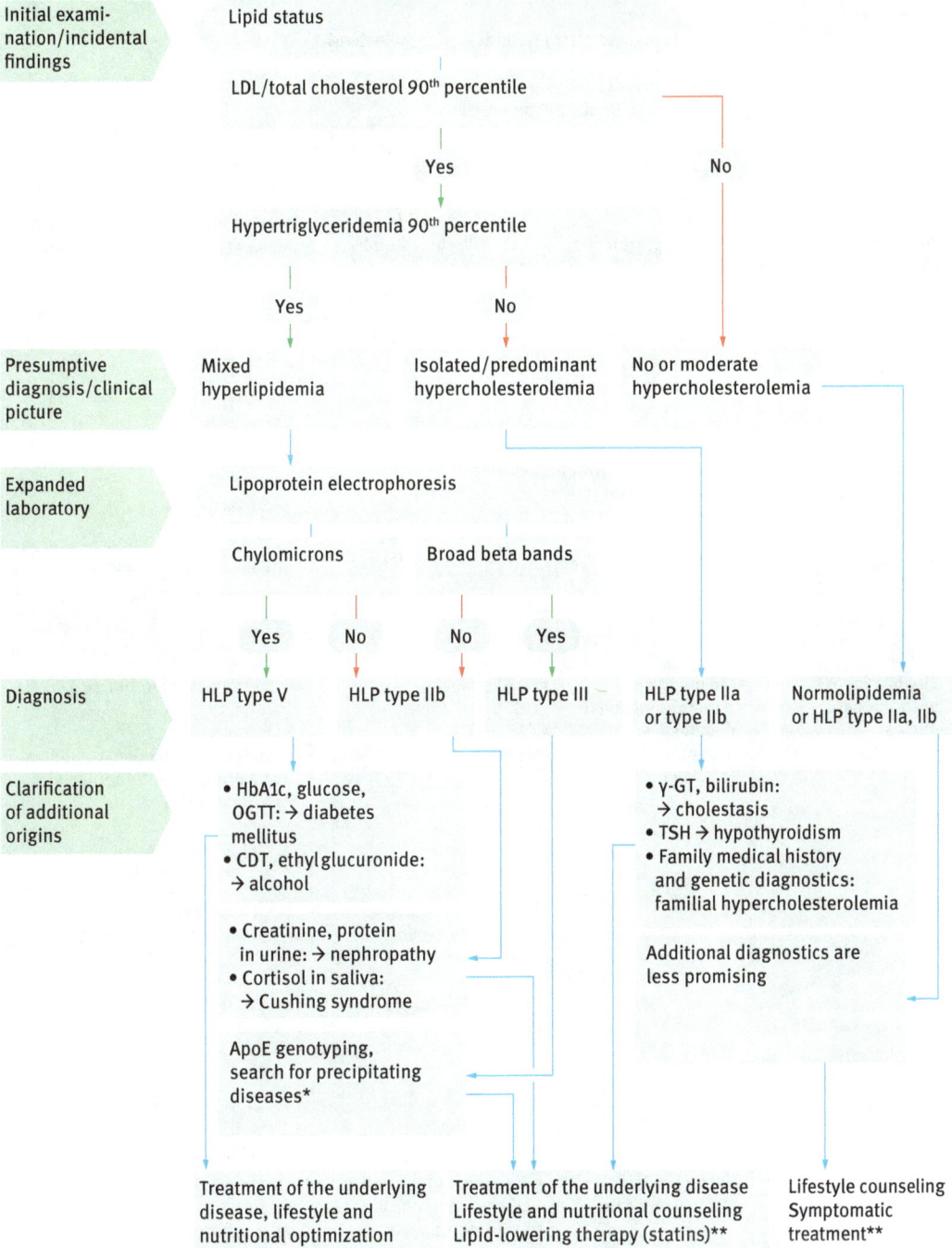

Initial examination/incidental findings

Lipid status

LDL/total cholesterol 90th percentile

Yes — No

Hypertriglyceridemia 90th percentile

Yes — No

Presumptive diagnosis/clinical picture

Mixed hyperlipidemia | Isolated/predominant hypercholesterolemia | No or moderate hypercholesterolemia

Expanded laboratory

Lipoprotein electrophoresis

Chylomicrons | Broad beta bands

Yes — No | No — Yes

Diagnosis

HLP type V | HLP type IIb | HLP type III | HLP type IIa or type IIb | Normolipidemia or HLP type IIa, IIb

Clarification of additional origins

- HbA1c, glucose, OGTT: → diabetes mellitus
- CDT, ethyl glucuronide: → alcohol

- Creatinine, protein in urine: → nephropathy
- Cortisol in saliva: → Cushing syndrome

ApoE genotyping, search for precipitating diseases*

- γ-GT, bilirubin: → cholestasis
- TSH → hypothyroidism
- Family medical history and genetic diagnostics: familial hypercholesterolemia

Additional diagnostics are less promising

Treatment of the underlying disease, lifestyle and nutritional optimization | Treatment of the underlying disease Lifestyle and nutritional counseling Lipid-lowering therapy (statins)** | Lifestyle counseling Symptomatic treatment**

Figure 4.12 Flow diagram for the differential diagnosis of hypercholesterolemia; *: Typical type III hyperlipoproteinemia precipitating diseases in apoE2 homozygosity are diabetes mellitus, hypothyroidism, hemochromatosis; **: Procedures as described in Figures 4.7, 4.8 or 4.9 and 4.16; Percentile limits, see Table 4.18; HLP = hyperlipoproteinemia (type names by Fredrickson), apoE = apolipoprotein E, CDT = carbohydrate deficient transferrin, TSH = thyroid-stimulating hormone.

Clarification of Hypertriglyceridemia and Hypoalphalipoproteinemia

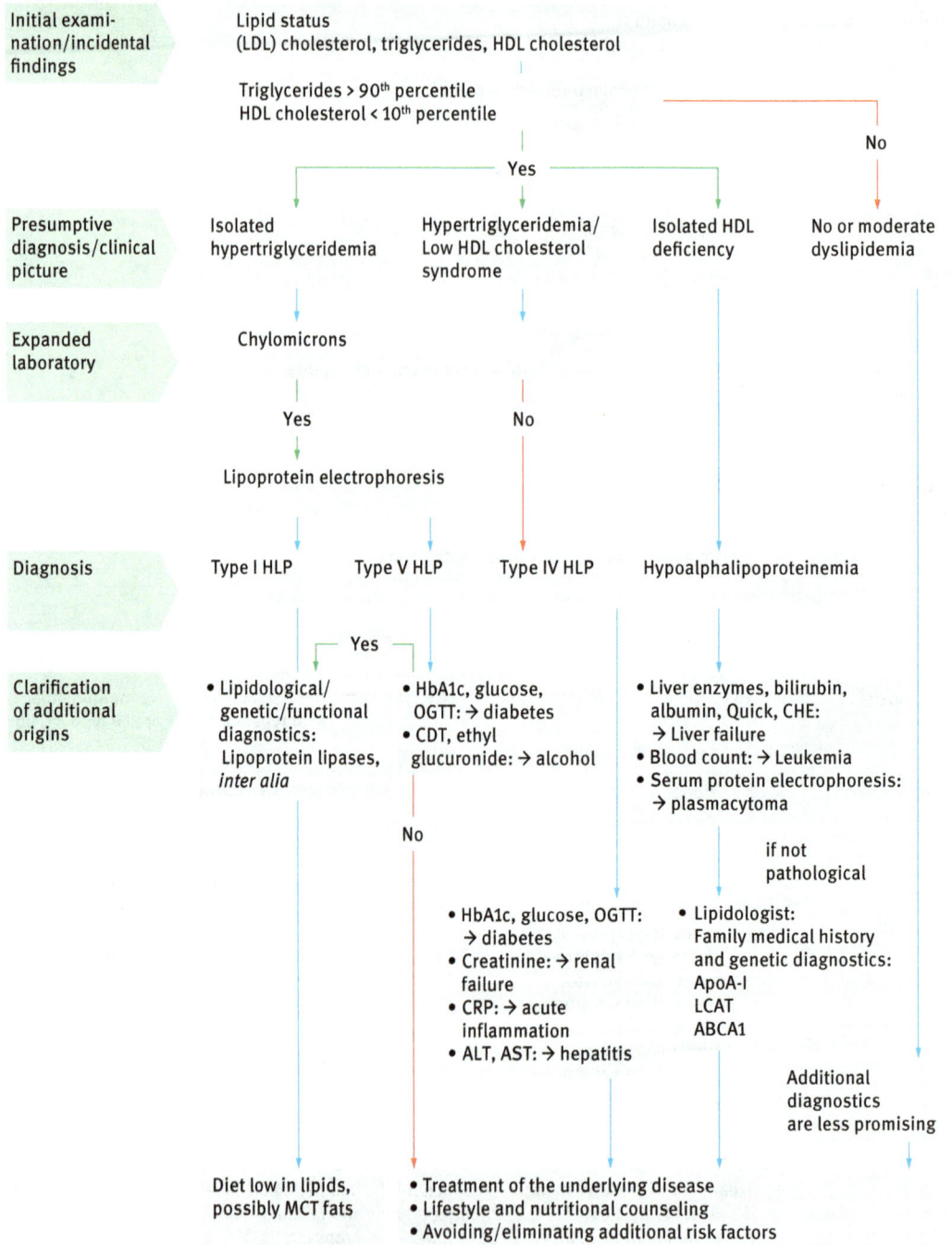

Initial examination/incidental findings

Lipid status
(LDL) cholesterol, triglycerides, HDL cholesterol

Triglycerides > 90th percentile
HDL cholesterol < 10th percentile

No

Yes

Presumptive diagnosis/clinical picture

Isolated hypertriglyceridemia | Hypertriglyceridemia/ Low HDL cholesterol syndrome | Isolated HDL deficiency | No or moderate dyslipidemia

Expanded laboratory

Chylomicrons

Yes   No

Lipoprotein electrophoresis

Diagnosis

Type I HLP   Type V HLP   Type IV HLP   Hypoalphalipoproteinemia

Yes

Clarification of additional origins

- Lipidological/ genetic/functional diagnostics: Lipoprotein lipases, *inter alia*

- HbA1c, glucose, OGTT: → diabetes
- CDT, ethyl glucuronide: → alcohol

- Liver enzymes, bilirubin, albumin, Quick, CHE: → Liver failure
- Blood count: → Leukemia
- Serum protein electrophoresis: → plasmacytoma

if not pathological

No

- HbA1c, glucose, OGTT: → diabetes
- Creatinine: → renal failure
- CRP: → acute inflammation
- ALT, AST: → hepatitis

- Lipidologist: Family medical history and genetic diagnostics: ApoA-I LCAT ABCA1

Additional diagnostics are less promising

Diet low in lipids, possibly MCT fats

- Treatment of the underlying disease
- Lifestyle and nutritional counseling
- Avoiding/eliminating additional risk factors

Figure 4.13 Flow diagram for the differential diagnosis of hypertriglyceridemia and low HDL cholesterol; percentile limits, see Table 4.18; HLP = hyperlipoproteinemia (type names by Fredrickson), CDT = carbohydrate-deficient transferrin, OGTT = oral glucose tolerance test, CHE = cholinesterase, CRP = C-reactive protein, ALT = alanine-aminotransferase, AST = aspartate-aminotransferase, apoA-I = apolipoprotein A-I, ABCA1 = ATP-binding cassette-transporter A1, LCAT = lecithin-cholesterol acyltransferase.

measuring the PBG deaminase activity, running a plasma fluorescence scan, and determining stool porphyrins. The combination of these four tests will enable the diagnosis of acute porphyria with a sensitivity of about 90 %.

If unclarity remains, one must await a renewed attack of pain and then proceed again according to the scheme for symptomatic patients.

Family testing: In all cases of acute porphyria, we recommend an assessment for porphyria

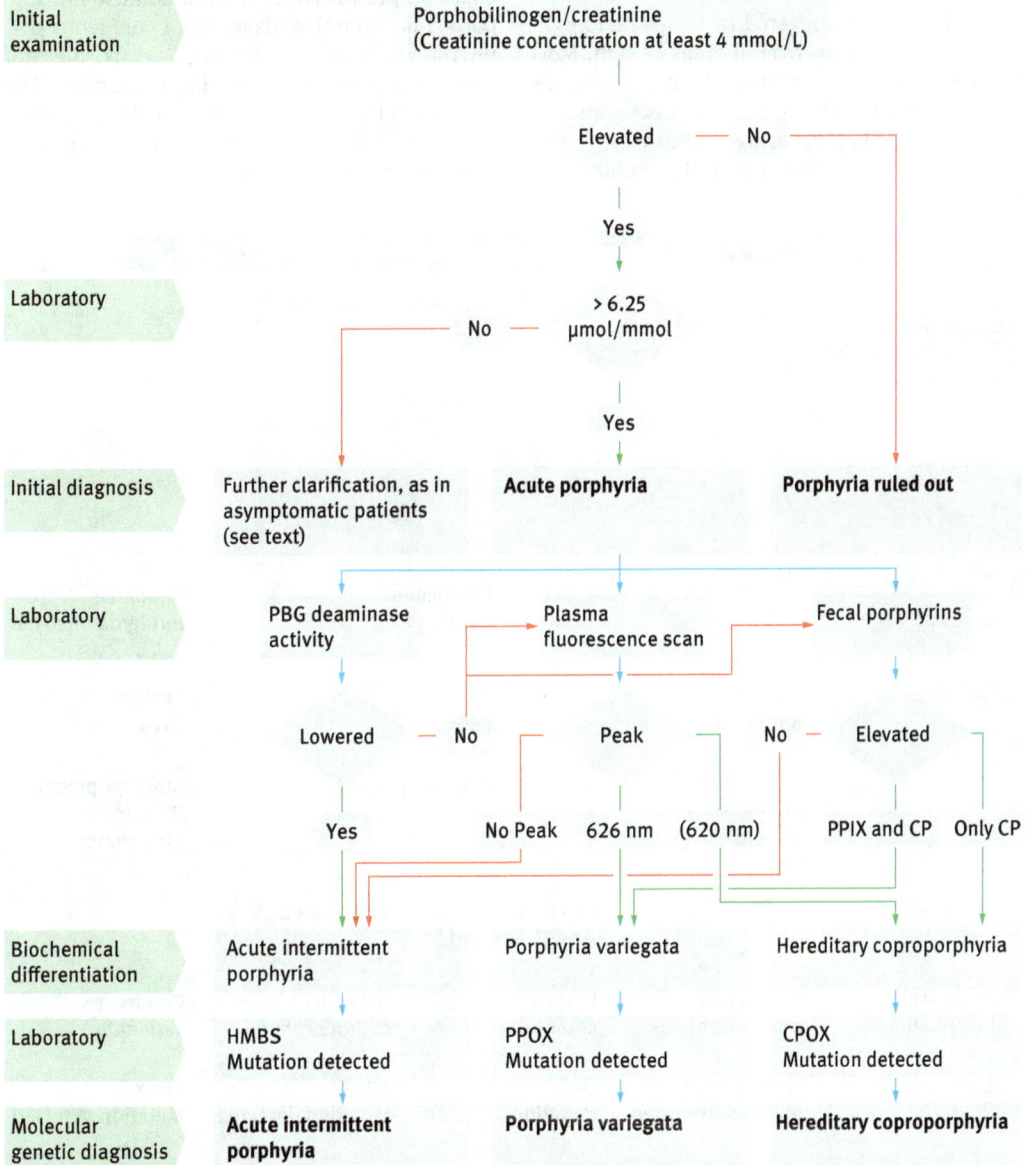

Figure 4.14 Flow diagram for the differential diagnosis of porphyrias accompanied by abdominal colic; PBG: porphobilinogen, CP: coproporphyrin, PPIX: proto- porphyrin IX, HMBS: hydroxymethylbilane synthase, PPOX: protoporphyrinogen oxidase, CPOX: coproporphyrinogen oxidase.

among all blood relatives of the index patient, and implementation of preventive measures for those affected. Blood relatives have a 50 % risk of also having inherited porphyria. The most reliable results are obtained by genetic testing for the mutation present the index patient.

4.2.3.2 Photodermatoses

This skin diseases triggered by exposure to light are limited to the uncovered areas of skin. Most often affected are the back of the hands and the face. Two disease pictures can be distinguished: The better known, blistering skin disease (▶ Figure 4.16a) manifests itself primarily in adulthood;

and second the acute and severely painfull photodermatosis (▶ Figure 4.16b) usually first appearing in childhood, and persisting into adulthood.

A simple screening test for cutaneous porphyrias is the plasma fluorescence scan. Porphyrins present in the plasma are excited at a wavelength of 410 nm, and the emission spectrum between 500 and 700 nm is measured. The presence of an emission peak between 615 nm and 636 nm supports a presumptive diagnosis of cutaneous porphyria, while the absence of this peak rules out cutaneous porphyria with high probability. The location of the peak maximum provides a certain amount of differentiation between the porphyria: a maximum at 626 nm is characteristic of porphy-

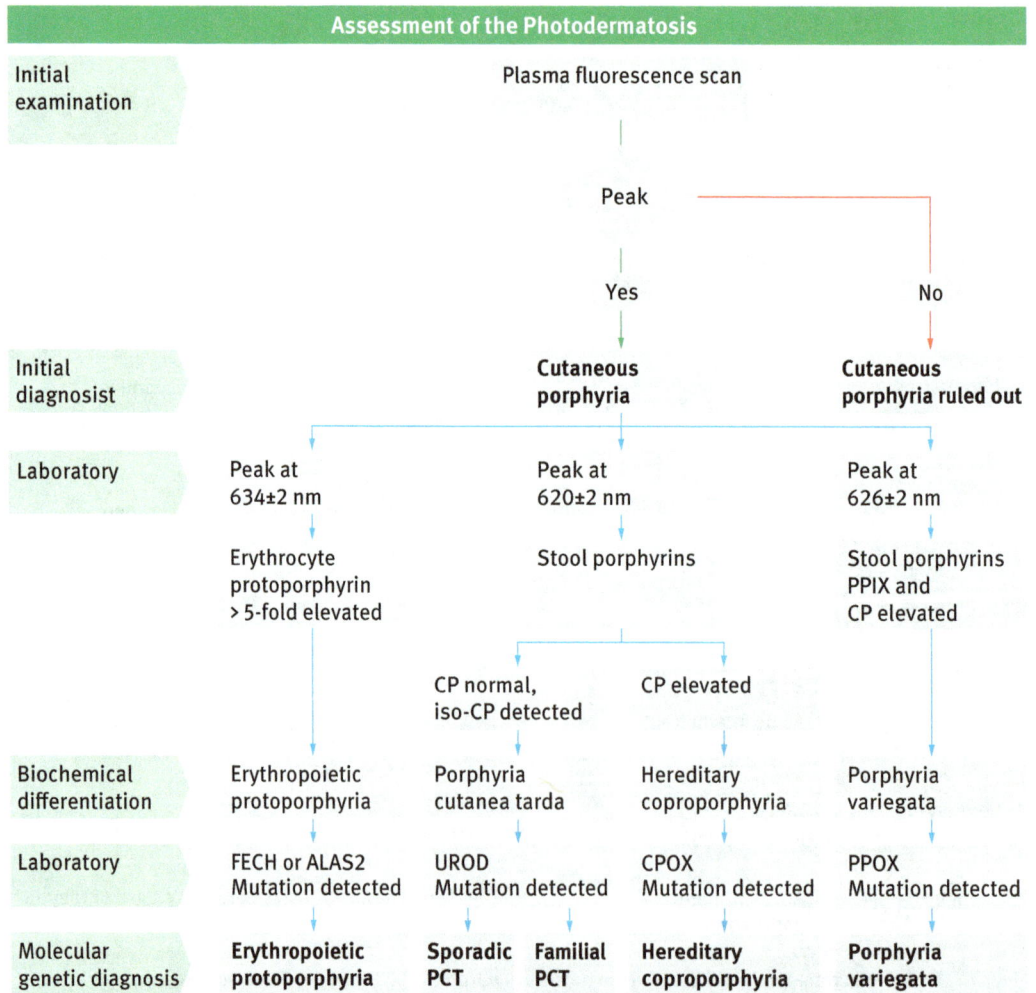

Assessment of the Photodermatosis			
Initial examination	Plasma fluorescence scan		
	Peak		
	Yes		No
Initial diagnosist	**Cutaneous porphyria**		**Cutaneous porphyria ruled out**
Laboratory	Peak at 634±2 nm	Peak at 620±2 nm	Peak at 626±2 nm
	Erythrocyte protoporphyrin > 5-fold elevated	Stool porphyrins	Stool porphyrins PPIX and CP elevated
		CP normal, iso-CP detected / CP elevated	
Biochemical differentiation	Erythropoietic protoporphyria	Porphyria cutanea tarda / Hereditary coproporphyria	Porphyria variegata
Laboratory	FECH or ALAS2 Mutation detected	UROD Mutation detected / CPOX Mutation detected	PPOX Mutation detected
Molecular genetic diagnosis	**Erythropoietic protoporphyria**	**Sporadic PCT** / **Familial PCT** / **Hereditary coproporphyria**	**Porphyria variegata**

Figure 4.15 Flow diagram for the differential diagnosis of photodermatoses accompanied by porphyria.

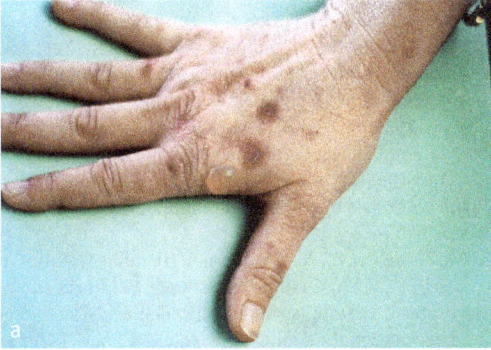

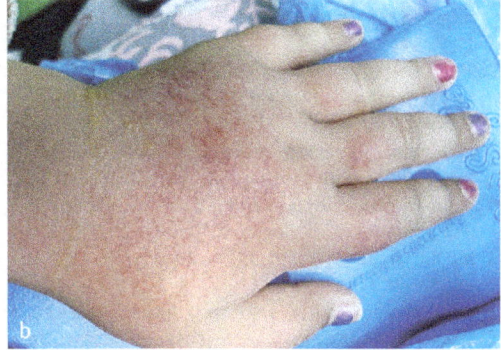

Abb. 4.16a, b Photodermatoses in porphyria.

ria variegata, while a maximum at 635 nm indicates erythropoietic protoporphyria. However, a peak maximum at 620 nm could be caused by more than one type of porphyria. The most frequent of these are porphyria cutanea tarda and hereditary coproporphyria. These two types of porphyria can be differentiated by examining the fecal porphyrins: The former is characterized by the presence of isocoproporphyrin, while the latter is associated with an increased coproporphyrin value. Other types of porphyria that exhibit a peak maximum at 620 nm, which were not included in the clarification scheme because of their rarity, are congenital erythropoietic porphyria and the acute intermittent porphyria with the complication of renal failure requiring dialysis. Congenital erythropoietic porphyria is characterized by the dominant occurrence of isomer I porphyrins in all body fluids. Acute intermittent porphyria with renal failure can be recognized by the presence of normal stool porphyrins. Due to the complicated hematological status in renal failure, the PBG deaminase activity usually decreased in this type of porphyria can show a falsely normal activity. Porphyria variegata likewise can be confirmed by fecal porphyrin measurements, which will show elevated coproporphyrin and elevated protoporphyrin. By contrast, erythropoietic protoporphyria exhibits an erythrocyte protoporphyrin level that is increased by at least 5-fold.

Genetic analysis can confirm the diagnoses. In the familial form of porphyria cutanea tarda, a mutation in the UROD gen is present, but no mutation is found in sporadic porphyria cutanea tarda. The type of mutation in erythropoietic protoporphyria can affect the risk of complicating,

protoporphyrin-related liver disease. In both acute porphyrias, hereditary coproporphyria and porphyria variegata, mutation screening in the index patient is recommended to facilitate the family screening as discussed above.

Literature

Alberti KG, Eckel RH, Grundy SM, Zimmet PZ, Cleeman JI, Donato KA, Fruchart JC, James WP, Loria CM, Smith SC Jr; International Diabetes Federation Task Force on Epidemiology and Prevention; Hational Heart, Lung, and Blood Institute; American Heart Association; World Heart Federation; International Atherosclerosis Society; International Association for the Study of Obesity. Harmonizing the metabolic syndrome: a joint interim statement of the International Diabetes Federation Task Force on Epidemiology and Prevention; National Heart, Lung, and Blood Institute; American Heart Association; World Heart Federation; International Atherosclerosis Society; and International Association for the Study of Obesity. Circulation. 2009 Oct 20; 120(16): 1640–5.

American Diabetes Association. Report of the Expert Committee on the Diagnosis and Classification of Diabetes Mellitus. Diabetes Care 1997; 20: 1183–1197.

American Diabetes Association. Standards of medical care in diabetes-2012. Diabetes Care. 2012 Jan; 35 Suppl 1: 11–63.38.

Anderson KE, Bloomer JR, Bonkovsky HL, Kushner JP, Pierach CA, Pimstone NR, Desnick RJ. Recommendations for the diagnosis and treatment of the acute porphyrias. Ann Intern Med. 2005 15; 142 (6): 439–50.

Assmann G, Cullen P, Fruchart JC, Greten H, Naruszewicz M, Olsson A, Paoletti R, Riesen W, Stoll M, Tikkanen M, von Eckardstein A; for the International Task Force for Prevention of Coronary Heart Disease. Implications of emerging risk factors for therapeutic intervention. Nutr Metab Cardiovasc Dis. 2005 Oct; 15(5): 373–81.

Blankenberg S, Zeller T, Saarela O, Havulinna AS, Kee F, Tunstall-Pedoe H, Kuulasmaa K, Yarnell J, Schnabel RB, Wild PS, Munzel TF, Lackner KJ, Tiret L, Evans A, Salomaa V; MORGAM Project. Contribution of 30 biomarkers to 10-year cardiovascular risk estimation in 2 population cohorts: the MONICA, risk, genetics, archiving, and monograph (MORGAM) biomarker project. Circulation. 2010 Jun 8; 121(22): 2388–97

Brown A, Reynolds LR, Bruemmer D. Intensive glycemic control and cardiovascular disease: an update. Nat Rev Cardiol. 2010 Jul; 7(7): 369–75

Castorino KN, Jovonivic L. Pregnancy and diabetes management: Advances and Controversies. Clin. Chem. 2011, 57(2): 221–30

Cholesterol Treatment Trialists' (CTT) Collaborators, Kearney PM, Blackwell L, Collins R, Keech A, Simes J, Peto R, Armitage J, Baigent C. Efficacy of cholesterol-lowering therapy in 18,686 people with diabetes in 14 randomised trials of statins: a meta-analysis. Lancet. 2008 Jan 12; 371(9607): 117–25.

Cholesterol Treatment Trialists' (CTT) Collaboration, Baigent C, Blackwell L, Emberson J, Holland LE, Reith C, Bhala N, Peto R, Barnes EH, Keech A, Simes J, Collins R. Efficacy and safety of more intensive lowering of LDL cholesterol: a meta-analysis of data from 170,000 participants in 26 randomised trials. Lancet. 2010 Nov 13; 376(9753): 1670–81

Currie CJ, Peters JR, Tynan A, Evans M, Heine RJ, Bracco OL, Zagar T, Poole CD. Survival as a function of HbA(1c) in people with type 2 diabetes: a retrospective cohort study. Lancet. 2010 Feb 6; 375(9713): 481–9.

Ekelund M, Shaat N, Almgren P, Groop L, Berntorp K. Prediction of postpartum diabetes in women with gestational diabetes mellitus. Diabetologia. 2010 Mar; 53(3): 452–7

Emerging Risk Factors Collaboration, Di Angelantonio E, Sarwar N, Perry P, Kaptoge S, Ray KK, Thompson A, Wood AM, Lewington S, Sattar N, Packard CJ, Collins R, Thompson SG, Danesh J. Major lipids, apolipoproteins, and risk of vascular disease. JAMA. 2009 Nov 11; 302(18): 1993–2000

Fioretto P, Dodson PM, Ziegler D, Rosenson RS. Residual microvascular risk in diabetes: unmet needs and future directions. Nat Rev Endocrinol. 2010 Jan; 6(1): 19–25.

Hersberger M, Rohrer L, von Eckardstein A (2008). Lipoproteins In: Blau N, Duran M, Gibson KM, editors. Physicians Guide to the Methods in Biochemical Genetics, Heidelberg Springer Verlag 2008

International Association of Diabetes and Pregnancy Study Groups Consensus Panel, Metzger BE, Gabbe SG, Persson B, Buchanan TA, Catalano PA, Damm P, Dyer AR, Leiva A, Hod M, Kitzmiler JL, Lowe LP,

McIntyre HD, Oats JJ, Omori Y, Schmidt MI. International association of diabetes and pregnancy study groups recommendations on the diagnosis and classification of hyperglycemia in pregnancy. Diabetes Care. 2010 Mar; 33(3): 676–82.

International Expert Committee. International Expert Committee report on the role of the A1c assay in the diagnosis of diabetes. Diabetes Care 2009; 32: 1327–1334

Jun M, Foote C, Lv J, Neal B, Patel A, Nicholls SJ, Grobbee DE, Cass A, Chalmers J, Perkovic V. Effects of fibrates on cardiovascular outcomes: a systematic review and meta-analysis. Lancet. 2010 May 29; 375(9729): 1875–84

Keil U, Fitzgerald AP, Gohlke H, Wellmann J, Hense HW. RisikoAbschätzung tödlicher Herz-Kreislauf-Erkrankungen: Die neuen SCORE-Deutschland-Tabellen für die Primärpravention. Deutsches Arzteblatt 102, A-1808-A1812. 2005

Kerner W, Bruckel J. Definition, Klassifikation und Diagnostik. Diabetologie 2010; 5: S 109–S 112

Lenters-Westra E, Slingerland RJ. Six of eight hemoglobin A1c point-of-care instruments do not meet the general accepted analytical performance criteria. Clin Chem. 2010 Jan; 56(1): 44–52.

Matthaei S, Bierwirth R, Fritsche A, Gallwitz B, Haring H-U, Joost H-G, Kellerer M, Kloos C, Kunt T, Nauck M, Schernthaner G, Siegel E, Thienel F. Behandlung des Diabetes mellitus Typ 2. Diabetologie 2010; 5: S 127–S 132

Minder EI, Schneider X. Porphyrins, Porphobilinogen and d-Aminolevulinic Acid. In: Blau N, Duran M, Gibson KM, editors. Physicians Guide to the Methods in Biochemical Genetics, Heidelberg Springer Verlag 2008: 751–780.

National Diabetes Data Group. Classification and diagnosis of diabetes mellitus and other categories of glucose intolerance. National Diabetes Data Group. Diabetes 1979; 28: 1039–1057.

Nordestgaard BG, Chapman MJ, Ray K, Boren J, Andreotti F, Watts GF, Ginsberg H, Amarenco P, Catapano A, Descamps OS, Fisher E, Kovanen PT, Kuivenhoven JA, Lesnik P, Masana L, Reiner Z, Taskinen MR, Tokgozoglu L, Tybjarg-Hansen A; European Atherosclerosis Society Consensus Panel Lipoprotein(a) as a cardiovascular risk factor: current status. Eur Heart J. 2010 Dec; 31(23): 2844–53.

Rathmann W, Kowall B, Tamayo T, Giani G, Holle R, Thorand B, Heier M, Huth C, Meisinger C Hemoglobin A1c and glucose criteria identify different subjects as having type 2 diabetes in middle-aged and older populations: The KORA S4/F4 Study. Ann Med. 2010 Nov 22. (Epub ahead of print)

Schulze MB, Hoffmann K, Boeing H, Linseisen J, Rohrmann S, Mohlig M, Pfeiffer AF, Spranger J, Thamer C, Haring HU, Fritsche A, Joost HG. An accurate risk score based on anthropometric, dietary, and lifestyle factors to predict the development of type 2 diabetes. Diabetes Care 30, 510–5, 2007

The Task Force for the management of dyslipidaemias. ESC/EAS Guidelines for the management of dyslipidaemias. European Heart Journal (2011) 32, 1769–1818

von Eckardstein A, Schulte H, Assmann G. Vergleich internationaler Konsensus-Empfehlungen zur Erkennung des prasymptomatischen Hochrisikopatienten für den Herzinfarkt in Deutschland. Z Kardiol. 2005 Jan; 94(1): 52–60.

World Health Organization. Definition, diagnosis and classification of diabetes mellitus and its complications: report of a WHO consultation. Part 1: diagnosis and classification of diabetes mellitus 1999 World Health Organization Geneva

Max G. Bachem, Thomas Seufferlein, Marco Siech

4.3 Liver and Pancreatic Disorders

4.3.1 Hepatobiliary Disorders (Figure 4.17)

Hepatobiliary diseases can be classified according to their origin, their appearance and their laboratory picture as follows:

- Diseases accompanied by hepatocellular damage
- Cholestatic diseases
- Mixed hepatocellular/cholestatic diseases
- Diseases with reduced synthesis capacity and detoxification function

Clinically, hepatobiliary disease can expressed as abdominal pain in the right upper quadrant, where a persistent or colicky pain can be found. In addition, there might be jaundice. In many cases, however, hepatobiliary disease is noted as an incidental finding through elevated transaminases or gamma-glutamyl transpeptidase (gamma-GT).

Medical history

With suspected hepatobiliary disease, medical history questions should especially solicit possible signs of liver disease. Fatigue, expressed through increased need for sleep, lethargy, weakness, and malaise, is the most common symptom of liver disease.

If pain is reported in the right upper abdomen, ask about the nature and duration of the pain. Furthermore, inquiry should be made into whether pruritus is present, whether the color of the stool and urine has changed, what is the extent of alcohol consumption, whether the patient has been in contact with individuals who have jaundice, whether gallstones are present, whether there has been a recent weight loss, whether the patient is aware of any inflammatory bowel disease, whether an autoimmune disease is present, whether the patient has recently been abroad, which medications is the patient currently on, and whether any parenteral drugs are being taken. With regard to sexually transmitted viral hepatitis, the patient should also be asked about sexual activity. For individuals who work in the medical field, an infection via needlestick injury should be ruled out.

Physical examination

The physical examination is often not particularly effective in patients with hepatobiliary disease. However, acute cases, severe progressive forms, and advanced liver disease can be detected by the presence of jaundice, abdominal pain in the liver region, enlargement of the liver or spleen, and possibly ascites, collateral circulation, or "fetor hepaticus". Special attention should also be given in the physical examination to signs of chronic alcohol abuse. The presence of hyperpigmentation could indicate increased iron or copper deposition (Kayser-Fleischer ring).

Ultrasound

Items to note in the abdominal ultrasound include the sizes of the liver and spleen, the texture and structure of the liver, any focal lesions, signs of liver cirrhosis, the presence of gallstones, bile ducts dilated as in cholestasis, and the presence of ascites, a mass lesion, or vascular disorders. The ultrasound findings can also yield evidence of a fatty liver.

Laboratory Diagnostics (Figure 4.17)

The basic laboratory diagnosis comprises the determination of electrolytes (sodium, potassium, calcium), glucose, creatinine, total and direct bilirubin, ALT, AST, AP, γ-GT, and lipase activity; CRP concentration, the basic coagulation parameters PT and PTT, the blood count with leukocyte differentiation, and urinalysis, where particular

Clinical picture: Abdominal pain in the right upper quadrant (colicky or persistent pain) and/or jaundice

Examination items: Jaundice? Liver size? Spider naevi? Hyperpigmentation? Collateral circulation? Distended abdomen? Pain on pressure? Ascites? Signs of alcohol abuse? Temperature?

Medical history items: Pains in the right upper abdomen? Alcohol? Pruritus? Colored stool or urine? Fatigue? Medications? Drugs? Contact with people having jaundice? Gallstones? Weight loss? Inflammatory bowel disease? Time spent abroad?

Presumptive diagnosis	**Hepatobiliary Disorders**

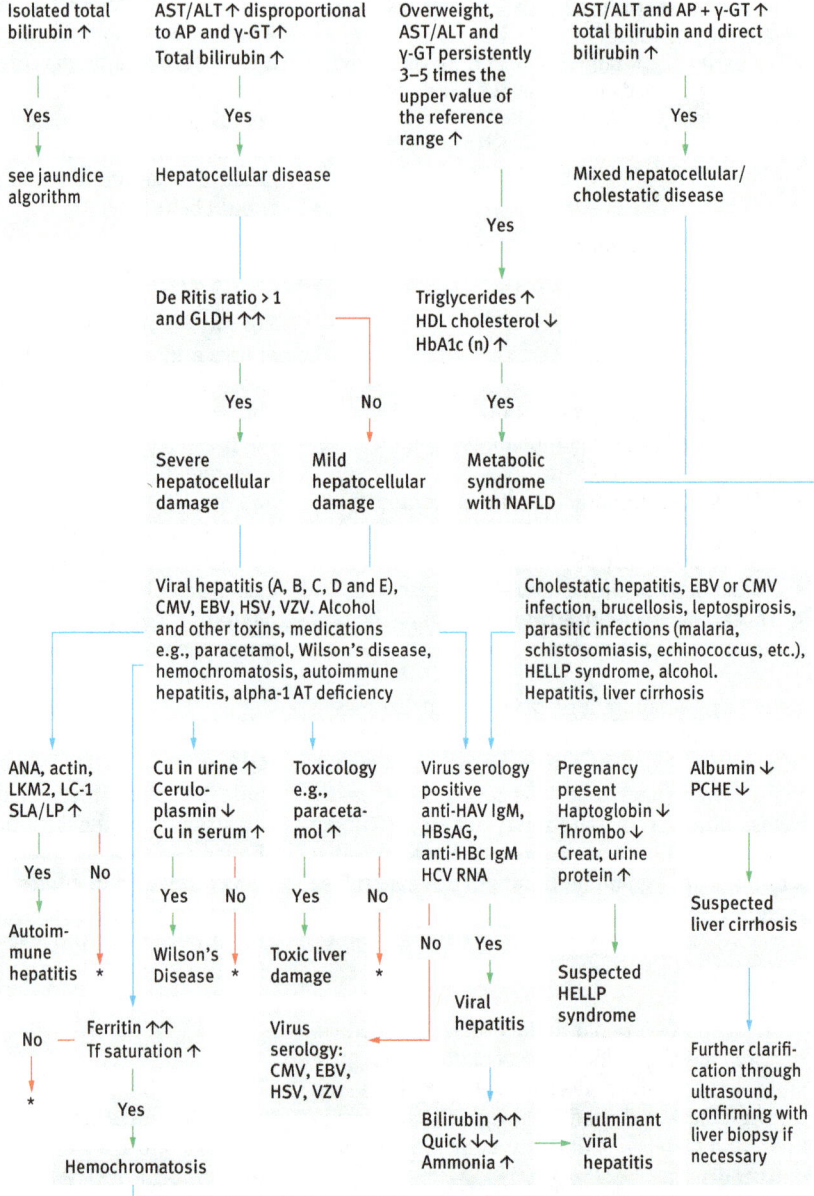

Basic laboratory diagnostics

Electrolytes, glucose, creatinine, total bilirubin, direct bilirubin, ALT, AST, AP, γ-GT, Lipase, CRP, PT (Quick value), PTT, blood count + differential, urinalysis + bilirubin + UBG

Isolated total bilirubin ↑ → Yes → see jaundice algorithm

AST/ALT ↑ disproportional to AP and γ-GT ↑
Total bilirubin ↑ → Yes → Hepatocellular disease

Overweight, AST/ALT and γ-GT persistently 3–5 times the upper value of the reference range ↑ → Yes

AST/ALT and AP + γ-GT ↑ total bilirubin and direct bilirubin ↑ → Yes → Mixed hepatocellular/cholestatic disease

Expanded laboratory

GLDH, albumin, PCHE, triglycerides, cholesterol, HDL cholesterol, HbA1c Serum electrophoresis

De Ritis ratio > 1 and GLDH ↑↑
→ Yes → Severe hepatocellular damage
→ No → Mild hepatocellular damage

Triglycerides ↑ HDL cholesterol ↓ HbA1c (n) ↑ → Yes → Metabolic syndrome with NAFLD

Ultrasound

Differential diagnosis

Viral hepatitis (A, B, C, D and E), CMV, EBV, HSV, VZV. Alcohol and other toxins, medications e.g., paracetamol, Wilson's disease, hemochromatosis, autoimmune hepatitis, alpha-1 AT deficiency

Cholestatic hepatitis, EBV or CMV infection, brucellosis, leptospirosis, parasitic infections (malaria, schistosomiasis, echinococcus, etc.), HELLP syndrome, alcohol. Hepatitis, liver cirrhosis

Further procedures

Specialized laboratory diagnostics

Virus serology: anti-HAV IgM, anti-HCV HBsAG, anti-HBc IgM HCV RNA, CMV, EBV

Ceruloplasmin, Cu in serum, Cu in urine, ferritin, Tf saturation, haptoglobin, ammonia

IgG, IgA, IgM Autoantibodies: ANA, AMA, LKM, Actin, LC-1, SLA/LP, pANCA

ANA, actin, LKM2, LC-1 SLA/LP ↑
→ Yes → Autoimmune hepatitis *
→ No → Ferritin ↑↑ Tf saturation ↑
  → No → *
  → Yes → Hemochromatosis

Cu in urine ↑ Ceruloplasmin ↓ Cu in serum ↑
→ Yes → Wilson's Disease *
→ No

Toxicology e.g., paracetamol ↑
→ Yes → Toxic liver damage *
→ No → Virus serology: CMV, EBV, HSV, VZV

Virus serology positive anti-HAV IgM, HBsAG, anti-HBc IgM HCV RNA
→ No
→ Yes → Viral hepatitis

Bilirubin ↑↑ Quick ↓↓ Ammonia ↑ → Fulminant viral hepatitis

Pregnancy present Haptoglobin ↓ Thrombo ↓ Creat, urine protein ↑ → Suspected HELLP syndrome

Albumin ↓ PCHE ↓ → Suspected liver cirrhosis → Further clarification through ultrasound, confirming with liver biopsy if necessary

Figure 4.17 epatobiliary Disorders. Clinical picture: Abdominal pains in the right upper quadrant (colicky or persistent pain) and/or jaundice or incidental finding (elevated ALT/AST or γ-GT).

or Incidental Finding (elevated ALT/AST or γ-GT)

Ultrasound items: Liver size? Structure, texture? Focal lesions? Cirrhosis? Gallstones? Cholestasis? Ascites? Mass lesion? Vascular disorders?

AP ↑↑, γ-GT ↑↑ direct bilirubin > 15% of the total bilirubin

AST/ALT n (↑), AP n (↑) Quick value ↓

Yes

Cholestatic disease

Ultrasound + MRCP Obstructed bile ducts

Albumin ↓
No — PCHE ↓

Yes

No liver cirrhosis

No

Intrahepatic cholestasis

Extrahepatic cholestasis

Yes

Liver cirrhosis

Choledocholi- thiasis?

No

Liver metastases, PBC, PSC, medications such as steroids, Budd-Chiari syndrome, pregnancy cholestasis

Rule out malignant tumor, such as pancreatic carcinoma.

Determine the Child-Pugh score

ANA, AMA AMA-M2, M4, M9, nuclear dots positive

PANCA positive centro- mere B

Medication history Possibly liver biopsy Possibly angio. MRI

Further clarifi- cation through ultrasound, confirming with liver biopsy if necessary

Yes

Yes

Suspected PBC

Suspected PSC

Liver biopsy

* search for other causes

attention should be paid to the bilirubin and the urobilinogen (UBG) fields in the urine test strip.

These basic laboratory diagnostic methods can be used to assess whether, for example, the isolated total bilirubin is increased, and to recognize the presence of a hepatocellular disease, a cholestatic disease, a mixed hepatocellular/cholestatic disease, or if there is evidence of insufficient synthesis.

If, among the basic laboratory diagnostic parameters, only the total bilirubin in serum/plasma is found to be increased and the measured parameters are otherwise normal, further clarification should be done according to the "jaundice" algorithm (▶ Figure 4.19). These cases might involve Gilbert's syndrome, hemolysis, ineffective erythropoiesis, drug effects, or Crigler-Najjar syndrome.

Diseases that can lead to hepatocellular damage

An AST/ALT value that is disproportionately increased compared to the activity of AP and gamma-GT indicates hepatocellular injury. In such a case, determining the GLDH activity and De Ritis ratios should clarify whether mild or severe hepatocellular injury is present. A De Ritis ratio >1 and a significantly increased GLDH are indications of severe hepatocellular injury. The most common origin of hepatocellular injury is viral hepatitis, which can be detected through virus serology by measuring the specific virus antibodies, viral antigens, or RNA (see the "Acute Viral Hepatitis" algorithm) (▶ Figure 4.18). In addition to viral hepatitis, other factors that lead to hepatocellular damage include alcohol and other toxins, medications, deposition diseases such as Wilson's disease and hemochromatosis, an alpha-1 antitrypsin deficiency, or autoimmune hepatitis. Evidence of alcohol-related hepatitis or medicine/toxin-induced liver damage are best gleaned from the medical history, and in the case of alcohol abuse also from the physical examination. Paracetamol-induced severe hepatocellular injury is detected by measuring the serum paracetamol levels. In Wilson's disease, the ceruloplasmin and copper concentrations found in serum/plasma are lowered, while urinary copper excretion is increased. The serum ferritin and transferrin saturation are significantly increased in hemochromatosis. A mutation in the HFE gene can be detected by PCR and melting curve analysis. The extent of iron deposition in the liver and its impact on the liver microarchitecture can be assessed through a liver biopsy and a corresponding histology work-up (Fletcher, 2003).

The presence of autoimmune hepatitis can be detected by measurement of antinuclear antibodies (ANA), LKM 2 antibodies, and antibodies against actin, LC1, and SLA.

Evidence of an alpha-1 antitrypsin deficiency could already be evident from the medical history (lung involvement). The lack of an alpha-1 band in the serum electrophoresis as well as quantitative measurement of the serum/plasma alpha-1 antitrypsin concentration will provide final confirmation of an alpha-1 antitrypsin deficiency (Fregonese, 2008).

Cholestatic diseases

If alkaline phosphatase and gamma-GT activity is significantly elevated in the basic laboratory diagnostics, and moreover the direct bilirubin concentration is >15 % of total bilirubin and the of transaminase activity is not particularly pronounced relative to the AP and gamma-GT values, a cholestatic liver disease is present (Geier, 2003; Heathcote, 2007). An ultrasound and/or MRCP will help to recognize whether the bile ducts are obstructed and extrahepatic cholestasis is present. If no stones are detected, the cholestasis might be due to a malignant tumor, e.g., papillary or pancreatic head carcinoma. If not bile duct obstruction is evident in the ultrasound or MRCP, an intrahepatic cholestasis could be present. Intrahepatic cholestasis can be due to liver metastases (sonographically detectable), primary biliary cirrhosis (PBC), primary sclerosing cholangitis (PSC), various medications such as steroids, Budd-Chiari syndrome (also sonographically detectable), or a pregnancy. Primary biliary cirrhosis can be recognized if antimitochondrial antibodies (AMA, and AMA-M2, M4, M9) are detected (Leuschner, 2003). In this case, indirect immunofluorescence will provide evidence of antinuclear antibodies (ANA), wherein nuclear dots will show up positive. Antibodies to centromeres and pANCA will be detectable in primary sclerosing cholangitis. With a suspicion of drug-induced intrahepatic cholestasis, a detailed medication history should be taken, with a liver biopsy conducted if necessary, which could likewise be indicated for suspected PBC and PSC.

Mixed hepatocellular/cholestatic diseases (Figure 4.17)

If the activity of both the cholestasis-indicating enzymes AP and γ-GT is increased, as well as in the enzymes that indicate hepatocellular injury (AST/ALT), and moreover the total bilirubin and direct bilirubin are elevated, a mixed hepatocellular/cholestatic disease is present. This pattern of mixed hepatocellular and cholestatic laboratory parameters can originate from cholestatic hepatitis, infection with EBV, CMV, Brucella, Leptospira, various parasites such as malaria, schistosomiasis, echinococcus, and also from alcoholic hepatitis, cirrhosis of the liver, or HELLP syndrome during pregnancy.

In pregnant women with symptoms of pre-eclampsia (edema, elevated blood pressure) or eclampsia (tonic-clonic seizures), and corresponding changes in the liver function tests in addition to increased creatinine, proteinuria, and decreases in the haptoglobin concentration and platelet count, HELLP syndrome must be considered (Hay 2008). Patients with the mixed hepatocellular/cholestatic pattern of liver function test results, who additionally have decreased albumin and pseudocholinesterase activity, most likely have cirrhosis. For clarification, *inter alia*, ultrasound and possibly liver biopsy should be ordered. In cholestatic hepatitis, abnormalities in the virus serology are present, i.e., hepatitis IgM antibodies, HCV RNA, or HBsAg would be detectable in such patients. A case in which the Quick value drops significantly during the course of proven viral hepatitis, while the serum bilirubin concentration increases and the ammonia rises to within the pathological range, could signal fulminant viral hepatitis.

Impaired liver synthesis capacity

If neither the enzymes that signal hepatocellular damage nor those that signal cholestasis are not particularly increased in the basic laboratory diagnostics, but the prothrombin time is reduced, this indicate the presence of a chronic liver disease with synthesis impairment. In these patients, the reduction in the serum albumin concentration and the lowering of serum/plasma pseudocholinesterase activity as well as indications from the physical examination suggest liver cirrhosis. With proven cirrhosis, the patient's prognosis should be assessed by determining the Child-Pugh score. If the etiology of the cirrhosis is uncertain, this might be clarified through a liver biopsy and histology work-up.

4.3.1.1 Non-Alcoholic Fatty Liver Disease (NAFLD)

A special case of hepatobiliary disease is a metabolic syndrome with non-alcoholic fatty liver disease (NAFLD) (Barshop, 2009; Erickson, 2009; Loomba, 2009). These patients (sometimes even children) exhibit a persistent increase in the AST/ALT and γ-GT activity by three to five times the upper reference range value. Additionally present are obesity, increased of serum/plasma triglyceride concentrations, decreased HDL cholesterol, and often an increase in HbA1c. In patients with this constellation of findings, the other causes of hepatobiliary disease should be ruled out, and liver biopsy should be considered for further clarification.

4.3.1.2 Acute Viral Hepatitis (Figure 4.18)

Acute viral hepatitis is triggered either through one of the five hepatitis virus (HAV, HBV, HCV, HDV, and HEV) or by other viruses such as cytomegalovirus (CMV), Epstein-Barr virus (EBV), herpes simplex virus (HSV) or Varicella viruses (VZV). Although these viruses cause systemic infections, they mainly damage the liver. The clinical picture of acute viral hepatitis is often an acute disease with pain in the right upper abdomen accompanied by nausea and loss of appetite; occasionally fever and/or jaundice can be present. Hepatitis virus infections can also be inapparent (asymptomatic), and not until later be diagnosed from laboratory test abnormalities.

Indications of liver disease in terms of acute viral hepatitis can be obtained from a targeted medical history, an accurate physical examination, abnormalities in the ultrasound examination, and a few specific laboratory tests.

Medical history items: Particularly relevant items when taking the medical history include symptoms of liver disease, such as fatigue, nausea, loss of appetite, colored stool or urine, and pain in the right upper abdomen. Other important questions to ask are whether pruritus is present, what medications and/or drugs are being taken,

Clinical picture: acute disease picture with pain in the right upper abdomen, fatigue, nausea,

Medical history items: Fatigue? Nausea? Fever? Loss of appetite? Pruritus? Alcohol? Medications? Drugs? Colored stool or urine? Contact with people having jaundice? Time spent abroad? Sexual history? Exposure to blood? Needlestick injury? Pains in the right upper abdomen?

Examination items: Liver size? Jaundice? Pain on pressure? Resistance? Muscular defense? Bowel sounds? Signs of alcohol abuse? Tremors?

Presumptive diagnosis Acute Viral Hepatitis

Basic laboratory diagnostics

Electrolytes, urea, creatinine, glucose, total bilirubin, ALT, AST, AP, γ-GT PT (Quick value), blood count + differential, urinalysis + bilirubin + UBG

AST & ALT elevated disproportionally to AP & γ-GT, total bilirubin elevated, dark urine

| Yes

Hepatocellular disease

Expanded laboratory

GLDH, direct bilirubin Serum electrophoresis Albumin, PCHE

De Ritis ratio > 1 and GLDH ↑↑

Yes / No

Severe hepatocellular damage / Mild hepatocellular damage

Differential diagnosis

Viral hepatitis (A, B, C, D or E)

Further procedures Specialized laboratory diagnostics

| Anti-HAV IgM and IgG pos. | HBsAg pos. Anti-HBc IgM and IgG pos. | Exacerbation of chronic HBV infection | Anti-HCV pos. | Anti-HEV IgM pos. and HEV-RNA pos. |

Virus serology: anti-HAV-IgM, HBsAG, anti-HBc-IgM, anti-HCV, HCV-RNA, anti-HDV, HDV-RNA, anti-HEV, HEV-RNA

Yes / Yes

| **Acute hepatitis A** | **Acute hepatitis B *1** | Anti-HDV pos. HDV-RNA pos. | HCV RNA Detection pos. | **Acute hepatitis E** |

Yes / Yes

If no hepatitis virus detected, rule out acute CMV, EBV, HSV and VZV infection

Anti-HDV pos. HDV-RNA pos.

Acute HDV superinfection *1 | **Acute hepatitis C *2**

Yes

Simultaneous infection with HBV and HDV | Recheck in 4–6 weeks • HBsAg • Anti-HBc

Loss of appetite, possible fever, possible jaundice

Ultrasound items: Liver size? Structure, texture?
Focal lesions? Cirrhosis? Cholestasis?
Ascites? Mass lesion?
Vascular disorders?

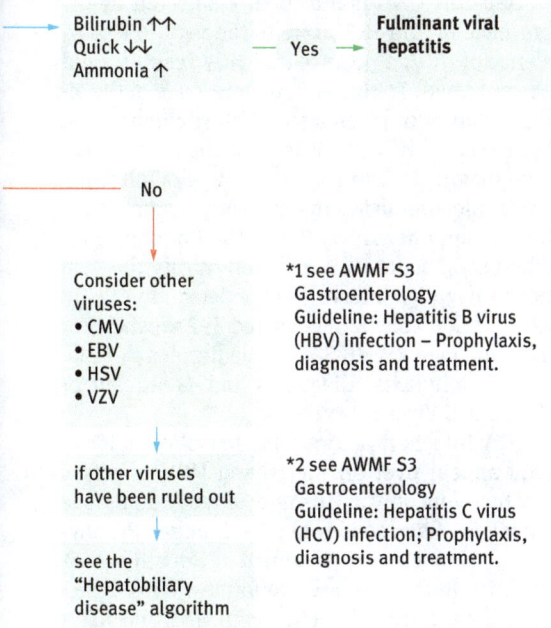

Bilirubin ↑↑
Quick ↓↓   — Yes →   **Fulminant viral
Ammonia ↑   hepatitis**

——————— No

Consider other   *1 see AWMF S3
viruses: Gastroenterology
• CMV   Guideline: Hepatitis B virus
• EBV   (HBV) infection – Prophylaxis,
• HSV   diagnosis and treatment.
• VZV

if other viruses   *2 see AWMF S3
have been ruled out   Gastroenterology
                         Guideline: Hepatitis C virus
                         (HCV) infection; Prophylaxis,
see the   diagnosis and treatment.
"Hepatobiliary
disease" algorithm

Figure 4.18 Acute viral hepatitis. Clinical picture:
acute disease picture with pain in the right upper
abdomen, fatigue, nausea, loss of appetite, possibly
fever, possibly jaundice.

how much alcohol is consumed, whether there has been any contact with persons who have hepatitis or jaundice, whether the patient has been abroad recently, for information on the patient's common sexual practices; particularly important for medical staff is the question of possible exposure to human blood, such as a needlestick injury.

Physical examination items: The physical examination should clarify if a generalized jaundice or scleral icterus is present, if the abdomen is painful to pressure, if resistance can be palpated and muscular guarding is present, if bowel sounds are present, and if any signs of alcohol abuse and chronic liver damage (collateral circulation, gynecomastia, any absence of secondary hair, ascites) are present.

Ultrasound items: The primary points of interest from ultrasound are the size, structure, and texture of the liver. Is there evidence of cirrhosis, cholestasis, ascites, mass lesions, or vascular disorders? Are vascular lesions present in the liver?

Laboratory Diagnostics items: Basic laboratory diagnostics includes the following determinations: Electrolytes, urea, creatinine, glucose, total serum/plasma bilirubin concentration, enzyme activities: ALT, AST, AP and γ-GT; PT (Quick value), blood count with differential count, and urinalysis. If a disproportionate increase in AST and ALT activity is observed as compared to AP and γ-GT, together with an increase in the total bilirubin and dark urine, hepatocellular disease is present. In this case, the laboratory diagnostics should be expanded, and the severity of hepatocellular damage evaluated by determining the GLDH and pseudocholinesterase (PCHE) activity along with the De-Ritis quotient. The transaminase levels correlate only moderately with the extent of hepatocellular damage. In addition, the bilirubin fractions should be determined by measurement of the direct serum bilirubin, a serum electrophoresis should be carried out, and the serum/plasma albumin concentration measured. A De-Ritis ratio > 1 with a significantly elevated GLDH indicates severe hepatocellular injury.

Differential diagnosis items: The most common origin of hepatocellular injury is viral hepatitis, followed by drug-induced liver damage, cholangitis, and alcoholic steatohepatitis.

If the non-viral diseases that cause hepatocellular damage are ruled out, the various hepatitis viruses are primarily detected by the presence of specific antibodies (Chevaliez, 2008; Chevaliez, 2009; Pawlotzky, 2007). Hepatitis A infection (incubation time: approx. 4 weeks) is detected by the presence of anti-hepatitis A virus IgM (Anti-HAV IgM). The IgM antibodies can persist in the circulation for several months. During convalescence, the anti-hepatitis A virus antibodies are predominantly of the IgG class. The excretion of HAV in the stool can be found only at the beginning of the icteric phase of the disease.

Acute hepatitis B is detected from HBsAg and the presence of anti-HBc IgM antibodies. In contrast to the other hepatitis viruses, hepatitis B virus is a DNA Virus. Antibodies are formed against HBsAg (anti-HBs), against the HBc antigen (anti-HBc), and against the HBe antigen (anti-HBe). In chronic hepatitis B, HBsAg, HBcAg, anti-HBc, and HBV/DNA can be detected in the serum. In cases of confirmed acute hepatitis B, a recheck for HBsAg and anti-HBc should be done 4–6 weeks later (see AWMF S3 Gastroenterology Guideline: Prophylaxis, Diagnosis and Course of Hepatitis B Virus Infection).

Hepatitis C virus infection is detected by the presence of anti-HCV. Due to the very low prevalence of HCV, a positive anti-HCV result should be confirmed. To this end, the presence of the virus in serum or plasma should be demonstrated by means of HCV RNA amplification. Since the "serodiagnostic window" is 7–8 weeks following acute infection using the currently available anti-HCV immunoassays, the method of choice for diagnosing acute HCV infection during the "antibody-negative interval" is the detection of HCV RNA, which can be recognized 1–2 weeks after infection (see AWMF S3 Gastroenterology Guideline: Prophylaxis, Diagnosis and Treatment of Hepatitis C Virus Infection).

HDV infection cannot occur in isolation, it can only appear over an underlying HBV infection and therefore only in HBsAg-positive patients (see AWMF S3 Gastroenterology Guideline: Prophylaxis, Diagnosis and Treatment of Hepatitis B Virus Infection). There are two forms of HDV infection: simultaneous infection with HBV and HDV, and an HDV superinfection over a chronic HBV infection. Evidence of acute or extant HBV infection is obtained by from an anti-HDV antibody determination as a screening test case. With a positive anti-HDV result, the blood (serum/plasma) HDV RNA should be determined. HDV RNA quantification can be use in monitoring therapy. Chronic HDV infection is characterized by the persistence of HDV RNA for at least 6 months.

Hepatitis E is a zoonotic disease, which is very rare in non-endemic areas such as the USA and Germany (prevalence < 2%). The transmission of hepatitis E (fecal/oral) is similar to that of hepatitis A.

A viral hepatitis complication that causes concern is the development of fulminant liver failure, which most commonly occurs in hepatitis B and D, as well as hepatitis E. The development of fulminant liver failure is rare with hepatitis A and C. Acute liver failure occurs in hepatitis E in a total of about 2% of patients, and in up to 20% of cases in pregnant women during their last trimester. The fulminant liver failure is also found with severe paracetamol poisoning, in pregnancy (the HELLP syndrome), and concomitant to vascular damage. Clinical signs include the development of hepatic encephalopathy to hepatic coma, a rapidly decreasing Quick value (PT), and increasing serum bilirubin concentrations (Heneghan, 2003). The lethality of fulminant hepatic failure following viral hepatitis is extremely high at 80%.

If none of the hepatitis viruses A–E are detected in the special laboratory diagnostics and virus serology, other viruses such as CMV, EBV, HSV, and VZV should be considered (Crum, 2006). If likewise none of these are detected, another cause of the hepatobiliary disease must be considered (see the "Hepatobiliary disease" algorithm) (▶ Figure 4.17).

4.3.1.3 Jaundice (Figure 4.19)

Jaundice or icterus refers to a yellowish discoloration of the skin and sclera as a result of bilirubin deposition due to an increase in the serum bilirubin concentration (Roche, 2004). Scleral icterus occurs when the serum bilirubin concentration is at least 3 mg/dL (51 mol/L). Higher serum bilirubin concentrations eventually lead to a yellowish discoloration of the skin, which changes to a greenish color as the bilirubin undergoes oxidation. Jaundice can occur with or without pain symptoms. Frequently the urine and stool are also markedly colored. If conjugated bilirubin is excreted via the kidneys, the urine will have a beer brown to cola color. Somewhat pale stools

indicates cholestasis as the cause of the hyperbilirubinemia.

Medical history items: Important information can be obtained from the medical history regarding the origin or a differential diagnosis of a jaundice case. The patient should be questioned in detail with regard to ingested medications, drugs, alcohol, and exposure to chemicals. Additionally, the patient should be questioned about any transfusions, tattoos, and sexual behaviors. With regard to extant hepatitis, important factors include a travel history, contact with patients who have jaundice and the duration of that jaundice, along with the presence of accompanying symptoms such as fever, pruritus, changes in the urine and/or stool, arthralgias, weight loss, abdominal pain and exanthem. Sudden pain in right upper abdomen followed by jaundice gives an indication of choledocholithiasis. Moreover, the presence of chills raises the possibility of ascending cholangitis.

Physical examination items: Signs such as spider naevi, palmar erythema, conspicuous secondary hair, gynecomastia, liver size, tenderness, collateral circulation, and inflow congestion indicate a chronic liver disease. A right-side pleural effusion can be observed in advanced liver cirrhosis. Ascites is also expected in such a case. On examination of the abdomen, of particular interest is the size and consistency of the liver, the size of the spleen, and the presence of ascites.

Ultrasound items: In the ultrasound as well, particular attention should be given to the liver size, structure and texture, the presence of gallstones or obstruction in the sense of cholestasis, the presence of ascites, evidence of cirrhosis, and the presence of a mass lesion in the region of liver, hepatic portal, or pancreatic head.

Laboratory Diagnostics items: The basic laboratory diagnostics involves determining the electrolytes, glucose, creatinine, total bilirubin, ALT, AST, AP, the basic coagulation parameters: Quick value (PT) and the PTT; blood count and differential, reticulocyte count, and the urinalysis. Of particular interest in the urinalysis are the bilirubin and urobilinogen findings. If only the total bilirubin is increased, and the AST/ALT, AP and PT are all within their reference ranges, this points

Clinical picture: Jaundice

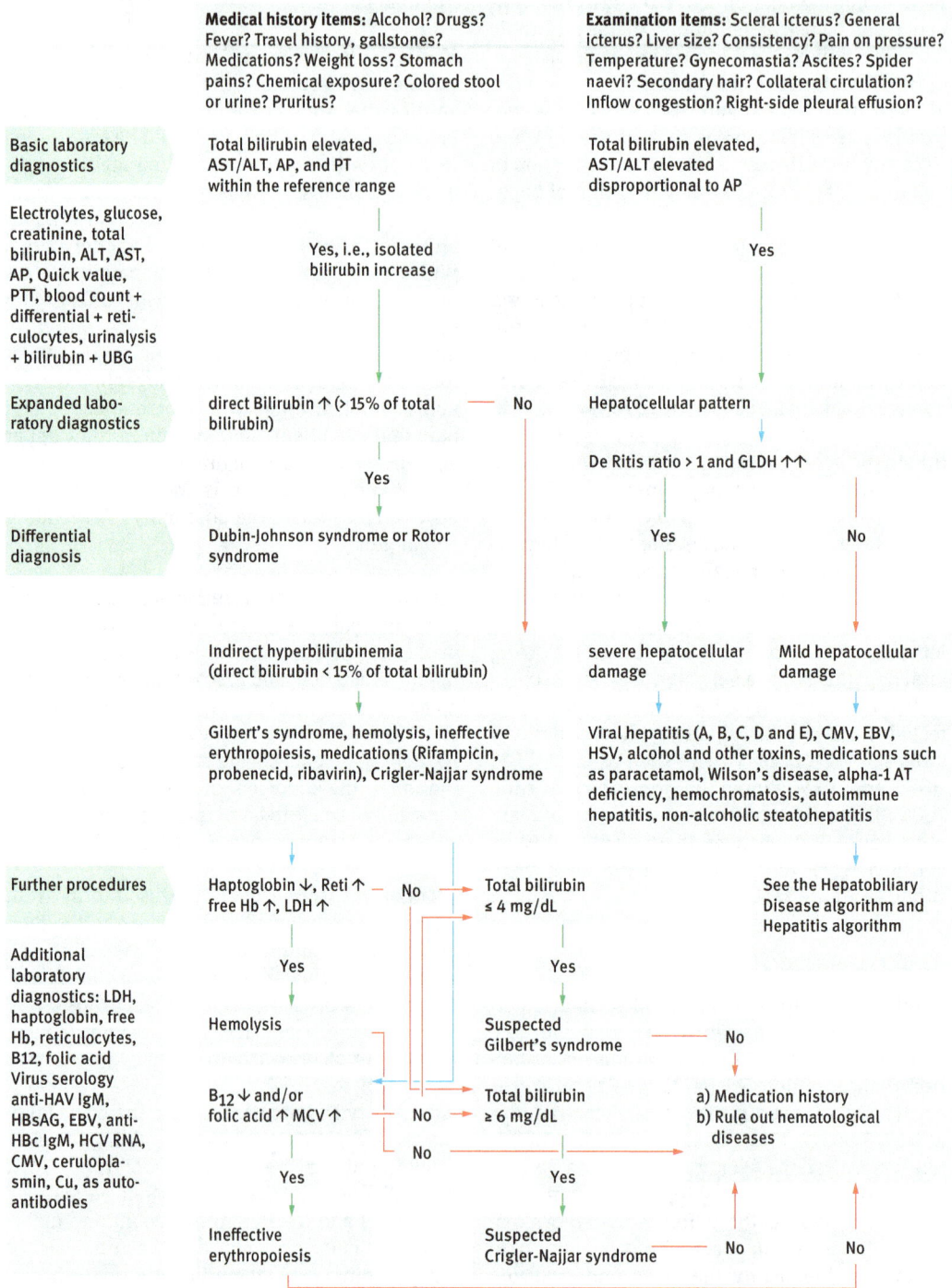

Medical history items: Alcohol? Drugs? Fever? Travel history, gallstones? Medications? Weight loss? Stomach pains? Chemical exposure? Colored stool or urine? Pruritus?

Examination items: Scleral icterus? General icterus? Liver size? Consistency? Pain on pressure? Temperature? Gynecomastia? Ascites? Spider naevi? Secondary hair? Collateral circulation? Inflow congestion? Right-side pleural effusion?

Basic laboratory diagnostics

Electrolytes, glucose, creatinine, total bilirubin, ALT, AST, AP, Quick value, PTT, blood count + differential + reticulocytes, urinalysis + bilirubin + UBG

Total bilirubin elevated, AST/ALT, AP, and PT within the reference range

Total bilirubin elevated, AST/ALT elevated disproportional to AP

Yes, i.e., isolated bilirubin increase

Yes

Expanded laboratory diagnostics

direct Bilirubin ↑ (> 15% of total bilirubin) — No

Hepatocellular pattern

De Ritis ratio > 1 and GLDH ↑↑

Yes

Differential diagnosis

Dubin-Johnson syndrome or Rotor syndrome

Yes   No

Indirect hyperbilirubinemia (direct bilirubin < 15% of total bilirubin)

severe hepatocellular damage

Mild hepatocellular damage

Gilbert's syndrome, hemolysis, ineffective erythropoiesis, medications (Rifampicin, probenecid, ribavirin), Crigler-Najjar syndrome

Viral hepatitis (A, B, C, D and E), CMV, EBV, HSV, alcohol and other toxins, medications such as paracetamol, Wilson's disease, alpha-1 AT deficiency, hemochromatosis, autoimmune hepatitis, non-alcoholic steatohepatitis

Further procedures

Additional laboratory diagnostics: LDH, haptoglobin, free Hb, reticulocytes, B12, folic acid Virus serology anti-HAV IgM, HBsAG, EBV, anti-HBc IgM, HCV RNA, CMV, ceruloplasmin, Cu, as auto-antibodies

Haptoglobin ↓, Reti ↑ free Hb ↑, LDH ↑ — No → Total bilirubin ≤ 4 mg/dL

See the Hepatobiliary Disease algorithm and Hepatitis algorithm

Yes

Hemolysis

Yes

Suspected Gilbert's syndrome — No

B12 ↓ and/or folic acid ↑ MCV ↑ — No

Total bilirubin ≥ 6 mg/dL

No

a) Medication history
b) Rule out hematological diseases

Yes

Yes

Ineffective erythropoiesis

Suspected Crigler-Najjar syndrome — No   No

Figure 4.19 Clinical picture: Jaundice.

Ultrasound items: Liver size? Structure,
texture? Cirrhosis? Gallstones? Cholestasis?
Intracanalicular/extracanalicular? Ascites?
Vascular disorders?

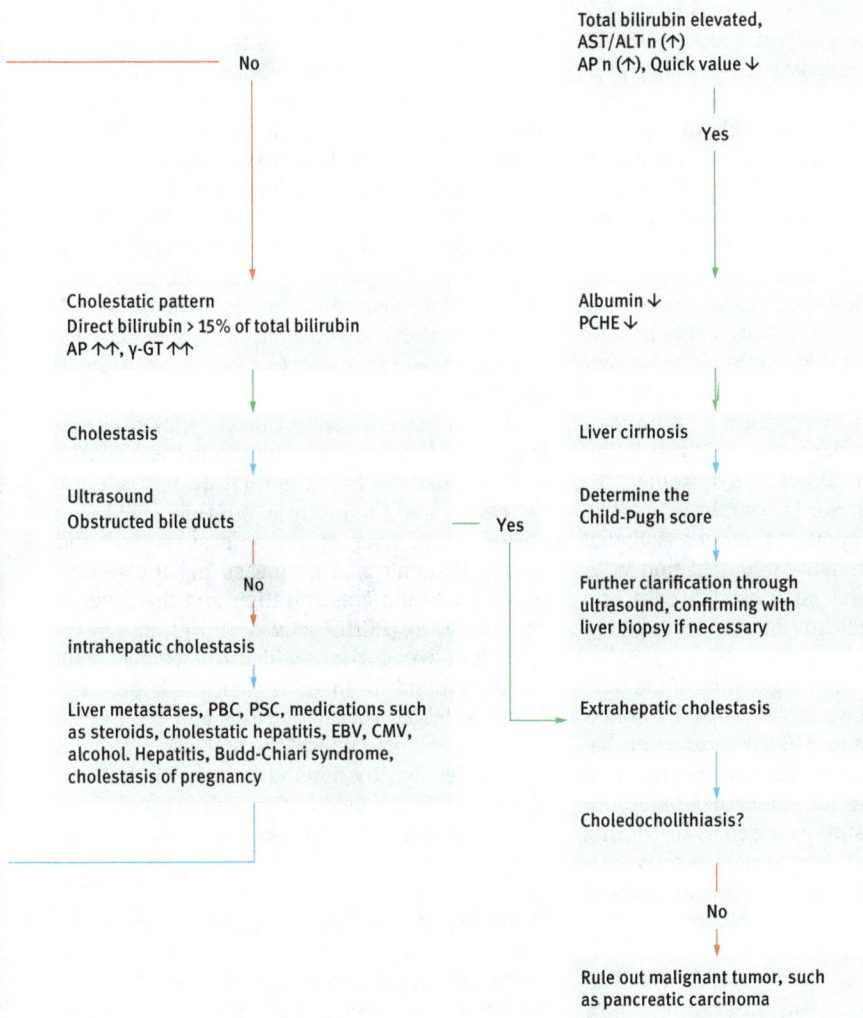

Total bilirubin elevated,
AST/ALT n (↑)
AP n (↑), Quick value ↓

No

Yes

Cholestatic pattern
Direct bilirubin > 15% of total bilirubin
AP ↑↑, γ-GT ↑↑

Albumin ↓
PCHE ↓

Cholestasis

Liver cirrhosis

Ultrasound
Obstructed bile ducts

Yes

Determine the
Child-Pugh score

No

Further clarification through
ultrasound, confirming with
liver biopsy if necessary

intrahepatic cholestasis

Liver metastases, PBC, PSC, medications such
as steroids, cholestatic hepatitis, EBV, CMV,
alcohol. Hepatitis, Budd-Chiari syndrome,
cholestasis of pregnancy

Extrahepatic cholestasis

Choledocholithiasis?

No

Rule out malignant tumor, such
as pancreatic carcinoma

to an isolated bilirubin increase. In this case, the direct bilirubin should also be measured, and if it is above 15 % of the total bilirubin, Dubin-Johnson syndrome or Rotor syndrome should be considered. A direct bilirubin value that is less than 15 % of the total bilirubin points to an indirect hyperbilirubinemia, which could be caused by the following diseases: Gilbert's syndrome, hemolysis, ineffective erythropoiesis, drug-induced hyperbilirubinemia, and Crigler-Najjar syndrome. In this case, the first step is to measure the serum/plasma haptoglobin concentration, reticulocyte count, free hemoglobin, and LDH activity. A lowered haptoglobin concentration and increased free hemoglobin and LDH points to acute hemolysis. If in addition the reticulocyte count is increased, this means that the hemolysis has already been present for a certain time. The hemolysis parameters being normal and a total bilirubin value < 4 mg/dL raises a suspicion of Gilbert's syndrome. The hemolysis parameters being normal and a total bilirubin value > 6 mg/dL points to Crigler-Najjar syndrome. If neither Gilbert's syndrome, Crigler-Najjar syndrome, nor is hemolysis present, and ineffective erythropoiesis has been excluded by measuring the vitamin B_{12}, folic acid, and MCV, this rules out another hematological disease, and an even more detailed drug history must be obtained.

In the basic laboratory diagnostics, if the total bilirubin is increased while AST and ALT are increased in proportion to AP, this presents a hepatocellular pattern of pathological liver function test results. In this case, the extent of hepatocellular damage should first be assessed by measuring the GLDH activity and determining the De Ritis ratio. Significantly increased GLDH activity and a De Ritis ratio > 1 points to severe hepatocellular damage. If the De Ritis ratio < 1 and the GLDH is only slightly increased, the hepatocellular damage is milder. There are many possible origins of the hepatocyte damage, including viral hepatitis (A, B, C, D, E, CMV, EBV, or HSV), alcohol and other toxins, drugs such as paracetamol, deposition diseases such as Wilson's disease and hemochromatosis, an alpha-1 antitrypsin deficiency, autoimmune hepatitis, and non-alcoholic steatohepatitis.

A cholestatic pattern is present in the liver-specific laboratory diagnostic assessment when the total bilirubin is elevated while the AST and ALT are not increased disproportionately compared to

AP. In such a case, the direct bilirubin would be > 15 % of total bilirubin, and the AP and γ-GT would also be significantly increased. A presumptive diagnosis of "cholestasis" made from this pattern of findings should be further differentiated through ultrasound. Extrahepatic cholestasis is characterized by obstructed bile ducts. Intrahepatic cholestasis can occur in the following diseases: liver metastases, primary biliary cirrhosis (PBC), primary sclerosing cholangitis (PSC), cholestasis-inducing drugs such as steroids, cholestatic hepatitis, alcoholic hepatitis, Budd-Chiari syndrome, and cholestasis of pregnancy. The differential diagnosis of these diseases is shown in the algorithms for "Hepatobiliary diseases" (▶ Figure 4.17) and "Hepatitis" (▶ Figure 4.18). In extrahepatic cholestasis, ultrasound should be used to clarify whether choledocholithiasis or cholestasis due to a malignant tumor (e.g., a pancreatic head carcinoma) is responsible.

If, in the basis laboratory diagnostics, a pattern is found of increased total bilirubin, the AST/ALT and AP enzymes being normal or only slightly increased, and the prothrombin time (PT) being pathological, liver cirrhosis is suspected and should be confirmed by measuring the serum/plasma albumin concentration and the pseudocholinesterase (PCHE) activity. A presumptive diagnosis of liver cirrhosis will also be evident from the ultrasound findings. If cirrhosis is detected from the laboratory diagnostics and ultrasound findings presented above, the patient's prognosis can be decided by determining the Child-Pugh score, and if the origin of the cirrhosis is unclear, further diagnostics would possibly include a liver biopsy.

Summary: As has been shown in the foregoing, the origin of a patient's jaundice can be discovered through the use of appropriate laboratory parameters, a targeted medical history, physical examination, and ultrasound (Roche, 2004). The first step is to find out whether an isolated hyperbilirubinemia is present, and if so, whether the conjugated or unconjugated fraction is increased. If no isolated bilirubin increase is present, clarification is needed whether abnormalities are present in other liver enzyme value, and whether the pattern is points more toward a hepatocellular or a cholestatic disease. With a cholestatic pattern, the next question is whether that cholestasis is intra- or extrahepatic. In addition to the bilirubin, if the liver synthesis parameters in particular are pathological, and ultrasound provides appropriate indication, cirrhosis must be considered.

Literature

AWMF, S3 Leitlinie Gastroenterologie: Hepatitis B-Virusinfektion – Prophylaxe, Diagnostik und Therapie. http://www.awmf.org/en/clinical-practice-guidelines/detail/ll/021-011.html

AWMF, S3 Leitlinie Gastroenterologie: Hepatitis C-Virus (HCV)-Infektion; Prophylaxe, Diagnostik und Therapie. http://www.awmf.org/en/clinical-practice-guidelines/detail/ll/021-012.html

Barshop NJ, Francis CS, Schwimmer JB, Lavine JE. Nonalcoholic fatty liver disease as a comorbidity of childhood obesity. Ped Health 2009; 3: 271–281.

Bjornsson E. The natural history of drug-induced liver injury. Semin Liver Dis 2009; 29: 357–63. Review.

Chevaliez S, Pawlotsky JM. Diagnosis and management of chronic viral hepatitis: antigens, antibodies and viral genomes. Best Pract Res Clin Gastroenterol. 2008; 22: 1031–48. Review.

Chevaliez S, Pawlotsky JM. Virological techniques for the diagnosis and monitoring of hepatitis B and C. Ann Hepatol. 2009; 8: 7–12. Review.

Crum NF. Epstein Barr virus hepatitis: case series and review. South Med J 2006; 99: 544–7. Review.

Erickson SK. Nonalcoholic fatty liver disease. J Lipid Res 2009; 50 Suppl: S412–6. Review.

Floreani A. Liver disorders in the elderly. Best Pract Res Clin Gastroenterol 2009; 23: 909–17. Review.

Fletcher LM, Powell LW. Hemochromatosis and alcoholic liver disease. Alcohol 2003; 30: 131–6. Review.

Fregonese L, Stolk J. Hereditary alpha-1-antitrypsin deficiency and its clinical consequences. Orphanet J Rare Dis 2008; 3: 16. Review.

Geier A, Gartung C, Dietrich CG, Lammert F, Wasmuth HE, Matern S. Diagnosis of cholestatic disorders. Med Klin (Munich) 2003; 98: 499–509. Review. German.

Hay JE. Liver disease in pregnancy. Hepatology 2008; 47: 1067–76. Review.

Heathcote EJ. Diagnosis and management of cholestatic liver disease. Clin Gastroenterol Hepatol 2007; 5: 776–82. Review.

Heneghan MA, Lara LL. Fulminant hepatic failure. Semin Gastrointest Dis 2003; 14: 87–100. Review.

Leuschner U. Primary biliary cirrhosis-presentation and diagnosis. Clin Liver Dis 2003; 7: 741–58. Review.

Loomba R, Sirlin CB, Schwimmer JB, Lavine JE. Advances in pediatric nonalcoholic fatty liver disease. Hepatology 2009; 50: 1282–93. Review.

Pawlotsky JM, Dusheiko G, Hatzakis A, Lau D, Lau G, Liang TJ, Locarnini S, Martin P, Richman DD,

Zoulim F. Virologic monitoring of hepatitis B virus therapy in clinical trials and practice: recommendations for a standardized approach. Gastroenterology. 2008; 134: 05–15. Review.

Roche SP, Kobos R. Jaundice in the adult patient. Am Fam Physician 2004; 69: 299–304. Review.

4.3.2 Pancreatic Diseases

4.3.2.1 Acute Pancreatitis (Figure 4.20)

The cardinal symptoms of acute pancreatitis (AP) are radiating, persistent epigastric pain, often radiating to the back, but can also project into the thorax, abdomen, and on both sides (Whitcomb, 2006). Since being supine intensifies the pain, patients are eager to sit. In this way, they bend the torso and draw up the knees. Nausea, vomiting and bloating can also occur.

Medical history items: The patient should be asked about the nature and duration of the pain while the medical history is being taken. Since gallstones (40–50 %) and alcohol (30–40 %) are the main causes of acute pancreatitis (Khan, 2010; Perez-Mateo, 2006), the patient should be asked about the presence of gallstones and whether alcohol is consumed regularly. Since acute pancreatitis can also be triggered by many drugs (furosemide, thiazides, tetracyclines, valproate, CSA), a detailed drug history should be taken (Khan, 2010). In addition, the patient should be asked about any recent viral infections, whether pancreatitis is prevalent in the family (indication for hereditary pancreatitis), and whether any autoimmune disorders are known (vasculitis, autoimmune pancreatitis).

Physical examination items: Low-grade fever, tachycardia, and hypotension are frequently observed during the physical examination of patients with acute pancreatitis. If jaundice is present, this can be due to:
- A gallstone located in the bile duct, or;
- Compression of the distal bile duct due to an edematous swelling of the pancreatic head.

A basal rale and a predominantly left-sided pleural effusion suggest pulmonary involvement. The abdominal wall will be stretched significantly due to the intense pain. Bowel sounds will be reduced or completely absent (paralytic ileus). In severe (necrotizing) pancreatitis, discoloration is occa-

Clinical picture: acute pain in the middle-left upper abdomen

Medical history items: Type and duration of pain? Alcohol? Gallstones? Medications? Infections (HIV, mumps)? Family medical history *1

Examination items: RR/pulse? Lung auscultation, temperature? Jaundice? Pain on pressure? Muscular defense? Bowel sounds?

Presumptive diagnosis

Acute Pancreatitis

Rule out myocardial infarction (ECG and laboratory) (see also diagram for "Acute abdomen")

Laboratory

Electrolytes, glucose, CRP, blood count, creatinine, ALT, AST, urinalysis, lipase (p-amylase)

Lipase (serum/plasma p-amylase) > 3 time the upper reference range value within 48–72 h after pain begins

No ——— Troponin I or (T)

No | Yes | Elevated

Diagnosis

No acute pancreatitis | **Acute Pancreatitis** | **Acute coronary syndrome**

Discrimination

Mild pancreatitis versus severe pancreatitis

Criteria for assessing degree of severity in pancreatitis

CRP > 150 mg/L | Leukocytes > 15.0×10^9/L | Creatinine > 170 µmol/L
pO_2 < 60 mmHg | Calcium < 2.0 mmol/L | Albumin < 32 g/L
LDH > 600 U/L | AST/ALT > 100 U/L | Glucose > 300 mg/dL
Age > 55 yrs | BMI > 30 kg/m^2 | Hematocrit > 0.44 L/L

Differentiation

Biliary/non-biliary pancreatitis

Each criterion met contributes one point.

Expanded laboratory

Calcium, PT, PTT, LDH, bilirubin, blood gas analysis (pO_2), albumin, AP, γ-GT

< 4 points | ≥ 4 points

Diagnosis

Mild pancreatitis | **Severe pancreatitis**

Further procedures

Frequent clinical and medical laboratory testing

Daily monitoring of CRP, calcium and leukocytes until pain is gone

Daily clinical and laboratory monitoring of CRP, Ca, leukocytes, pO_2, glucose and creatinine.

Drops in CRP and leukocytes within the reference ranges ——— No

Normalization of the laboratory values, clinical improvement

Yes

New increases in CRP and/ or leukocytes and/or LDH

Yes

Mild pancreatitis with an uncomplicated course

Development of severe pancreatitis

Sterile necrosis Severe pancreatitis with an uncomplicated course

Confirm with ultrasound, possibly CT or MRI

Ultrasound items: Gallstones? Cholestasis? Fluidity? Pancreatic edema?
Ascites? Mass lesion?

*1 With a remarkable family medical
history, molecular genetic clarification
of hereditary pancreatitis
(trypsin mutation, SPINK mutation,
CFTR mutation)

*2 With CRP < 81 mg/L and leukocytes
< 13×10^9/L, infected necrosis is
unlikely

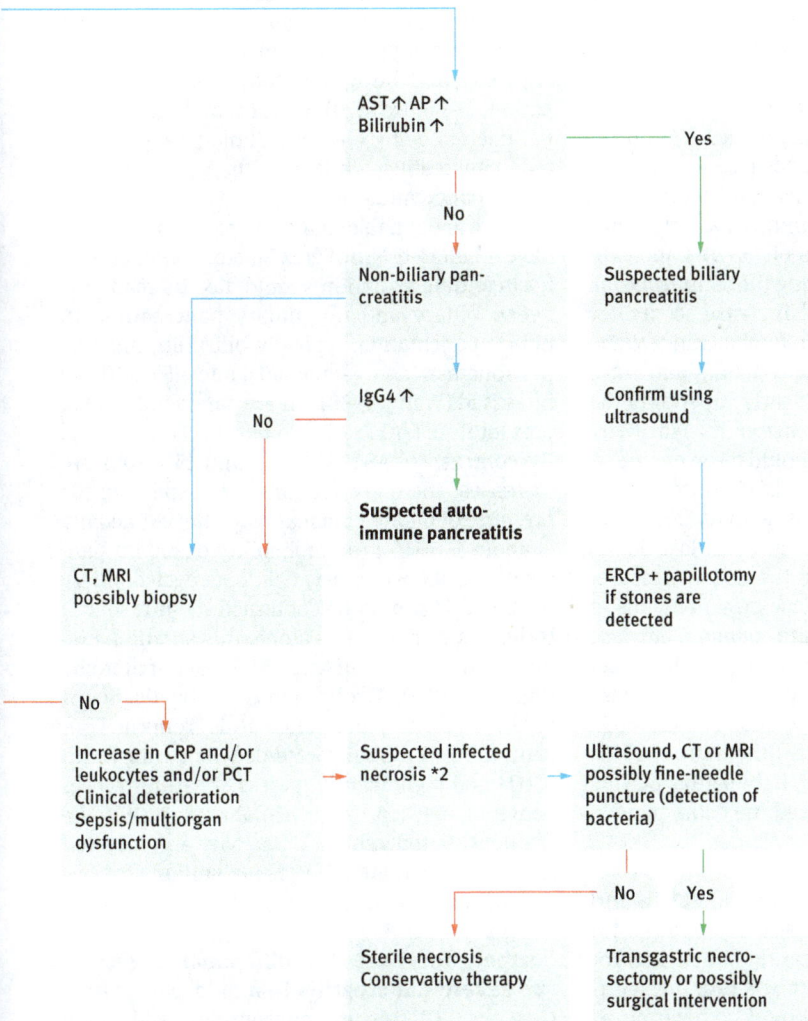

AST ↑ AP ↑
Bilirubin ↑

Yes

No

Non-biliary pan-
creatitis

Suspected biliary
pancreatitis

IgG4 ↑

No

Confirm using
ultrasound

**Suspected auto-
immune pancreatitis**

CT, MRI
possibly biopsy

ERCP + papillotomy
if stones are
detected

No

Increase in CRP and/or
leukocytes and/or PCT
Clinical deterioration
Sepsis/multiorgan
dysfunction

Suspected infected
necrosis *2

Ultrasound, CT or MRI
possibly fine-needle
puncture (detection of
bacteria)

No   Yes

Sterile necrosis
Conservative therapy

Transgastric necro-
sectomy or possibly
surgical intervention

Figure 4.20 Acute Pancreatitis. Clinical picture:
acute middle-left upper
abdominal pain.

sionally observed in the periumbilical or flank region (Cullen's sign, Grey-Turner's sign).

Ultrasound items: In the ultrasound examination, special attention should be paid to the presence of gallstones. Bile duct dilatation, pancreatic edema, the presence of peripancreatic fluid, or ascites can be further evidence of acute pancreatitis. A mass lesion, due to a pancreatic cyst or malignancy, should also be ruled out by ultrasound.

Laboratory Diagnostics items: A presumptive diagnosis of "acute pancreatitis" can be made from the medical history, and the results of the physical examination, and possibly ultrasound findings (Wang, 1988). Especially since the pain symptoms can be similar to those for acute myocardial infarction, acute coronary syndrome should be ruled out by an ECG and determining of troponin I or T at an early stage.

The basic laboratory diagnostics should include the electrolytes, glucose concentration; ALT, AST, and lipase activity; CRP level, blood count, urinalysis, and creatinine concentration.

A presumptive diagnosis of "acute pancreatitis" is confirmed by measuring the serum/plasma lipase activity, which will increase to greater than three times the upper reference range value within 48–72 hours after the onset of pain. Since the lipase measurement is clearly superior to the amylase measurement because of its sensitivity and specificity, the former should be given preference over the latter (Kiriyama, 2010; Sutton, 2009; Chase, 1996). Simultaneous activity measurements for lipase and amylase or P-amylase do not offer higher sensitivity than the lipase measurement alone. Although amylase measurements in serum and urine are still quite common, amylase increases should be interpreted with caution because of their low specificity, since the amylase activity can increase under various conditions in the absence of acute pancreatitis (Sutton, 2009; Kiriyama, 2010; Chase, 1996). If the serum/plasma lipase activity is not increased, no acute pancreatitis is present.

Discrimination between mild pancreatitis and severe pancreatitis Because the prognosis for mild pancreatitis is significantly better than for severe pancreatitis (Whitcomb, 2006), the severity in a pancreatitis case should be determined at an early stage in the course of the disease. The severity cannot be assessed from the magnitude of the enzyme activity for lipase (or amylase). It is possible to observe moderately increased enzyme activity in severe (necrotizing) pancreatitis, as well as very high lipase and amylase values in mild (edematous) pancreatitis. Various scoring schemes are recommended for determining the severity in a pancreatitis case (BISAP, Ranson score, Imrie score, Glasgow criteria, Apache II score); these essentially take into account changes in several laboratory parameters, and the patient's age and body mass index (Papachristou, 2010; Imrie, 2003; Dambrauskas, 2010). One scoring scheme we commonly use considers, for example, the CRP concentration, WBC, creatinine concentration, current oxygen partial pressure (pO_2), calcium concentration, albumin concentration; LDH, AST and ALT activity; glucose concentration, hematocrit value, and the age and body mass index of the patient (▶ Figure 4.20). Fewer than four of these parameters being clearly pathological points to mild pancreatitis, while more than four indicates severe pancreatitis.

Since about half of our acute pancreatitis cases have a biliary origin (Perez-Mateo, 2006), an early-stage differentiation should also be made between biliary and non-biliary pancreatitis. In biliary pancreatitis, typically bilirubin, alkaline phosphatase (and gamma-GT), and AST/ALT are increased (Wang, 1988). Biliary pancreatitis is not present if AST/ALT, AP and bilirubin are normal. By contrast, if AST/ALT, AP and bilirubin are increases, there are grounds for suspecting the presence of biliary pancreatitis. If the ALT activity is about 150 U/L, the probability of biliary pancreatitis is 95 % (Tenner, 1994). Suspected biliary pancreatitis should be confirmed by ultrasound. If there is evidence of a stone, this should be removed in conjunction with ERCP and papillotomy (Sharma, 1999). Alcohol abuse can be diagnosed as the origin of acute pancreatitis from the concentration of carbohydrate-deficient transferrin (CDT) and significantly increased serum trypsin activity (Aparicio, 2001; Al-Bahrani, 2005). The frequently used gamma-GT activity and elevated erythrocyte volume (MCV) is not suitable for this purpose (Jaakkola, 1994).

Further procedures for mild pancreatitis versus severe pancreatitis In a mild pancreatitis case, the CRP, calcium concentration, and leukocyte count should be checked daily until the pain is gone. Mild pancreatitis cases in which these parameters fall back into the reference range within a few days will follow an uncomplicated course. By contrast, if the CRP concentration and leukocyte count do not return to the reference range, or there are further increases in the CRP level and/or leukocyte count and/or serum/plasma LDH activity, this is an indication that severe pancreatitis has developed (Dambrauskas, 2007). This suspicion should be confirmed through diagnostic imaging such as ultrasound, CT or MRI (also known as MRT). Often the severe acute pancreatitis frequently develops from mild AP within the first 5–7 days after hospital admission.

In a case of severe pancreatitis, the CRP concentration, serum calcium concentration, leukocyte count, arterial oxygen pressure (pO_2), and glucose and creatinine concentrations should be measured daily to detect further complications. Normalization of these laboratory values over the following few days or weeks points to an uncomplicated course of severe pancreatitis. Any necrosis in this case will be sterile. However, if further increases occur in the CRP concentration (Al-Bahrani, 2005) and/or leukocyte count and/or procalcitonin concentration (Mofidi, 2009; Rau, 2007), and/or a deterioration of the clinical status occurs with development of sepsis or multiple organ failure (MOF), it is highly likely that the severe acute pancreatitis is complicated by infected necrosis. If the CRP concentration is below 81 mg/L and the leukocyte count does not exceed 13×10^9/L, infected necrosis is unlikely (Dambrauskas, 2007). If infected necrosis is suspected in a case of severe pancreatitis, this should be confirmed by imaging methods (air detection) or if necessary fine-needle aspiration (evidence of bacteria). If no bacteria are detected which points to the necrosis being sterile, conservative treatment should be continued. If bacteria are detected, the necrosis must be removed by surgical intervention; more recently, this can also be done using transgastric or minimally invasive necrosectomy. In the absence of these measures, a patient with infected necrosis or an abscess has little chance of survival.

4.3.2.2 Chronic Pancreatitis (Figure 4.21)

Chronic pancreatitis (CP) is an inflammatory disease of the pancreas with advancing acinar cell destruction, leukocyte infiltration, gait irregularities, and increasing fibrosis (Steer, 1995). The consequence for the patient is exocrine pancreatic insufficiency with maldigestion and steatorrhea, later also endocrine insufficiency with development of diabetes mellitus. The cardinal symptom of CP is epigastric pain lasting for weeks to months, radiating to the back, and also nausea and vomiting (Lankisch, 2000). Since food intake often intensifies the pain, the patient is afraid to eat and thus experiences weight loss.

About 20 % of patients with CP exhibit signs of exocrine and/or endocrine dysfunction without pain symptoms (Layer, 1995). The exocrine insufficiency leads to diarrhea, steatorrhea and weight loss.

Medical history items: When taking the medical history, the patient should be asked about the nature and duration of the pains (are the pains always present, or relapsing, radiating, radiating into the back, or colicky?). Since chronic alcohol abuse is the most common cause of chronic pancreatitis in adults in the Western industrialized countries (Pezzilli, 2008), ask about the level of alcohol consumption. It is furthermore relevant to ask whether nicotine abuse is present and what medications are being taken. Symptoms of maldigestion (weight loss, diarrhea, loss of appetite, nausea) should also be discussed. In younger patients, evidence of hereditary chronic pancreatitis can be obtained from the family medical history (Pezzilli, 2006).

Physical examination items: The physical examination findings are often relatively unremarkable in patients with chronic pancreatitis. Pain on pressure, muscular defense, resistance, and jaundice can be present. Pay special attention to signs of alcohol abuse (spider naevi, palmar erythema, gynecomastia, absence of secondary hair, or tremors).

Ultrasound items: Evidence of chronic pancreatitis to be found during the ultrasound examination includes calcifications in the pancreas region, dilated pancreatic ducts, possible cholestasis, pancreatic cysts, and enlargement of the pancreatic head.

Laboratory Diagnostics items: A presumptive diagnosis of chronic pancreatitis can be made from the clinical symptoms, a typical medical history and the ultrasound findings. This clinical

Clinical picture: nonspecific upper abdominal pain, postprandial pain, food (fat) intolerance,

Medical history items: Type and duration of pain: Recurring?, Radiating?, Radiating into the back?, Colicky? Alcohol? Medications? Weight loss? Loss of appetite? Diarrhea? Nausea? Nicotine abuse? (especially in young patients) → Family medical history *2

Examination items: Jaundice? Pain on pressure? Resistance? Muscular defense? Bowel sounds? Signs of alcohol abuse? Gynecomastia? Tremors? Palmar erythema? Secondary hair?

Presumptive diagnosis	**Chronic pancreatitis (CP)**	**Rule out peptic ulcer disease, gastric carcinoma** Medical history – Ultrasound – Gastroscopy
Differential diagnosis	Serum/plasma lipase > 3 times the upper reference range value	Characteristic medical history (dull, nonspecific, recurring upper abdominal pains ± weight loss, ± diarrhea, ± alcohol abuse) ± Pancreatic calcification (X-ray or ultrasound)
Basic laboratory diagnostics	Characteristic medical history and typical ultrasound findings	

Differential diagnosis — No

Na, K, Ca, glucose, blood count, CRP, creatinine, ALT, AST, bilirubin, lipase, urinalysis

| Yes | Yes | | Yes |

Acute or recurring pancreatitis — No

Suspected chronic pancreatitis (CP) ├─ Differentiation quite difficult ──────

Eliciting the etiology of CP

Yes

Suspected acute attack of chronic pancreatitis

Origin of CP:	Clarification through:
Alcohol (75%)	→ Medical history, CDT
Hypercalcemia	→ S/P calcium concentration
Medications	→ Medical history
Idiopathic	→ Medical history
Genetic (15%)	→ Mutation analysis *2
Autoimmune	→ IgG4, ANA, RF
Recurring AP	→ Medical history, lipase
Obstructive	→ Medical history, ultrasound

After normalization of lipase

Further procedures

see diagram "Acute pancreatitis"

Determination of the extent of exocrine pancreatic insufficiency:

specialized laboratory diagnostics

Direct function tests: Pathological secretin-pancreozymin test pathway or pathological Lundh test result

Indirect function tests: Elastase conc. in stool ↓ or chymotrypsin activity in stool ↓

Secretin-pancreozymin test or elastase conc. in stool or chymotrypsin activity in stool

Tedious, invasive, expensive

Simple, non-invasive, inexpensive

| No | Yes | Yes | No |

OGTT Test blood glucose daily HbA1c

If the secretin-pancreozymin test is normal, exocrine insufficiency is ruled out

Chronic pancreatitis with exocrine insufficiency

Chronic pancreatitis with exocrine insufficiency

If the chymotrypsin activity is normal, exocrine insufficiency is either mild or absent

*1 possible weight loss, possibly jaundice, possible insulin-deficient diabetes
*2 With a remarkable family medical history, molecular genetic clarification of a hereditary origin of CP
   (trypsin mutation, SPINK mutation, CFTR mutation)

dyspepsia complaints, maldigestion *1

Ultrasound items: Gallstones? Cholestasis? Pancreatic duct dilatation? Fluidity? Ascites? Pancreas size? Mass lesion? Pseudocysts? Pancreatic calcification?

Mass lesion, non-specific upper abdominal or back pains, loss of appetite, weight loss, nausea, possibly jaundice

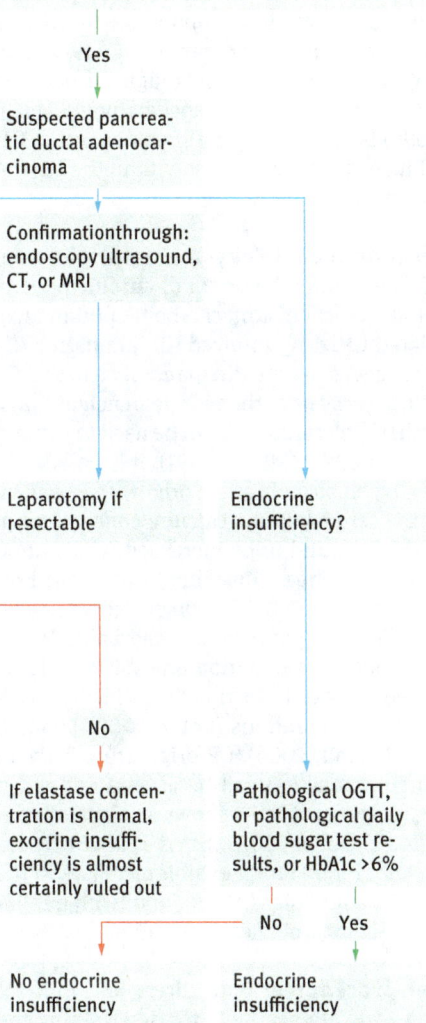

Yes

Suspected pancreatic ductal adenocarcinoma

Confirmationthrough: endoscopy ultrasound, CT, or MRI

Laparotomy if resectable

Endocrine insufficiency?

No

If elastase concentration is normal, exocrine insufficiency is almost certainly ruled out

Pathological OGTT, or pathological daily blood sugar test results, or HbA1c >6%

No   Yes

No endocrine insufficiency

Endocrine insufficiency

Figure 4.21 Chronic pancreatitis. Clinical picture: non-specific upper abdominal pain, postprandial pain, food (fat) intolerance, dyspepsia complaints, maldigestion, possible weight loss, possible jaundice, possible insulin-deficient diabetes.

symptomatology is characterized by nonspecific epigastric pain, often intensified postprandially, food (fat) intolerance, dyspepsia complaints, signs of maldigestion with weight loss, and possibly the presence of jaundice.

The basic laboratory diagnostic items to be determined include the following parameters: sodium, potassium, calcium, glucose, blood count, CRP, creatinine, bilirubin, ALT, AST, lipase and urinalysis.

Peptic ulcer disease or gastric carcinoma should be ruled out by evidence from the medical history, ultrasound, and possibly gastroscopy.

Pain symptoms that are more acute and serum/plasma lipase activity that is greater than 3 times the upper reference range value could point either to acute pancreatitis or an acute exacerbation of chronic pancreatitis. In this case, the further procedures outlined in the laboratory diagnostic pathway "Acute pancreatitis" (▶ Figure 4.20) should be followed. In chronic pancreatitis the serum/plasma lipase activity is usually less than 3 times the upper reference range value assuming that acute exacerbation of chronic pancreatitis is not present.

Differentiation between chronic pancreatitis and pancreatic ductal adenocarcinoma can be difficult (Buxbaum, 2010). Both diseases are not infrequently characterized by a mass lesion in the pancreatic head. However, patients with chronic pancreatitis are usually younger (i.e., 40 years) than patients with pancreatic cancer. Patients with CP had often already had several acute pancreatitis attacks. Male patients are affected far more frequently, and alcohol abuse is present in a high percentage of these patients. The diagnostic imaging procedures often identify calcification.

By contrast, patients with pancreatic head tumors due to adenocarcinoma are usually older, between 60 and 80 years. Risk factors for pancreatic cancer include hereditary pancreatitis, chronic pancreatitis, smoking and a family medical history (Buxbaum, 2010). Patients with pancreatic cancer seek medical attention when a painless jaundice is noticed, or because of abdominal pain radiating to the back pain (with no jaundice). 75 % of patients with pancreatic cancer exhibit increases in the cholestasis-indicating parameters, such as direct bilirubin, alkaline phosphatase (AP), and gamma glutamyl transferase (gamma-GT). These patients also often have mild anemia. The imaging results generally show no calcification of the tumor in pancreatic cancer cases. Hardly any differentiation between chronic pancreatitis and pancreatic cancer is possible through measurements of the tumor markers CA 19-9 or CEA (Nazli, 2000; Okusaka, 2006). Several studies have shown that CA 19-9 measurements have a sensitivity of 70–90 % and a specificity of 70–98 % with respect to diagnosing pancreatic cancer (Okusaka, 2006). The serum/plasma CA19-9 concentration can be above the reference range both in patients with pancreatic cancer as well as those with CP. If a cut-off value of 37 KU/L is chosen, a pPV of 72 % and an nPV of 96 % are found for CA 19-9 with respect to pancreatic cancer. Note also that about 10 % of the European and American populations are Lewis negative, and hence do not produce Ca 19-9 (Goggins, 2005). In the differential diagnosis between CP and pancreatic ductal adenocarcinoma, imaging methods such as endo-ultrasonography, CT, or MRI have a higher sensitivity than the laboratory diagnostics.

Clarification the etiology of chronic pancreatitis: To determine the origin of chronic pancreatitis, the medical history can be helpful in alcohol-related CP, drug-induced CP, idiopathic CP, recurrent acute pancreatitis, and obstructive CP (Pezzilli, 2008). The carbohydrate-deficient transferrin (CDT) determination can be used to confirm alcohol-related CP (Stibler, 1991). It is possible to identify hypercalcemia as the origin of CP by measuring the serum/plasma calcium concentration, and if this is found to be increased, verification is obtained by measuring the parathyroid hormone concentration. With a suspected genetically-based CP (younger patient, remarkable family medical history), a mutation analysis should be performed to search for trypsin-, SPINK- possibly CFTR-type mutations (Cohn, 2000; Etemad, 2001; Whitcomb, 2004). CP originating from an autoimmune reaction can be ascertained when the measurement of IgG-4 shows an elevated concentration (Pearson, 2003; Snyder, 2008). These patients not infrequently exhibit increases in the antinuclear antibodies (ANAs), and (with qualifications) a rheumatoid factor elevation.

Further procedures: Both direct and indirect function tests are available for determining the degree of exocrine pancreatic insufficiency in chronic pancreatitis. In the direct method, which is tedious, invasive, expensive, pancreatic secretions are suctioned out before after stimulation in the course of a gastro-duodenoscopy, and from this sample the bicarbonate, lipase, amylase, and trypsin values are measured. In the procedure known as the secretin-pancreozymin test, the concentration and amount of bicarbonate is measured after stimulation with secretin, and then the enzyme concentrations and amount are measured again after stimulation with cholecystokinin (pancreozymin) (Lankisch, 2000; Somogyi, 2003). The Lundt test is carried out by applying endogenous stimulation of the pancreas with a test meal that contains defined percentages of carbohydrates, proteins and fats, and then measuring the pancreatic enzymes.

The secretin-pancreozymin test is considered the currently most sensitive diagnostic method for confirming or ruling out exocrine pancreatic insufficiency. If the secretin-pancreozymin test result is normal, exocrine insufficiency is ruled out. The disadvantage of the direct pancreatic function tests is that they are tedious for both the patient and the examiner, they are invasive, and due to the numerous measurements and the cost of the pancreatic stimulation, they are expensive.

By contrast, the indirect pancreatic function tests are simple, non-invasive and relatively inexpensive (Lankisch, 2000). It has been shown that the immunological measurement of elastase concentration in the stool has higher sensitivity and specificity than does measurement of chymotrypsin activity in the stool (Gupta, 2005). Compared to the secretin-pancreozymin test, the elastase concentration measurement has virtually identical sensitivity and specificity with respect to detecting exocrine pancreatic insufficiency.

If the value from measuring chymotrypsin activity in the stool is normal, either no or only mild exocrine pancreatic insufficiency is present. It should be noted that falsely pathological stool chymotrypsin determination results can be obtained due to diarrhea, celiac disease, cachexia due to chronic inflammatory diseases or tumors, and obstructive jaundice (Lankisch, 2000). Moreover, the immunological measurement of elastase concentration is not reliable in the presence of diarrhea. If the stool elastase concentration is normal and diarrhea is not present, exocrine insufficiency is almost certainly ruled out.

The measurement of stool fat excretion for the detection of exocrine pancreatic insufficiency, or for clarifying whether enzyme replacement is necessary, is hardly ever performed nowadays. The fecal fat determination is not very sensitive, and is labor-intensive. Increased fat excretion is indicated when the stimulated lipase concentration result in the secretin-pancreozymin test is 10 % below normal. The easily accomplished stool weight determination is consistent with the stool fat analysis in 3/4 of the patients.

Diagnosis of endocrine pancreatic insufficiency: Endocrine pancreatic function can be investigated with an oral glucose tolerance test, daily blood sugar monitoring, or an HbA1c concentration measurement. If the HbA1c concentration > 6 % and/or the oral glucose tolerance test is abnormal, endocrine pancreatic insufficiency is present.

Literature

Al-Bahrani AZ, Ammori BJ. Clinical laboratory assessment of acute pancreatitis. Clin Chim Acta 2005; 362: 26–48.

Aparicio JR, Viedma JA, Aparisi L, Navarro S, Martinez J, Perez-Mateo M. Usefulness of carbohydrate-deficient transferrin and trypsin activity in the diagnosis of acute alcoholic pancreatitis. Am J Gastroenterol 2001; 96: 1777–81.

Buxbaum JL, Eloubeidi MA. Molecular and clinical markers of pancreas cancer. JOP. J Pancreas 2010; 11: 536–544.

Chase CW, Barker DE, Russell WL, Burns RP. Serum amylase and lipase in the evaluation of acute abdominal pain. Am Surg 1996; 62: 1028–33.

Dambrauskas Z, Gulbinas A, Pundzius J, Barauskas G. Value of routine clinical tests in predicting the development of infected pancreatic necrosis in severe acute pancreatitis. Scand J Gastroenterol 2007; 2: 1256–1264.

Dambrauskas Z, Gulbinas A, Pundzius J, Barauskas G. Value of the different prognostic systems and biological markers for predicting severity and progression of acute pancreatitis. Scand J Gastroenterol. 2010; 45: 959–70.

Etemad B, Whitcomb DC: Chronic pancreatitis: diagnosis, classification, and new genetic developments. Gastroenterology 2001; 120: 682–707.

Goggins MG. The molecular diagnosis of pancreatic cancer. In: Von Hoff DD, Evans DB, Hruban RH. Eds. Pancreatic Cancer. 1st ed. Sudbury: Jones and Bartlett Publishers, 2005: 251–264.

Gupta V, Toskes PP. Diagnosis and management of chronic pancreatitis. Postgrad Med J 2005; 81: 491–497.

Imrie CW. Prognostic indicators in acute pancreatitis. Can J Gastroenterol. 2003; 17: 325–8. Review.

Jaakkola M, Sillanaukee P, Lof K, Koivula T, Nordback I. Blood tests for detection of alcoholic cause of acute pancreatitis. Lancet 1994; 343: 1328–9.

Khan AS, Latif SU, Eloubeidi MA. Controversies in the Etiologies of Acute Pancreatitis. JOP. J Pancreas 2010; 11: 545–552.

Kiriyama S, Gabata T, Takada T, Hirata K, Yoshida M, Mayumi T, Hirota M, Kadoya M, Yamanouchi E, Hattori T, Takeda K, Kimura Y, Amano H, Wada K, Sekimoto M, Arata S, Yokoe M, Hirota M. New diagnostic criteria of acute pancreatitis. J Hepatobiliary Pancreat Sci 2010; 17: 24–36.

Lankisch PG, Layer P. Chronische Pankreatitis, Diagnostik und Therapie. Deutsches Arzteblatt 2000; 97: 2169–2177.

Mofidi R, Suttie SA, Patil PV, Ogston S, Parks RW. The value of procalcitonin at predicting the severity of acute pancreatitis and development of infected pancreatic necrosis: systematic review. Surgery 2009; 146: 72–81.

Nazli O, Bozdag AD, Tansug T, Kir R, Kaymak E. The diagnostic importance of CEA and CA 19–9 for the early diagnosis of pancreatic carcinoma. Hepatogastroenterology 2000; 47: 1750–2.

Okusaka T, Yamada T, Maekawa M. Serum tumor markers for pancreatic cancer: the dawn of new era? JOP, Journal of the Pancreas 2006;7 : 332–336.

Papachristou GI, Muddana V, Yadav D, O'Connell M, Sanders MK, Slivka A, Whitcomb DC. Comparison of BISAP, ranson's, APACHE-II and CTSI scores in predicting organ failure, complications and mortality in acute pancreatitis. Am J Gastroenterol 2010; 105: 435–441.

Pearson RK, Longnecker DS, Chari ST, Smyrk TC, Okazaki K, Frulloni L, Cavallini G. Controversies in clinical pancreatology: autoimmune pancreatitis: does it exist? Pancreas 2003; 27: 1–13

Perez-Mateo M. How we predict the etiology of acute pancreatitis. Journal of the Pancreas 2006; 7: 257–261.

Pezzilli R, Lioce A, Frulloni L. Chronic Pancreatitis: A Changing Etiology? JOP. J Pancreas 2008; 9: 588–592.

Rau BM, Kemppainen EA, Gumbs AA, Buchler MW, Wegscheider K, Bassi C, Puolakkainen PA, Beger HG. Early assessment of pancreatic infections and overall prognosis in severe acute pancreatitis by procalcitonin (PCT): a prospective international multicenter study. Ann Surg 2007; 245: 745–54.

Sharma VK, Howden CW. Metaanalysis of randomized controlled trials of endoscopic retrograde cholangiography and endoscopic sphincterotomy for the treatment of acute biliary pancreatitis. Am J Gastroenterol 1999; 94: 3211–4.

Smith RC, Southwell-Keely J, Chesher D. Should serum pancreatic lipase replace serum amylase as a biomarker of acute pancreatitis? ANZ J Surg 2005; 75: 399–404.

Snyder MC, Cappell MS. Clinical presentation, diagnosis and management of autoimmune pancreatitis. Minerva Gastroenterol Dietol 2008; 54: 389–405.

Steinberg W, Tenner S. Acute Pancreatitis. The New England Journal of Medicine 1994; 330: 1198–1210.

Stibler H. Carbohydrate-deficient transferrin in serum: a new marker of potentially harmful alcohol consumption reviewed. Clin Chem. 1991; 37: 2029–37.

Sutton PA, Humes DJ, Purcell G, Smith JK, Whiting F, Wright T, Morgan L, Lobo DN. The role of routine assays of serum amylase and lipase for the diagnosis of acute abdominal pain. Ann R Coll Surg Engl 2009; 91: 381–4.

Tenner S, Dubner H, Steinberg W. Predicting gallstone pancreatitis with laboratory parameters: a meta-analysis. Am J Gastroenterol. 1994; 89: 1863–6.

Wang SS, Lin XZ, Tsai YT, Lee SD, Pan HB, Chou YH, et al., Clinical significance of ultrasonography, computed tomography and biochemical tests in the rapid diagnosis of gallstone-related pancreatitis: a prospective study. Pancreas 1988; 3: 153–8.

Whitcomb DC. Clinical practice. Acute pancreatitis. N Engl J Med 2006; 354: 2142–50.

Whitcomb DC: Value of genetic testing in management of pancreatitis. Gut 2004; 53: 1710–1717.

Whitcomb DC, Yadav D, Adam S, Hawes RH, Brand RE, Anderson MA, Money ME, Banks PA, Bishop MD, Baillie J, Sherman S, DiSario J, Burton FR, Gardner TB, Amann ST, Gelrud A, Lo SK, DeMeo MT, Steinberg WM, Kochman ML, Etemad B, Forsmark CE, Elinoff B, Greer JB, O'Connell M, Lamb J, Barmada MM. Multicenter approach to recurrent acute and chronic pancreatitis in the United States: The North American Pancreatitis Study 2 (NAPS2). Pancreatology 2008; 8: 520–531.

Walter Hofmann, Jochen H.H. Ehrich, Walter G. Guder, Frieder Keller, Jürgen Scherberich

4.4 Kidneys and Efferent Urinary Tract

For those affected, many acquired and hereditary kidney diseases harbor the risk of remaining undiagnosed because of asymptomatic initial courses, and then later lead to renal failure that requires dialysis. This situation has repeatedly been picked up by the lay press, which have dubbed it with epithets such as the "silent tragedy" or the "insidious death". In the year 2009, more than 60,000 patients in Germany underwent dialysis due to stage 5 chronic kidney disease (CKD V), and their number has increased in subsequent years. At more than 60 %, patients with diabetes and/or hypertension represent the majority of these patients. Approximately 10 % of all German adults have grade III CKD, which in addition to the renal complications also carries an increased cardiovascular risk. To counteract this threatening development in the area of public health, more diagnostic concepts should be developed for the early detection of nephropathy.

Ideally, nephrology laboratory diagnostics in children and adults should

1. Filter out affected patients through targeted screening or mass screening;
2. Through standardized initial diagnostics, specify measures with stepwise escalation of invasiveness to uncover the localization, cause, and degree of severity of kidney disease, and
3. In the course of the diagnostics, identify the progression, remission, or recurrence of kidney damage.

"Diagnostic pathways" should make a constructive contribution to this effort, and both demonstrate the analytical problems, including costs, as well as approaches to solutions.

The currently available recommendations for detecting and differentiating kidney diseases (Hofmann and Schmolke 2009) should be appropriately structured, and the basics of an EDP-supported design for use in the clinic (Hofmann, et al., 2009) be made available or requesTable.

4.4.1 Ruling out Disorders of the Kidneys and Efferent Urinary Tract

4.4.1.1 Medical History and Clinical Picture

In the majority of kidney disease cases, the clinical picture is unremarkable and uncharacteristic. For this reason, basic diagnostics are indicated for ruling out kidney disease in all medical examinations. There are a few main symptoms, such as hematuria, which point to a kidney disease or involvement that can be acute or chronic, and functional or structural (▶ Table 4.19). The precise medical history of the patient and patient's family and a thorough physical examination of the patient will help structure the somewhat elaborate laboratory diagnostics, which in turn can be expanded through imaging and histopathology studies to enable a complete diagnosis.

4.4.1.2 Pre- and Post-analytical Principles

Blood tests and urine analyses should be carried out in parallel on the same day. The blood sample can be done at any time of day. For urine tests, the second midstream morning urine has proved particularly favorable, but urine from any other part of the day can also be used, i.e., there should be no diagnostic delay. To reduce sources of pre-analysis error (e.g., through bacterial decomposition), the basic recommendation is to use freshly produced spontaneous urine without stabilizing additives.

Table 4.19 Clinical symptoms and signs and medical history findings in kidney disease.

General symptoms	Polydipsia, loss of appetite, paleness, listlessness/drop in performance, fever, edema, dehydration, palpable upper/lower abdominal tumor that shifts during breathing, gastrointestinal symptoms, skin changes, arterial hypertension, hearing impairment
Urine, urination	Oliguria/anuria, polyuria, (macro)hematuria, foamy urine (proteinuria), dysuria, pollakiuria, nocturia, enuresis/incontinence, urinary retention
Endocrinology	Hyposomia, failure to thrive
Neurology	Acute attacks (syncope, seizures), blurred vision, headaches
Pains	Abdominal pain, flank pain, bone pain
Conspicuous stigmata	Congenital external malformations on the ears (dysmorphic ears and hearing disability), eyes (retinopathy, visual disability), face, hands (hexadactyly), legs (missing patella), and spine (egg shaped vertebra); small stature, etc.
Indications from the medical history	Positive family medical history for kidney disease; patient's medical history: pathologic fetal ultrasound, oligohydramnios, polyhydramnios, preterm delivery, "small for date" (fetal programming, Barker hypothesis), growth retardation, blurred visual and hearing impairment, recurrent urinary tract infections, etc.

Data with information on the stability of blood and urine components have been published (Guder, et al., 2012). This source defines the maximum transport and storage times that do not extend the overall error for the tests beyond the validity guidelines set by the German Medical Association.

For quantification, for excreted cells and chemical substances are traditionally standardized as the values per one liter of urine. To compensate for the effect of different urine concentrations on the substance concentrations, it is recommended in addition to specify the value for a urine volume-independent reference parameter for which the total excretion per day is constant. Generally, creatinine is selected as this reference parameter, giving rise to what is known as the urine ratio, i.e., specifying the substance/creatinine ratio in units of mol substance/mmol creatinine, or mg substance/g creatinine. The implementation of a 24-hour urine collection and calculating the substance excretion per day is no longer required in most cases.

4.4.1.3 Basic diagnostic approach

In addition to urinalysis using test strip as markers for proteinuria, leukocyturia and hematuria, a blood count is obtained along with the analysis of electrolytes, Na^+, K^+, glucose, C-reactive protein, and the plasma or serum creatinine as the basis for the GFR formula calculation. These studies represent stage 1 of addressing the question of "ruling out kidney disease". In cases of doubt, (e.g., in the absence of muscle mass), the plasma/serum cystatin C value can be determined as a particularly sensitive marker of incipient renal failure. Particularly good methods to rule out incipient renal damage are those that can rule out microalbuminuria, i.e., albumin excretion below the detection limit of conventional urine protein test strip. Either an isolated test strip result that is positive for protein, leukocytes and blood, or an isolated elevation in creatinine or cystatin C, indicate that extending the diagnostics to the next stage is required, to wit microscopic examination of the urine. A test strip positive for protein or albumin must be clarified through quantification and differentiation (albumin, α_1-microglobulin) using the urine protein/creatinine ratio.

In addition to measuring the amount of urine and inspecting turbidity and color, modern urinalysis includes chemical test sets ("expert systems")

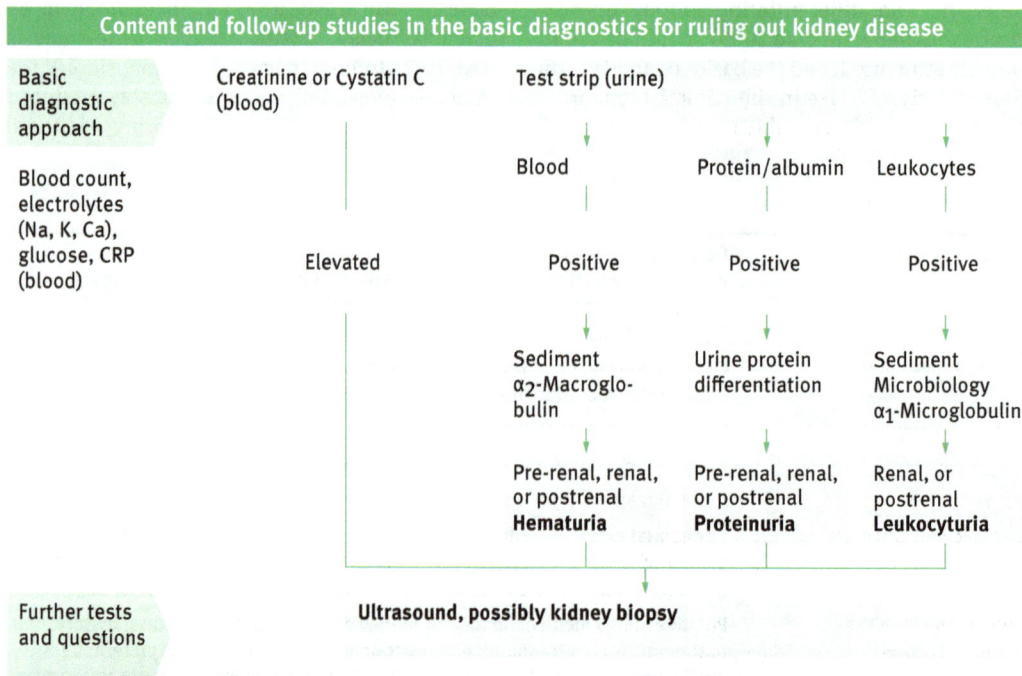

Content and follow-up studies in the basic diagnostics for ruling out kidney disease				
Basic diagnostic approach	Creatinine or Cystatin C (blood)	Test strip (urine)		
		↓	↓	↓
Blood count, electrolytes (Na, K, Ca), glucose, CRP (blood)		Blood	Protein/albumin	Leukocytes
		│	│	│
	Elevated	Positive	Positive	Positive
		↓	↓	↓
		Sediment α_2-Macroglobulin	Urine protein differentiation	Sediment Microbiology α_1-Microglobulin
		↓	↓	↓
		Pre-renal, renal, or postrenal **Hematuria**	Pre-renal, renal, or postrenal **Proteinuria**	Renal, or postrenal **Leukocyturia**
		↓		
Further tests and questions	**Ultrasound, possibly kidney biopsy**			

Figure 4.22 Content and follow-up studies in the basic diagnostics for ruling out kidney disease.

after the use of test strip, and possibly automatic examination of the morphological components of the urine ("automated cell counting"). Since modern test strip recognize many components of urine sediment (e.g., leukocytes, erythrocytes, nitrite for bacteriuria), it is recommended that urine sediment only be analyzed in positive test strip fields (test strip sieve). This is further recommended for ruling out kidney disease in the examination of asymptomatic patients, while urine sediment should always be investigated in patients with test indications (e.g., suspected urinary calculus, diabetes mellitus) and in high-risk patients (e.g., hereditary predisposition for kidney disease or hypertension).

If the basic diagnostics are pathological, and especially if "active sediment" is present, a nephrologist should become involved as soon as possible.

Pre-analytics: Any urine sample can be used for urinalysis during the screening stage. Concentration effects in a specific gravity (cation concentration) or conductivity measurement or can be compensated by reference to urine creatinine.

In any case, midstream urine should be collected after cleaning the external genitalia with physiological saline or water (no disinfectant) to avoid contamination of the urine sample by cells, bacteria and protein. If spontaneous urine cannot be obtained, catheter urine or bladder puncture urine can also be used for the urinalysis studies. The timing and type of urine collection should be recorded.

4.4.1.4 Analysis

Test strip

The main test strip detection methods are summarized in ▶ Table 4.20. Regarding the methods, automated readers are increasingly being used, partly to better facilitate semi-quantitative reading of test strip by avoiding subjective interpretation. In this connection, some devices determine the conductivity of the urine as a measure of the urine density.

Urine sediment testing is always indicated when the following issues or findings are present:
- Suspected kidney disease or disorders of the urinary tract;
- Positive test strip box for blood, leukocytes, or protein;
- To rule out pathogenic crystal formations and infections in the course of urinary calculus metaphylaxis.

The following components should always be examined by microscope: erythrocytes to identify dysmorphic acanthocytes when erythrocyte counts are elevated; epithelial cells, leukocytes, casts, and crystals where relevant (cystine).

Figure 4.20 Test strip fields for urinalysis for diseases of the kidney and urinary tract, with measuring principles, measurement ranges, and reference ranges (after Guder, 2009).

Test strip field	Measurement principle	Detection limits / measurement range	Normal findings (reference range)
Protein	Absence of detection	ca. 300 mg/L albumin	Negative
Albumin	Absence of detection, immune reaction	ca. 20–80 mg/L albumin	Negative (< 20 mg/L)
Blood, hemoglobin, myoglobin	Pseudoperoxidase activity	ca. 1.5–6 mg Hb/L	Negative (< 8×10^6/L)
Leukocytes	Indoxyl esterase activity	ca. 5–10 × 10^6 granulocytes/L	Negative (< 5–8 × 10^6/L)
Glucose	Glucose oxidase activity	ca. 1000 mg/L (5.2 mmol/L)	Negative (< 2 mmol/L)
Nitrite	Griess test	0.6–1 mg/L nitrite	Negative
pH	Color indicators	pH 5–9	pH 5–7.5
Concentration, "specific gravity"	Polyelectrolyte detection of cations	Corresponds to 1000–1030	1010–1042 (corresponds to 300–1400 mOsmol/kg water)
Creatinine	Chemical	0.88/26.5 mmol/L (0.1–3 g/L)	4.5–13 mmol/L (0.5–1.5 g/L)

Extensive compilations have been published on the evaluation of urine sediments (Atlas of Urine Sediments, 2003; Fogazzi, et al., 1999). An erythrocyte cast indicates a renal (glomerular) origin for hematuria. Cystine crystals point to cystinuria, while any other crystals have no diagnostic significance, since their occurrence varies greatly depending on pH and nutrition.

4.4.2 Stepwise Diagnostics of the Glomerular Filtration Rate

4.4.2.1 Stages of Chronic Renal failure

The glomerular filtration rate (= GFR) is the paramount measure of kidney function. An estimate of the GFR is necessary for:

- Testing whether impaired renal function is present; for
- Staging of chronic renal failure (▶ Table 4.21), for
- Dosage adjustment of medications, and for
- Assessing the progression of kidney disease.

The classification of acute kidney injury (AKI) into stages is based on the increase in serum creatinine and diuresis (▶ Table 4.21). By contrast, the classification of chronic kidney disease (CKD) into stages is based on the glomerular filtration rate (GFR).

4.4.2.2 Analysis and Calculation of the Glomerular Filtration Rate

At present, the creatinine clearance (CL_{creat} = GFR) that measures renal function can be calculated from the plasma/serum levels according to the MDRD (Modification of Diet in Renal Disease) formula (Levey, et al., 2007), or the Cockcroft-Gault formula (Cockcroft and Gault, 1976; Walser, 1998). A supplementary parameter that offers better information in individual collectives (e.g., pediatrics, geriatrics) is the measurement of cystatin C instead of creatinine (Stevens, et al., 2008).

Cystatin C is a serum proteinase inhibitor that is present in the blood in almost constant amounts, and freely undergoes glomerular filtration due to its low molecular mass. The substantial independence of the plasma cystatin C concentration from extrarenal factors means that its clearance can be estimated directly from the plasma cystatin C

concentration using formulas. Compared to creatinine, cystatin C offers the following advantages: Practically no dependence on muscle mass, and very little on the patient's sex and other extrarenal factors. With minimal interindividual variation, an increase in the blood concentration already occurs with a GFR < 80 mL/min. The increase in cystatin C due to renal failure is steeper and more rapid than with creatinine. Thus, it gives an earlier indication of incipient renal impairment in a case of acute kidney injury. Cystatin C is therefore particularly suitable for the early detection of acute kidney injury (AKI) (Nejat, et al., 2010; Herget-Rosenthal, et al., 2007) (▶ Table 4.21).

Various methods are used to calculate the GFR (▶ Table 4.22).

The **inulin clearance** has to be measured under standard conditions, and requires continuous infusion of insulin until a steady state has been achieved. Inulin is no longer available in many places (Tsinalis and Thiel, 2009).

As is the case with the the the **Cr51-EDTA clearance** test for measuring GFR, renal plasma flow is measured by Hippuran or MAG3 clearance tests which can only be performed when a nuclear medicine laboratory is available.

Among bona fide mGFR markers, the **iohexol clearance** test is often referred to as the gold standard. The problem with intravenous bolus injections is the inevitable distribution phase, which is why iohexol clearance calculations from the area under the curve (AUC) measured over at less than 3 half-lives can easily yield falsely low values.

The traditionally used measure of mGFR was **endogenous creatinine clearance**, but this method is very unreliable due to the cumulative error (Walser, 1998).

The Modification of Diet in Renal Disease (MDRD) formula for eGFR takes into account the serum/plasma creatinine (S/P_{creat}, in mg/dL), age (years), gender, and ethnic origin (Froissart, et al., 2005). The MDRD GFR formula applies is valid for a standard body surface area of 1.73 m² and was originally developed for serum creatinine determination using the old Jaffe method. Quite recently, the reference methods were redefined based on enzymatic methods (Myers, 2008; Levey, et al., 2007). Additionally, a conversion formula ($S_{creat\_Jaffe} \times 0.95 = S_{creat\_enzym}$) was recommended for when the creatinine is determined enzymatically and calibrated by isotope dilution mass spectrometry (IDMS) (Levey, et al., 2005).

Table 4.21 Stages of acute kidney injury according to the Acute Kidney Injury Network (AKIN) criteria, and stages of chronic kidney disease (CKD). The AKI stages are creatinine- and diuresis-based (Murrey, et al., 2008), while the CKD stages are GFR-based (Levey, et al., 2005).

Acute Kidney Injury Network (AKIN)			Chronic kidney disease (CKD)	
AKI stage	Creatinine increase within 7 days	Diuresis	CKD stage	GFR
			I	< 120 mL/min
I	1.5 times = + 50 % or > 0.3 mg/dL	< 90 mL/h	II	< 90 mL/min
II	2 time = + 100 %	< 60 mL/h	III	< 60 mL/min
III	3 time = + 200 % or > 0.4 mg/dL	< 30 mL/h	IV	< 30 mL/min
	Oliguria > 24 h	= Dialysis	V	< 15 mL/min
	Anuria > 12 h		PD = dialysis	
			I–V, T	T = status post kidney transplant

Table 4.22 Formulas for calculation of glomerular filtration rate (GFR) as a measure of renal function.

Name	GFR formula
Endogenous creatinine clearance (GFR)	$GFR \approx CL_{creat} = U \cdot V/P$ $GFR = CreaUrine (\mu mol/L \cdot Urine\ volume\ collected\ (mL)/ [CreaSerum (\mu mol/L) \cdot Collection\ period\ (min)]$
Modification of Diet in Renal Disease formula (MDRD) (Froissart, et al., 2005)	Jaffe method $GFR = 186.3 \cdot Crea^{-1,154} \cdot Age^{-0,203} \cdot 0.741\ (female) \cdot 1.212\ (black)$ Reference method-based analysis $GFR = 175 \cdot Crea^{-1,154} \cdot Age^{-0,203} \cdot 0.741\ (female) \cdot 1.212\ (black)$
Chronic Kidney Disease Epidemiology Collaboration formula (CKD-EPI formula for creat > 0.7 mg/dL for females and creat > 0.9 mg/dL for males) (Levey, et al., 2009)	$GFR\text{-}female = 144 \cdot [Crea\ (\mu mol/L)/0.7]^{-1.209} \cdot (0.993)^{Age}$ $GFR\text{-}male = 141 \cdot [Crea\ (\mu mol/L)/0.9]^{-1.209} \cdot (0.993)^{Age}$
Cystatin C GFR (Filler, et al., 2012; Grubb, et al., 2005, Inker, et al., 2012)	$GFR = 84.69 \cdot Cystatin\ C^{-1.68}$ $(female: \times 0.85;\ in\ children < 14\ years: \times 1.384)$
Cockcroft-Gault formula (Cockcroft and Gault, 1976)	$GFR = [140 - Age(years)] /[0.8 \cdot Serum\text{-}Crea(\mu mol/L) \cdot Weight(kg)]$
Cockcroft-Gault GFR, newly calibrated creatinine (Tsinalis, 2009)	$GFR = [155 - Age\ (years)] / [Serum - Crea(\mu mol/L) \cdot Weight\ (kg) \cdot 0.85\ (female)]$

The MDRD equation has only been validated for GFR values < 60 mL/min. The CKD-EPI GFR formula is an improved MDRD equation that is based on new S_{creat} (mg/dL) measurement methods and indicated for all stages of renal failure (Levey, et al., 2009). The CKD-EPI formula classifies fewer patients as having kidney disease, and recognizes cardiovascular risk more accurately than does the MDR formula (Matsushita, 2012). The Cystatin C GFR can also be calculated from Cystatin C (nephelometrically, in mg/L), (Filler G, et al., 2012; Grubb A, et al., 2012; Inker LA, et al., 2012). The Oerebro formula for determining the Cystatin C GFR is independent of age, sex, weight, and race (Tidman, et al., 2008).

Assessment of a decreased GFR: GFR is age dependent and normale values have been established for 3 age groups: < 18 years, 18–65 years, and > 65 years (▶ Fig. 4.23).

The diagnostic procedure for patients over 65 years of age will be described as an example. A GFR > 90 mL/min is unremarkable. If the GFR value is below 90 mL/min, a urine test should

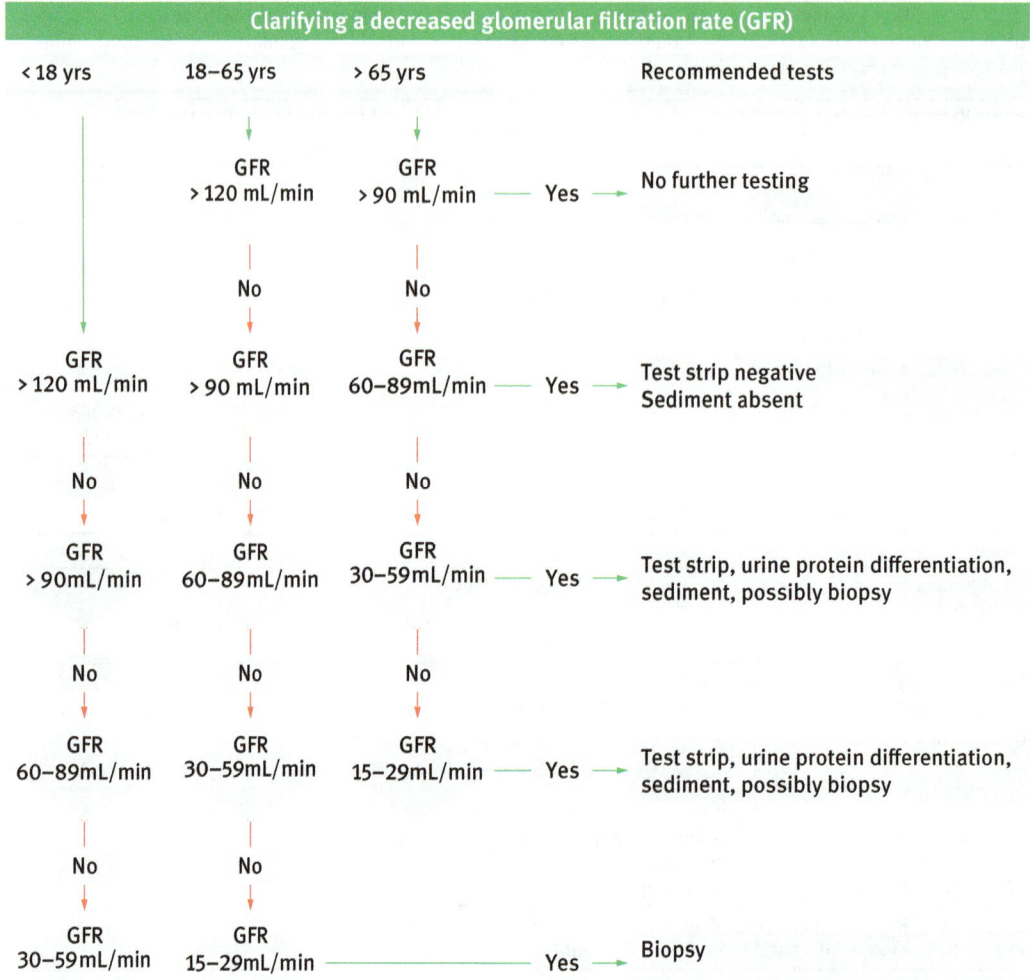

Clarifying a decreased glomerular filtration rate (GFR)			
< 18 yrs	18–65 yrs	> 65 yrs	Recommended tests
	GFR > 120 mL/min	GFR > 90 mL/min — Yes →	No further testing
	No	No	
GFR > 120 mL/min	GFR > 90 mL/min	GFR 60–89mL/min — Yes →	Test strip negative Sediment absent
No	No	No	
GFR > 90mL/min	GFR 60–89mL/min	GFR 30–59mL/min — Yes →	Test strip, urine protein differentiation, sediment, possibly biopsy
No	No	No	
GFR 60–89mL/min	GFR 30–59mL/min	GFR 15–29mL/min — Yes →	Test strip, urine protein differentiation, sediment, possibly biopsy
No	No		
GFR 30–59mL/min	GFR 15–29mL/min	— Yes →	Biopsy

Figure 4.23 Clarifying a decreased glomerular filtration rate (GFR) by measured (mGFR) or estimated GFR (eGFR).

also be done using a test strip. If the GFR is below 60 mL/min, an initial urine protein differentiation and a step wise increase of diagnostic invasiveness are indicated. If the GFR is below 30 mL/min (CKD IV, III AKI), a renal biopsy might be indicated for further clarification after pre- and post-renal origins have been ruled out.

Any decrease in the GFR requires clarification in younger patients (with the exception of infants).

Adjustment of medication dosages according to the GFR: The Cockcroft-Gault formula (Cockcroft and Gault, 1976; Dettli, 1976; Spruill, et al., 2008) is suitable for adapting the medication dosage to the level of kidney function, especially when "lean body weight" is taken into account for the weight (Han, et al., 2007). The Cockcroft-Gault formula has been modified for use with enzymatically calibrated creatinine measurements (Walser, 1998).

Estimating the progression of kidney failure: Estimating the progression of renal function loss is carried out as a linear regression analysis of the GFR as a function of time (t) (Kamper, 2007).

All calculations of the GFR – as well as the inulin and the isotope clearance – overestimate renal function in acute renal failure with rising creatinine values. Conversely, all GFR calculation formulas underestimate renal function during the restitution phase of acute renal failure with falling creatinine values. GFR estimates always lag behind reality, and most clearly so in the case of complete anuria.

4.4.3 Stepwise Diagnostics of Proteinuria

4.4.3.1 Forms of Proteinuria

Prerenal proteinuria: A high excretion rate of filterable small-molecule proteins, present to an increased extent in the plasma, is defined as prerenal proteinuria, e.g., Bence-Jones proteinuria in monoclonal gammopathy, myoglobinuria in rhabdomyolysis, or hemoglobinuria in hemolysis.

Bence-Jones proteinuria (free light chains): Immunofixation and quantification of free light chain both in serum/plasma as well as urine are used for the detection and differentiation of free light chains (kappa = κ, lambda = λ) in patients with monoclonal gammopathy. The quantitative determination in serum/plasma was more sensitive than in the urine (Hofmann, et al., 2004). A κ/λ ratio outside the specified reference range is another criterion for detecting monoclonal gammopathy.

Myoglobinuria and hemoglobinuria: Simultaneous detection of high creatine kinase activity in serum and myoglobunria in patients with acute renal failure indicate rhabdomyolysis or crush syndrome. Simultaneous detection of high LDH activity in serum and hemoglobinuria in patients with acute renal failure indicate hemolytic-uremic syndrome.

Glomerular proteinuria: High-molecular-weight proteins having a molecular weight of about 60 kD are used as markers for glomerular proteinuria, e.g., albumin, transferrin, IgG, which are filtered only in very small amounts under physiological conditions. Differentiation into selective and non-selective glomerular proteinuria as an indication of steroid sensitivity or resistance can be done based on the proportions of various high-molecular-weight proteins in the urine.

Tubular proteinuria Low-molecular-weight proteins (known as microproteins, such as α_1-microglobulin) have been recommended as markers of tubular injury (Boesken, et al., 2002), since they are freely filtered and normally reabsorbed in healthy kidneys. When tubular reabsorption is impaired they appear in elevated concentrations in the final urine.

Furthermore, enzymes from various parts of the tubules and tubular cell compartments (e.g. lysosomes) are used as markers of tubular damage (e.g., N-acetyl-β-D-glucosaminidase (β-NAG) from lysosomes, alanine aminopeptidase (ALAP), γ-glutamyltransferase (γ-GT), alkaline phosphatase (AP), and dipeptidyl peptidase IV (DPPIV) from the brush border of the proximal tubule epithelium (Scherberich, 1990, Scherberich et al., 1994)). In recent years, proteins such as neutrophil gelatinase-associated lipocalin (NGAL) (Devarajan, 2008; Decavele, et al., 2011) or kidney injury molecule-1 (KIM-1) (Bonventre, 2008) were recommended to detect early kidney damage. While elevated urine levels of tubule enzymes (β-NAG, ALAP, DPPIV, γ-GT, or AP) and tubule proteins indicate an acute degree of tubule damage, the rate of α_1-microglobulin excretion reflects the impaired reabsorption capacity of the tubule as an acute and chronic defect.

Tubular proteinuria is caused not only by tubulointerstitial inflammatory or toxic kidney disease, but also in response to functional overload of the proximal tubules, with strong glomerular proteinuria in the course of nephrotic syndrome. Also, a urologic origin has been reported for tubular proteinuria that accompanies increasing intratubular pressure (e.g., through renal obstruction in prostate hypertrophy) (Everaert, et al., 2000).

4.4.3.2 Decision Tree for Proteinuria

Pathological proteinuria is usually detected in routine diagnostic using test strip. The test strip only shows a positive for albumin when the total protein concentration reaches 250–300 mg/L (► Figure 4.24). With a pathological test strip result, a quantitative protein determination should be made; for further clarification (glomerulopathy, tubulopathy?), a urine protein differentiation is recommended.

4.4.3.3 Quantification of Proteinuria

Use of the total urine sample for a quantitative proteinuria determination is considered obsolete. As in the case of endogenous creatinine clearance, the cumulative error is too large and the

Basic clarification of proteinuria

Test strip for protein (Albumin > 30 mg/L)

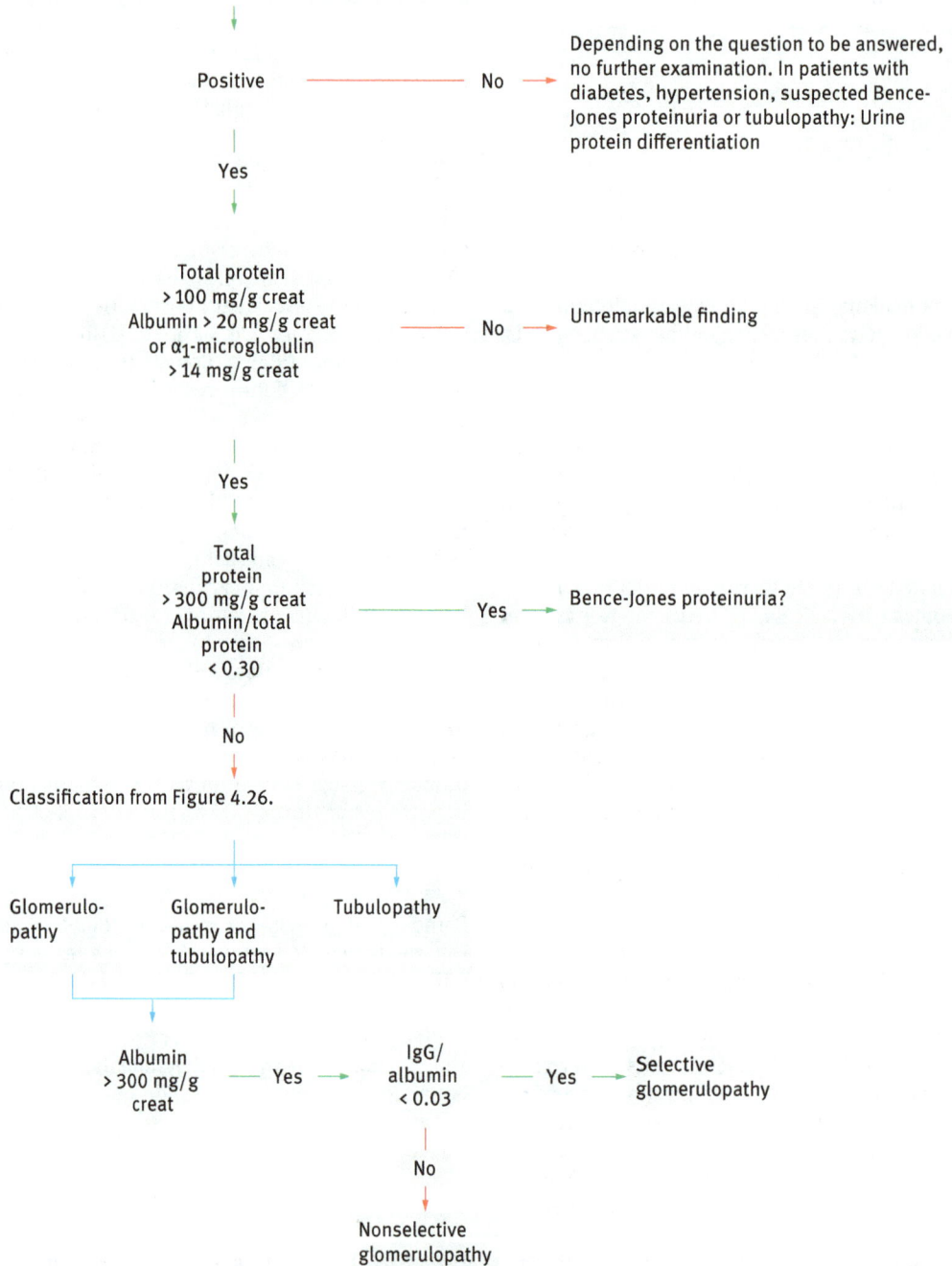

Positive —————— No → Depending on the question to be answered, no further examination. In patients with diabetes, hypertension, suspected Bence-Jones proteinuria or tubulopathy: Urine protein differentiation

Yes

Total protein
> 100 mg/g creat
Albumin > 20 mg/g creat
or α_1-microglobulin
> 14 mg/g creat —————— No → Unremarkable finding

Yes

Total
protein
> 300 mg/g creat
Albumin/total
protein
< 0.30 —————— Yes → Bence-Jones proteinuria?

No

Classification from Figure 4.26.

Glomerulo-pathy   Glomerulo-pathy and tubulopathy   Tubulopathy

Albumin
> 300 mg/g
creat —— Yes → IgG/albumin < 0.03 —— Yes → Selective glomerulopathy

No

Nonselective glomerulopathy

Figure 4.24 Decision tree after the initial examination for differentiation of proteinuria (prerenal, renal, postrenal).

result is delayed for 24 hours. The proteinuria/creatinine ratio is now a clearly established alternative, since creatinine excretion via the kidneys is constant at about 1.0 g per day (Ginsberg, 1983, Price, et al., 2005).

Proteinuria/day =
$Protein_{urine}(mg/L)/creatinine_{urine}(g/L)$

The protein/creatinine ratio in spontaneous urine (mg/g) corresponds quite precisely to the protein excretion in a 24-hour urine sample, and thus to the proteinuria/day (Antunes, et al., 2008).

Mild proteinuria in patients with diabetes or hypertension is not detected using the classical test strip. Thus, in such cases with a negative test strip result, a sensitive total protein determination or a urine protein differentiation with albumin and α_1-microglobulin should be performed.

Urinary protein differentiation (Hofmann, et al., 2001, Hofmann, et al., 2003) includes the determination of total protein, albumin, α_1-microglobulin, and creatinine in the urine. If the determined concentrations of total protein, albumin and α_1-microglobulin are within the reference range, the findings are unremarkable (▶ Figure 4.24). However, if the concentrations are found to be above the reference range limit, with an albumin concentration > 300 mg/g creatinine and in the presence of glomerulopathy, an IgG determination will permit a distinction between selective or nonselective proteinuria. Alternatively, if a discrepancy is found between the total protein (> 300 mg/g creatinine) and the albumin-total protein ratio (< 0.30), Bence Jones proteinuria might be present. The measurement of albumin and α_1-microglobulin and entry in the diagnostic diagram (▶ Figure 4. 26) permits the assignment of a clinical diagnosis (glomerulopathy, tubulopathy and glomerulopathy, or tubulopathy).

The expectation groups are allocated to the various forms of proteinuria (Scherberich, 2009) based on the proteinuria differentiation (Hofmann, et al., 2001; Hofmann, et al., 2003):

Predominantly selective glomerular proteinuria
- Minimal-change glomerulopathy
- Membranous glomerulonephritis, grade 1
- Focal segmental glomerulonephritis, grade 1
- IgA nephritis
- Stage III of diabetic nephropathy

Predominantly nonselective glomerular proteinuria
- Rapid progressive glomerulonephritis
- Proliferative glomerulonephritis (vasculitides)
- Membranoproliferative glomerulonephritis
- Membranous glomerulonephritis, grades 2 and 3
- Focal segmental glomerulonephritis, grades 2 and 3
- Stages III and IV of diabetic nephropathy
- Arterial hypertension, benign nephrosclerosis
- EPH gestosis

Predominantly nonselective glomerular and tubular proteinuria
- Renal amyloidosis
- Gold nephropathy, D-penicillamine glomerulonephritis
- Diabetic nephropathy (stages IV and V)
- Nephrosclerosis
- Membranoproliferative glomerulonephritis with renal failure
- Systemic vasculitides with kidney involvement
- Acute kidney transplant rejection

4.4.3.4 Further Diagnostics

Further examinations are used to differentiate between individual disease entities.

Creatinine (cystatin C) in the blood and/or α_1-microglobulin in urine should be monitored closely during the course. Based on the proteinuria differentiation, further tests are suggested (▶ Figure 4.25), including:
1. For selective or nonselective glomerular proteinuria and/or tubular proteinuria: complement C3, C4 (acute, postinfectious glomerulonephritis), c- and pANCA (Wegener's granulomatosis, idiopathic rapidly progressive glomerulonephritis), cryoglobulins (multiple myeloma), antinuclear antibodies (ANA) and their subgroups (lupus nephritis), anti-GBM antibody (anti-basal membrane glomerulonephritis). Pathological results in individual tests suggest consideration of doing a kidney biopsy.
2. For Bence-Jones proteinuria: serum electrophoresis, free light chains in the plasma/serum, immunofixation in the serum. Here again, pathological results in individual tests (Hofman, et al., 2004) suggest consideration of doing a bone marrow biopsy.

Further diagnostics for proteinuria		
Selective glomerular proteinuria Nonselective glomerular and/or tubular proteinuria	Bence-Jones proteinuria	Tubulopathy
↓	↓	↓
Complement C3, C4 ASL c-, p-ANCA Cryoglobulins, ANA, anti-GBM antibodies	Serum electrophoresis Free light chains in the serum Immunofixation in the serum	Urine sediment: Leukocyte casts Leukocytes Bacteria see Leukocyturia pathway
Yes	Yes	Yes
↓	↓	↓
Acute glomerulonephritis Rapid progressive glomerulo-nephritis Chronic glomerulonephritis Nephropathy in systemic disease (possibly kidney biopsy)	Multiple myeloma MGUS Lymphoma (possibly bone marrow biopsy)	Abacterial interstitial nephritis Acute pyelonephritis

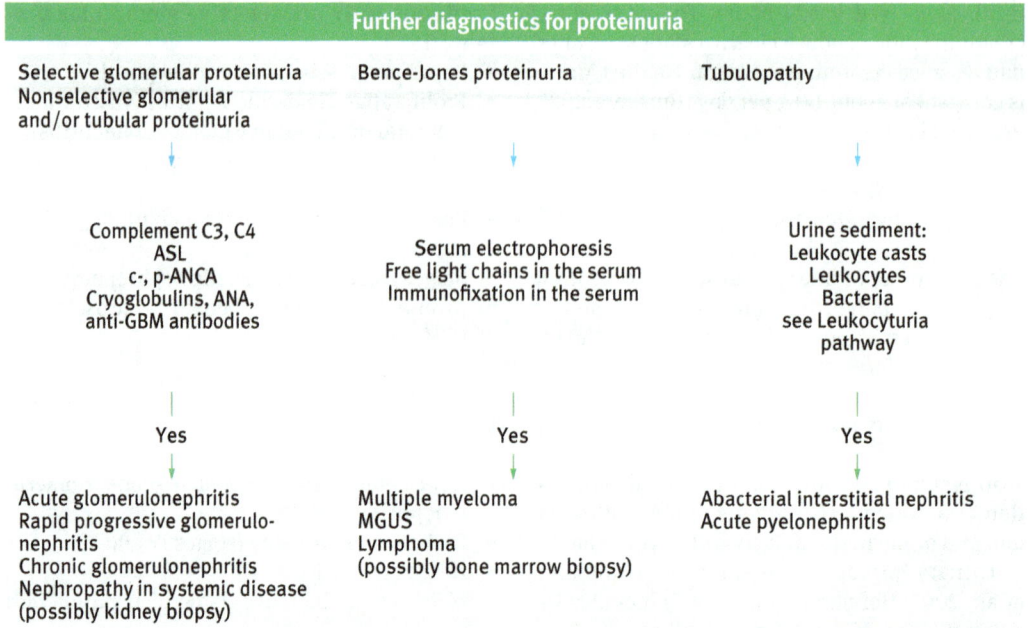

Figure 4.25 Further diagnostics for proteinuria.

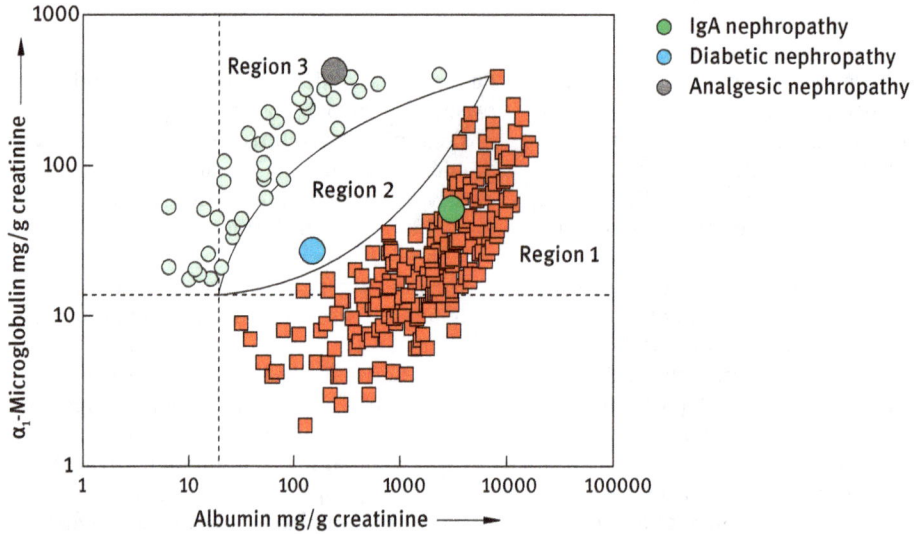

Figure 4.26 Distribution of albumin and α_1-microglobulin excretion in the urine in patients with primary glomerulopathy (Region 1, ■) and patients with tubulointerstitial nephropathy (Region 3, ○). In addition to the normal range limits for albumin (20 mg/g creatinine) and α_1-microglobulin (14 mg/g creatinine), curves are drawn for the calculated lower and upper separator functions for the two diagnostic groups registered. The overlap is labeled as the Region 2. Within this region are frequently found patients with diabetic nephropathy or nephrosclerosis. Note that the areas represent expectation groups and therefore cannot be interpreted as corresponding to diagnoses. Additionally shown is the excretion of albumin vs. α_1-microglobulin for a patient with IgA nephropathy ●, a patient with diabetic nephropathy ●, and a patient with analgesic nephropathy ●, (from Hofmann and Schmolke, 2009).

3. For tubulopathy: a sediment examination (leukocyte casts, bacteria, leukocytes). The expectation groups in different types of tubular proteinuria can be: pyelonephritis and interstitial nephritis attributable to:
   - Analgesic nephropathy;
   - Tubulotoxic nephropathy (aminoglycosides, cisplatin, cadmium, mercury lead, or lithium);
   - Fanconi syndrome(s), renal tubular acidosis (type II);
   - Myeloma kidney;
   - Chromoprotein kidney (malaria tropica, rhabdomyolysis)

4.4.3.5 Biomarkers and Proteomics

Proteome analysis of urine raises hope of investigating disease processes at the molecular level. Related to genome analysis for genetic diseases, this approach attempts to predict the disease course by determining which polypeptides and proteins undergo increased or decreased excretion in the urine.

The diagnostic targets achievable through the use of new urine biomarkers or proteome analysis include:
- Localization of the damage, and
- Assessing the degree of damage, which permit
- Differentiation between acute and chronic damage.

It is also possible to characterize the processes that have prognostic value over the course of the urinary tract injury.

The proteomic analysis of urine provides significant advantages over the analysis of blood. Approximately 70 % of the proteins and polypeptides in urine comes from the kidneys and urinary tract, while 30 % originate from other organs and have undergone glomerular filtration (Decramer, et al., 2008). A detailed description of all of the methods used in the proteomic analysis of urine can be found in recently published review articles (Decramer, et al., 2008; Mischak, et al., 2010). The complexity of the sample is reduced in a first step, prior to mass spectrometric detection. This can be done by electrophoresis, for example, using capillary electrophoresis (CE), 2-dimensional gel electrophoresis (2DE), or liquid chromatography (LC). In a second step, the masses and concentration of the previously separated proteins in the sample are identified using mass spectrometry (MS, MALDI-TOF). Differentiated proteomic analysis has been able to identify specific patterns in CKD cases, both for glomerulopathies and complex tubulopathies (Good, et al., 2010).

4.4.4 Stepwise Diagnostics for Hematuria

Forms and origins of hematuria: Hematuria is defined as a pathological proliferation of blood cells or blood pigments in the urine. The condition in which a red color is visible is called macrohematuria, while the condition that is only detectable from the hemoglobin or erythrocyte count ($< 10 \times 10^6$/L) using a test strip or sediment analysis is called microhematuria. The origin of hematuria can be prerenal (e.g., hemolysis), renal (e.g., glomerulonephritis), or post-renal (e.g., stones, cancer).

4.4.4.1 Decision Tree for Hematuria

As an initial examination of the question of "differentiation of hematuria", the finding is first confirmed in a morning urine/spontaneous urine sample using a test strip (▶ Abb.4.27). If the test strip is negative for the presence of blood, the result is normal. By contrast, if the test strip for detecting blood is positive, further tests are needed to clarify whether hemoglobinuria, erythrocyturia, or myoglobinuria is present. If no erythrocytes can be found in the sediment, it is necessary only to distinguish between hemoglobinuria (is free hemoglobin present in the blood?), myoglobinuria (is creatine kinase present in the blood?), or any other cause (e.g., are oxidants present in the urinary vessel?). If erythrocytes are found, on the other hand, the detection of erythrocyte casts (positive in only 30 % of all active glomerulonephritis cases) and/or deformed erythrocytes (dysmorphic erythrocytes), in particular acanthocytes (> 10 %, alternatively, > 10 per visual field) is proof of glomerular/renal hematuria. Post-renal hematuria is assumed if a high erythrocyte count is not accompanied by erythrocyte casts, or even more meaningfully if the acanthocyte count is less than 10 % of the erythrocyte count.

In parallel with the sediment analysis, urine protein differentiation with quantitative measurement of α_2-macroglobulin, IgG, and albumin also enables differentiation between prerenal and

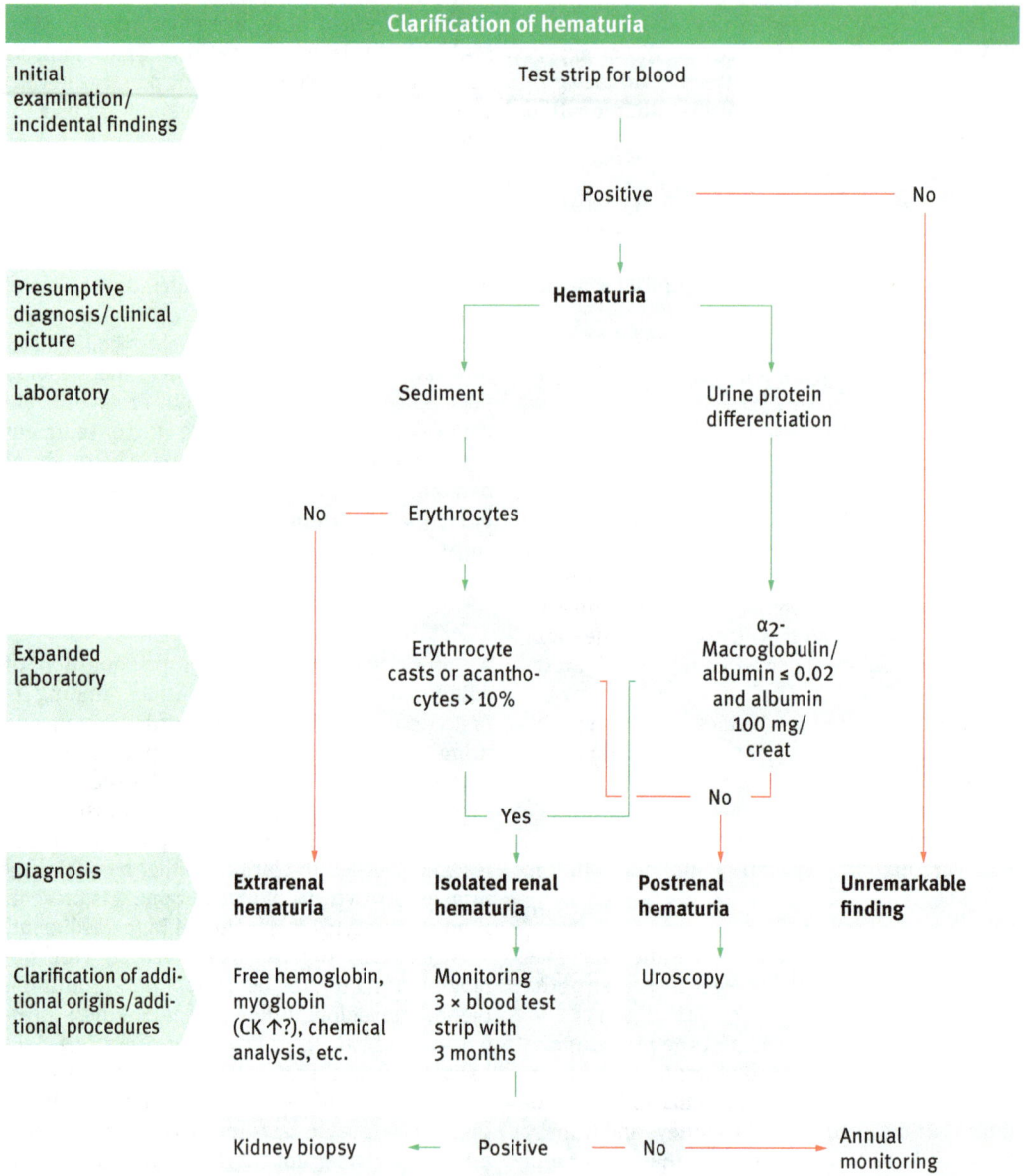

Figure 4.27 Clarification of hematuria.

postrenal hematuria when the albumin excretion is greater than 100 mg/g creatinine. An α_2-macroglobulin/albumin ratio greater than 0.02 and an IgG/albumin ratio above 0.2 points to postrenal hematuria, while a respective ratio less than 0.02 or 0.2 makes renal disease highly likely (▶ Figure 4.28). In general, postrenal hematuria should be further clarified from the urological perspective (uroscopy). In a case of renal hematuria with the test strip result repeatedly positive for blood (3 times within three months) is an indication for a kidney biopsy (▶ Figure 4.27).

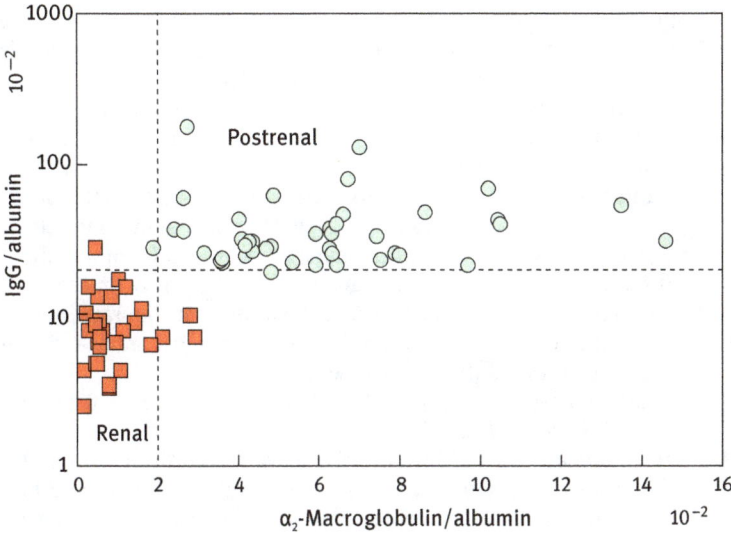

Figure 4.28 Differentiation of hematuria/erythrocyturia (Hofmann, et al., 2001).

Further differential diagnostic considerations and investigations:

In a case of **prerenal hematuria**, further distinction must be made:

hemolytic anemia (transfusion accident), thrombotic thrombocytopenic purpura, paroxysmal nocturnal hematuria, thalassemia minor, glucose-6-phosphate dehydrogenase deficiency.

In a case of **renal hematuria**, differentiation between the following origins must be made:

primary glomerulonephritis, such as IgA nephropathy, acute postinfectious glomerulonephritis, rapidly progressive glomerulonephritis, and membranoproliferative glomerulonephritis; and, secondary glomerulonephritis, such as lupus nephritis.

In, **postrenal hematuria** discussion should focus on the following origins, *inter alia*: stone disease and tumors in the efferent urinary tract.

4.4.5 Stepwise Diagnostics of Leukocyturia

Symptoms of infection of the kidneys and urinary tract: urinary tract infections (UTI) are the most common bacterial infections in humans (incidence: women: 4–5 %; elderly women: 10–12 %; rarely in men before age 50, after which the frequency increases due to the increasing number with prostate disease). The symptoms include urinary urgency, painful urination, and suprapubic pain in the foreground. The most prevalent

uropathogenic organism is *Escherichia coli*, which can be detected in 80–90 % of outpatients and more than 50 % of inpatients. *Proteus, Klebsiella, Enterobacter,* and enterococci are encountered more rarely. A "nitrit-positive" test strip is usually seen in cases with UTI mediated by *E. coli, Klebsiella,* or *Proteus mirabilis,* but may be negative in cases with enterococcae, *Pseudomonas aeruginosa,* or *Staphylococcus spp.*

4.4.5.1 Decision Tree for Leukocyturia

Chemical, microscopic, and microbiological examinations of the urine are the primary diagnostic approaches used (▶ Figure 4.29.):

Leukocytes and Bacteria: leukocyturia and/or bacteriuria is a common symptom of acute and chronic urinary tract infections (UTIs). The test strip detection of leukocytes based on the measurement of granulocyte esterase in urine (▶ Table 4.20). Since microscopic sediment examination finds only intact cells, the number of leukocytes detected will decrease on prolonged retention of urine, while conversely the number of positive test strip results will increase due to the additional formation of esterase. The cut-off between normal and pathologically elevated leukocyte excretion is defined in age-dependent terms, but generally a value of $10–20 \times 10^6$ leucocytes/L (= 10–20/µL) in native urine is suspicious and warrants monitoring, while values $> 20 \times 10^6$ leucocytes/L are pathological. This assumes that the urine sample was properly obtained.

The test strip detects only granulocytes by measuring an esterase produced by these cells. Neutrophil granulocytes are a component of leukocyturia, as they typically occur in urinary tract infections.

By contrast, lymphocytes and monocytes, and their soluble membrane proteins sCD14 and sCD30, frequently appear in cases of kidney transplant rejection. Eosinophil granulocytes also occur in the urine in cases of toxic-related (acute) interstitial nephropathy of an allergic origin. They are detection using Giemsa, Wright's, and Hansel staining. Eosinophiluria has a sensitivity and specificity of approximately 90 % (Hansel staining) for diagnosing acute interstitial nephritis. However, this can usually only be detected for a few hours up to a few days.

Leukocyturia that occurs together with leukocyte casts is an indication of involvement of the renal parenchyma.

Different clinical presumptive diagnoses are made depending on whether the leukocyturia is accompanied by the positive detection of pathogens (bacteria, viruses, fungi, protozoa), proteinuria, or an active urinary sediment (with erythrocyturia, casts).

Sterile leukocyturia (no positive bacteriological findings) is suggestive of genitourinary tuberculosis or adenovirus cystitis, a foreign body in the bladder, analgesic nephropathy (in the presence of tubular proteinuria), or – in rare cases – Kawasaki syndrome. Vulvitis, balanitis, and urolithiasis must be ruled out.

▶ Figure 4.29 shows the procedure for established leukocyturia.

With a positive leukocyte finding ($> 10 \times 10^6$/L) and simultaneous hematuria, proteinuria differentiation facilitates distinguishing between renal origins with no visible bacteriuria (analgesic nephropathy, chronic pyelonephritis, renal tuberculosis, urolithiasis, nephritis, rapid progressive glomerulonephritis), with bacteriuria (acute pyelonephritis), and postrenal origins (pyelitis,

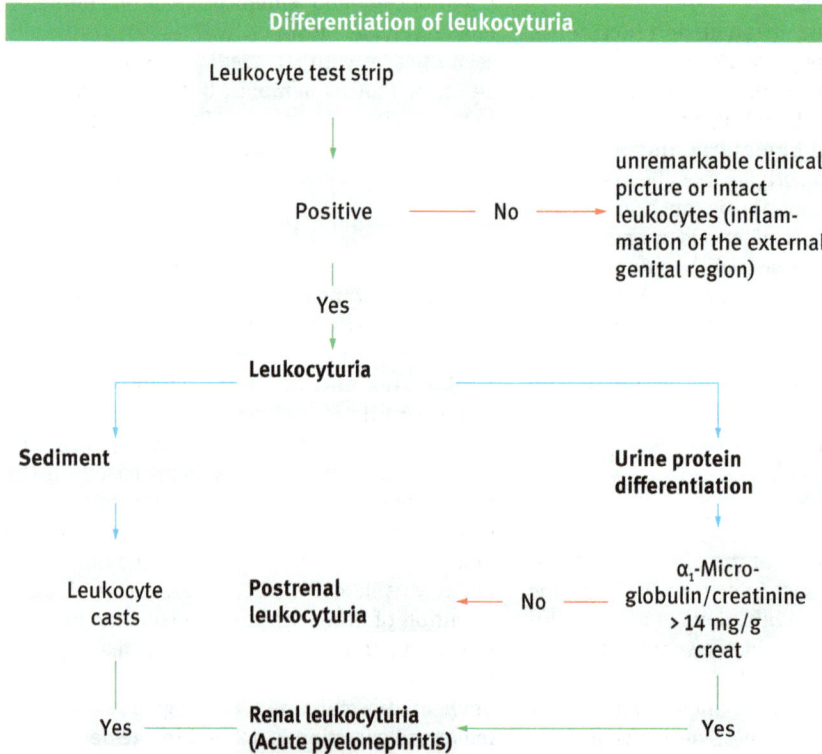

Figure 4.29 Differentiation of leukocyturia.

acute urethritis, cystitis, gonorrhea). Cases of renal origin exhibit a simultaneous increase in the tubular marker α_1-microglobulin, which is absent in cases of urological origin. An exception here would be kidney obstruction due to stones, inflammation of the efferent urinary tract, or prostate enlargement, which would result in increased α_1-microglobulin due elevated intratubular pressure (Everaert, et al., 2000).

Leukocyturia in the absence of hematuria and proteinuria also tends to favor cystitis or renal lymphoma, whereas urogenital TB and analgesic nephropathy are more associated with proteinuria. ▶ Table 4.23 shows the expected diagnoses in bacteria-positive and bacteria-negative leukocyturia cases.

4.4.5.2 Further Diagnostics

Urine microbial counts and the detection of antibacterial substances: The successful detection of bacteriuria requires that antibacterial therapy will have been discontinued for at least three days before the urine test. A microbial count of 10^7/L

(10,000/mL) can be expected with mid-stream and catheter urine, due to contamination. Microbial counts over 100,000/mL for freshly produced midstream urine point to significant bacteriuria. Follow-up monitoring is indicated for counts between 10^7/L and 10^8/L (10,000 and 100,000/mL). Chronic pyelonephritis can be present despite finding a microbial count $< 10^7$/L (10,000/mL), especially if the inflammation foci in the kidney are encapsulated, or if polyuria is present. With a clinical suspicion, further diagnostic clarification (leukocyturia or leukocyte casts) is required. The German Society for Hygiene and Microbiology (DGHM) recommends conducting a test to detect antibacterial substances each time a urine microbial count is made. Even when no inhibitors are expected from consideration of the patient's medication history, antibacterial substances are detected in up to 30 % of urine samples. Failure to detect these can lead to a misinterpretation of the microbial count. Only when the presence of inhibitors can be ruled out with certainty can the microbial count results be used without reservation.

Table 4.23 a, b Differentiation of leukocyturia.

a) Further distinctions in a case of renal hematuria:		
	Bacterial positive	Bacterial negative
Hematuria positive/negative	Acute pyelonephritis	Analgesic nephropathy
	Xanthogranulomatous pyelonephritis	Chronic pyelonephritis
		Urinary tract tuberculosis
		Urolithiasis
		Tubulointerstitial nephritis
		Rapid progressive glomerulonephritis
b) Further distinctions in a case of postrenal leukocyturia:		
	Hematuria positive	Hematuria negative
Bacterial positive	Gonorrhea	Chlamydia
	Cystitis	Urethritis
		Trichomoniasis
		Oxyuriasis
Bacteria positive/negative		Chronic prostatitis
		Urethritis, urolithiasis
Bacterial negative	Bladder diverticulitis	Pyelitis
	Bladder cancer	Acute urethritis
	Polyoma of the urogenital tract	
	Ureteral calculus, bladder stones	

4.4.5.3 Tubulointerstitial Kidney Disorders

Acute tubulointerstitial nephropathy can be distinguished from the chronic forms.

Acute tubulointerstitial nephropathy: This disease can be caused by viruses, bacterial infections and medications. In the foreground is a tubular proteinuria with increased secretion of the tubular marker α_1-microglobulin. An additional established hematuria can be further differentiated through sediment analysis. Acanthocytes have a higher specificity for glomerular diseases than do erythrocyte casts, which are also found in an interstitial nephritis. A typical scenario for hantavirus nephritis is thrombocytopenia with hemorrhage and renal failure.

Chronic tubulointerstitial nephropathy: Analgesic nephropathy is the classic representative of chronic interstitial nephritis. Pathogenetically, a chronic intake of mixed analgesics (acetylsalicylic acid (aspirin, ASA), paracetamol, caffeine) and pyrazolone-containing analgesics will be present. The disease develops after a cumulative intake of 2–5 kg over several years.

Acute and chronic pyelonephritis: Acute tubulointerstitial nephritis can result from a bacterial infection of the upper urinary tract. Dysuria complaints with percussion-sensitive pain in the kidney bed are characteristic symptoms. Leukocyte casts are pathognomonic for pyelonephritis. The pattern of protein excretion with tubular proteinuria (α_1-microglobulin) points to the genesis of the disease. It is not possible to differentiate between acute pyelonephritis and an acute episode of a chronic pyelonephritis (Scherberich, 2010).

4.4.6 Implementation of the Diagnostic Pathways in a Hospital and Laboratory Information System (HIS, LIS)

The present decision tree (▶ Figure 4.30) enables the launch of the diagnostic pathway in the laboratory computer or the hospital information system by means of the Order Entry system (paperless requests for laboratory tests). Input to the system can take the form of a symptom, e.g., clarification hematuria, or a question: "Rule out kidney disease". The result will be an annotated finding, such as "Renal hematuria is present" or "No

evidence of kidney disease", which ultimately represents the result from the diagnostic pathway. The graphical representation of the pathway enables the user to see immediately what tests were used, and understand how the final findings were obtained.

Literature

Antunes VV, Veronese FJ, Morales JV. Diagnostic accuracy of the protein/creatinine ratio in urine samples to estimate 24-h proteinuria in patients with primary glomerulopathies: a longitudinal study. Nephrol Dial Transplant. 2008; 23: 2242–6.

Atlas des Harnsediments CD-ROM Chronolab, Zug, Schweiz 2003.

Boesken WH, Berg C, Schneider T. Diagnostisches Vorgehen und Verlaufsbeobachtungen bei tubulointerstitiellen Erkrankungen. Nieren-/Hochdruck-Krankheiten 2002; 31: 329–335.

Bonventre JV. Kidney Injury Molecule-1 (KIM-1): A specific and sensitive biomarker of kidney injury. Scand J Clin Lab Invest 2008; 68: S241; 78–83.

Caubet C, Lacroix C, Decramer S, Drube J, Ehrich JHH, Mischak H, Bascands JL, Schanstra JP. Advances in urinary proteome analysis and biomarker discovery in pediatric renal disease. Pediatr Nephrol 2010; 25: 27–35.

Cockcroft DW, Gault MH. Prediction of creatinine clearance from serum creatinine. Nephron. 1976; 16: 31–41.

Decavele A, Dhondt L, De Buyzere ML, Delanghe JR. Increased urinary neutrophil gelatinase associated lipocalin in urinary tract infections and leukocyturia. Clin Chem Lab Med 2011; 49: 999–1003.

Decramer S, de Peredo AG, Breuil B, Mischak H, Monsarrat B Bascands JL, Schanstra JP. Urine in clinical Proteomics. Mol Cell Proteomics 2008; 7: 1850–1862.

Delanghe JR. How to establish glomerular filtration rate in children. Scan J Clin Lab Invest 2008; S241: 46–51.

Dettli L. Drug dosage in renal disease. Clin Pharmacokinet. 1976; 1: 126–34.

Devarajan P. Neutrophil gelatinase- associated lipocalin (NGAL): A new marker of kidney disease Scand J Clin Lab Invest 2008; 68: S241; 89–94.

Drube J, Schiffer E, Mischak H, Kemper MJ, Neuhaus T, Pape L, Lichtinghagen R, Ehrich JHH. Urinary proteome pattern in children with renal Fanconi syndrome. Nephrol Dial Transplant 2009; 24: 2161–2169.

Drube J, Zurbig P, Schiffer E, Lau E, Ure B, Gluer S, Kirschstein M, Pape L, Decramer S, Bascands JL, Schanstra JP, Mischak H, Ehrich JHH. Urinary proteome analysis identifies infants but not older children requiring pyeloplasty. Pediatr Nephrol 2010; 25: 1673–1678.

Everaert K, Hoebecke P, Delange J. A review on urinary proteins in outflow disease of the upper urinary tract. Clin Chim Acta 2000; 297: 183–9.

Filler G, Huang S-HS, Yain A. The usefulness of cystatin C and related formulae in pediatrics. Clin Chem lab Med 2012; 50: 2081–91.

Fogazzi GB, Ponticelli C, Ritz E. The Urinary Sediment, An Integrated View. 2nd ed. Oxford University Press 1999.

Froissart M, Rossert J, Jacquot C, Paillard M, Houillier P. Predictive performance of the modification of diet in renal disease and Cockcroft-Gault equations for estima ting renal function. J Am Soc Nephrol. 2005; 16: 763–73.

Ginsberg JM, Chang BS, Matarese RA, Garella S. Use of single voided urine samples to estimate quantitative proteinuria. N Engl J Med. 1983 22; 309: 1543–6.

Good DM, Zurbig P, Argiles A Bauer HW, Behrens G, Coon JJ, et al. Naturally occurring human urinary peptides for use in diagnosis of chronic kidney disease. Mol Cell Proteomics 2010 Nov. 9 (11) 2424–37.

Grubb A, Nyman U, Bjork J. Improved estimation of glomerular filtration rate (GFR) by comparison of eGFRcystatin C and eGRFcreatinine. Scan J Lab Invest (2012) 723 (1): 73–77.

Guder WG, da Fonseca Wollheim F, Heil W, Schmitt Y, Topfer G, Wisser H, Zawta B. Die Qualität diagnostischer Proben. Empfehlungen der Arbeitsgruppe Präanalytik der Deutschen Vereinten Gesellschaft für Klinische Chemie und Laboratoriumsmedizin. 7. Auflage, BD Heidelberg 2012.

Guder WG. Harnstatus (visuelle Betrachtung und Teststreifen und ggf. Harnsediment). In Guder WG, Nolte J. Das Laborbuch für Klinik und Praxis. Munchen Elsevier, Urban und Fischer 2. Aufl. 2009, pp 811–814.

Han PY, Duffull SB, Kirkpatrick CM, Green B. Dosing in obesity: a simple solution to a big problem. Clin Pharmacol Ther. 2007; 82: 505–8.

Haubitz M, Wittke S, Weissinger EM, Walden M, Rupprecht HD, Floege J, Haller H, Mischak H. Urine protein patterns can serve as diagnostic tools in patients with IgA nephropathy. Kidney Int 2005; 67: 2313–20.

Herget-Rosenthal St., Bokenkamp A. Hofmann W. How to estimate GFR-serum creatinine, serum cystatin C or equations? Clin. Biochem 2007; 40; 153–61.

Hofmann W, Aufenanger J, Renz H. Diagnostische Pfade – ein Ansatz zur Verbesserung klinischer Ablaufe? Klinikarzt 2009; 38: 264–5.

Hofmann W, Edel H, Guder W. G., Ivandic M, Scherberich J. E. Harnuntersuchungen zur differenzierten Diagnostik einer Proteinurie. Dtsch Arztebl 2001; 98: 756–763 (B637–B644).

Hofman W, Garbrecht M, Bradwell AR, Guder WG. A new concept for detection of Bence Jones proteinuria in patients with monoclonal nephropathy. Clin Lab 2004; 50: 181–5.

Hofmann W, Guder WG, Garbrecht M. Cystatin C as GFR marker in patients with monoclonal gammopathy, J Lab Med 2002; 26: 513.

Hofmann W, Ruth D, Guder WG. Urine protein differentiation and Protis, a new expert system for its interpretation. Riv Med lab-JLM 2003; 4: 67–8.

Hofmann W, Schmolke M. Niere und ableitende Harnwege, in Renz H.: Praktische Labordiagnostik., 2009 Berlin, Walter de Gruyter-Verlag pp 245–78.

Kamper AL. The importance of a correct evaluation of progression in studies on chronic kidney disease. Nephrol Dial Transplant. 2007; 22: 3–5.

Inker LA, Schmid CH, Tighiouart H, Eckfeldt JH, Feldman HI, Greene T, et al. Estimating glomerular filtration rate from serum creatinine and cystatin C. New Engl J Med 2012; 367: 20–9.

Kouri T, Fogazzi G, Gant V, Hallander H, Hofmann W, Guder WG. European Urinalysis Guidelines. Scand J Clin Lab Invest 2000; 60; Suppl 231.

Levey AS, Coresh J, Greene T, et al. Expressing the Modification of Diet in Renal Disease Study equation for estimating glomerular filtration rate with standardized serum creatinine values. Clin Chem 2007; 53: 766–72.

Levey AS, Eckardt KU, Tsukamoto Y, Levin A, Coresh J, Rossert J, et al. Definition and classification of chronic kidney disease: a position statement from Kidney Disease: Improving Global Outcomes (KDIGO). Kidney Int. 2005; 67: 2089–100.

Levey AS, Stevens LA, Schmid CH, Zhang YL, Castro AF 3rd, Feldman HI, et al. CKD-EPI (Chronic Kidney Disease Epidemiology Collaboration). A new equation to estimate glomerular filtration rate. Ann Intern Med. 2009; 150: 604–12.

Matsushita K, Mahmoodi BK, Wooward M, Emberson JR, Jafar TH et. al. Chronic Kidney Disease Prognosis Consortium. Comparison of risk prediction estimated glomerular filtration rate. JAMA, 2012; 307: 1941–51

Mischak H, Allmaier G, Apweiler R, Attwood T, Baumann M, Benigni A et al. Recommendations for biomarker identification and qualification in clinical proteomics. Sci Transl Med. 2010; 2: 46ps42.

Murray PT, Devarajan P, Levey AS, Eckardt KU, Bonventre JV, Lombardi R, Herget-Rosenthal S, Levin A. A framework and key research questions in AKI diagnosis and staging in different environments. Clin J Am Soc Nephrol. 2008 May; 3(3): 864–8.

Myers GL. Standardization of serum creatinine measurement: Theory and practice. Scand J Clin Lab Invest 2008; Suppl 241: 57–63

Nejat M, Pickering JW, Walker RJ, Endre ZH. Rapid detection of acute tubular injury. Nephrol Dial Transplant 2010; 25: 3283–9.

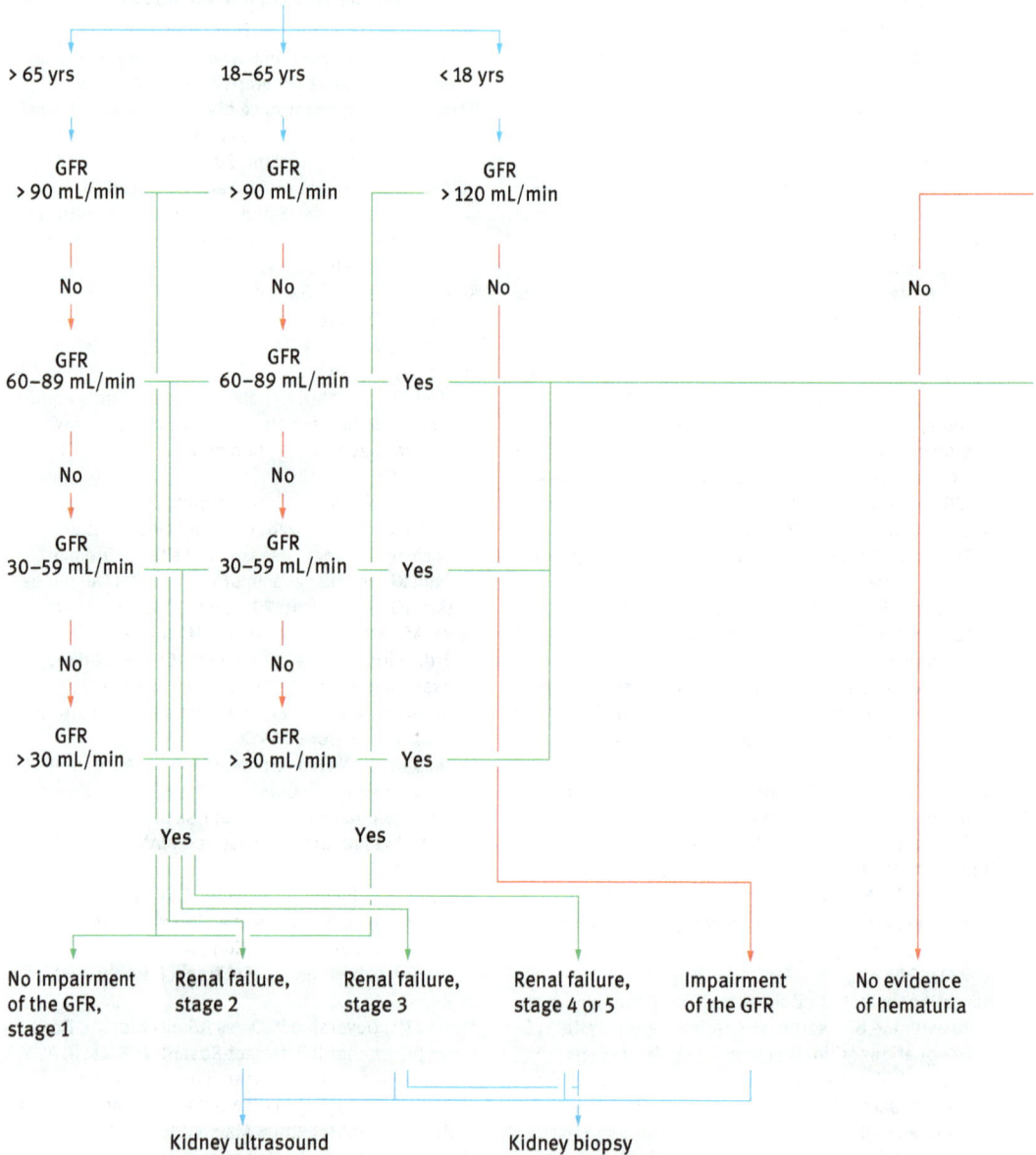

Figure 4.30 Decision tree for the kidney diagnostic pathway in a hospital information system (A. von Meyer, Munich).

Basic diagnostics
Blood count, sodium, potassium, glucose, total protein, albumin, CRP

Test strip (urine)

Test strip (blood)   Test strip (protein)   Test strip (leukocytes)

Positive   Positive   No   Positive   No   Yes

Yes   Yes   Sediment

Sediment   Urine protein quantification and differentiation

Erythrocyte casts

= 0   > 0

α₂-Macroglobulin/ albumin   < 0.02   Total protein 1000 mg/g creat

neg.   > 0.02

Acantho-cytes   pos. > 10%   Yes

Postrenal hematuria   Renal hematuria   see urine protein differentiation finding   No evidence for proteinuria   No evidence for urinary tract infection   Evidence for urinary tract infection

Uroscopy   Kidney biopsy   Microbiological examination of urine

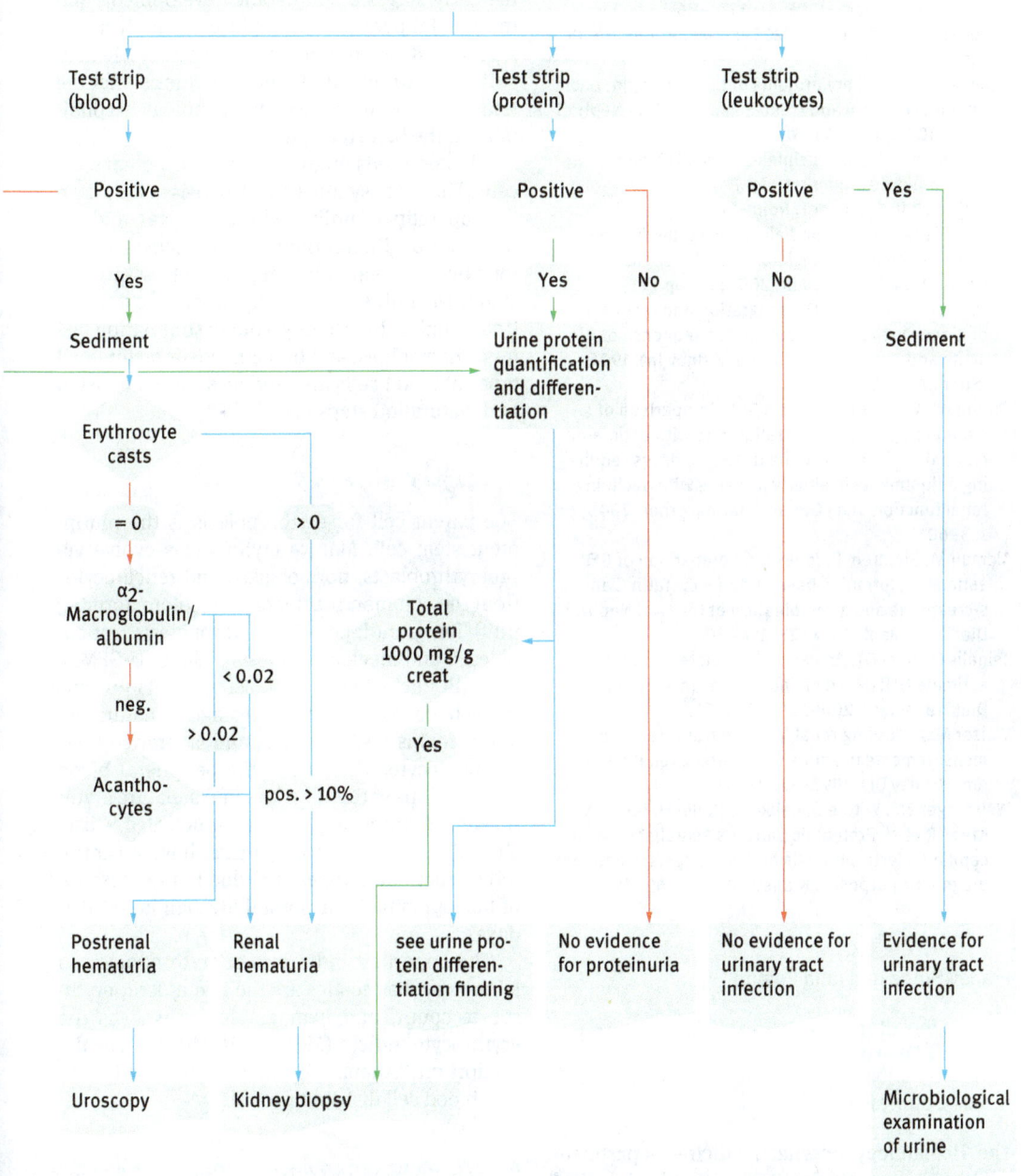

Patel SS, Kimmel PL, Singh A. New clinical practice guidelines for chronic kidney disease: a framework for K/DOQI. Semin Nephrol. 2002; 22: 449–58. Review.

Price CP, Newall RG, Boyd JC. Use of protein: creatinine ratio measurements on random urine samples for prediction of significant proteinuria: a systematic review. Clin Chem. 2005; 51: 1577–86.

Scherberich, JE Proteinurie 2009: www.proteinurie.de (under revision)

Scherberich JE Urinary proteins of tubular origin; basic immunochemical and clinical aspects. Am J Nephrol 1990; 10 Suppl. 1: 43–51.

Scherberich JE: Harnwegsinfektionen 2010: www.harnwegsinfekt.de (under revision)

Scherberich JE, Hammer F, Rolinski B. Impact of chronic renal failure and hemodialysis on serum free polyclonal immunoglobulin kappa/lambda light chains. Nephrol. Dial. Transplant. 2006; 21; pp 22.

Scherberich JE, Wolf G. Disintegration and recovery of kidney membrane proteins: consequence of acute and chronic renal failure. Kidney Int. 1994; (Suppl.47), S52–57.

Spruill WJ, Wade WE, Cobb HH 3rd. Comparison of estimated glomerular filtration rate with estimated creatinine clearance in the dosing of drugs requiring adjustments in elderly patients with declining renal function. Am J Geriatr Pharmacother. 2008; 6: 153–60.

Tidman M, Sjostrom P, Jones I. A Comparison of GFR estimating formulae based upon s-cystatin C and s-creatinine and a combination of the two. Nephrol Dial Transplant. 2008; 23: 154–60.

Tsinalis D, Thiel GT. An easy to calculate equation to estimate GFR based on inulin clearance. Nephrol Dial Transplant. 2009; 24: 3055–61.

Walser M. Assessing renal function from creatinine measurements in adults with chronic renal failure. Am J Kidney Dis. 1998; 32: 23–31.

Weissinger EM, Wittke S, Kaiser T, Haller H, Bartel S, Krebs R et al. Proteomic patterns established with capillary electrophoresis and mass spectrometry for diagnostic purposes. Kidney Int 2004; 65: 2426–34.

Pranav Sinha und Julia Poland

4.5 Hematology – Introduction and Overview

4.5.1 General Hematology

The Hematology internal medicine department deals with physiological and pathophysiological processes in the cellular components of blood (erythrocytes, leukocytes, platelets), hematopoiesis (blood formation), and the blood-forming organs.

Over 95 % of hematopoiesis occurs in the bone marrow, which is distributed throughout the body in the cavities of the bones (medullary hematopoiesis). This takes place in the yolk sac during the early stages of embryonic development, and in the fetal period it takes place in the liver and spleen (extramedullary hematopoiesis). Reactivation of extramedullary hematopoiesis after the fetal period occurs only under pathological conditions in the bone marrow.

All blood cells originate from pluripotent stem cells. Through asymmetric cell division, they have the capability of unlimited self-renewal, and the potential of differentiation and proliferation to form hematopoietic and lymphopoietic stem cells. Under the influence of many different cytokines (interleukins, interferons, colony stimulating factors, chemokines, and tumor necrosis factors), all types of blood cells are produced by cell division and maturation steps.

4.5.1.1 Erythropoiesis

The parent cell for erythropoiesis is the pluripotent stem cell. Mature erythrocytes evolve via proerythroblasts, normoblasts, and reticulocytes from the common precursor cell (colony forming unit) for granulopoiesis, erythropoiesis, monopoiesis, and megakariopoiesis – the CFU-GEMM. The still nucleated normoblast ejects its nucleus in the bone marrow. The next stage of maturation still contains RNA residues, and is referred to as a reticulocyte. This enters the peripheral blood and develops within 1–2 days into a mature erythrocyte. Erythrocytes are non-nucleated, disc-shaped, about 7 microns in size, have a central indentation, and appear red due to the presence of hemoglobin. Their normal lifespan is 100–120 days.

The important indicators of erythropoiesis in laboratory diagnostics are the hematocrit, erythrocyte count, and hemoglobin, as well as the erythrocyte indices (MCV, MCH, MCHC – see the section on "Anemia"), reticulocytes, and RDW (red blood cell distribution width).

4.5.1.2 Megakariopoiesis – Thrombopoiesis

As in the erythropoiesis process, under the influence of thrombopoietin, the pluripotent stem cells (via the CFU-GEMMs) first give rise to mega-karioblasts. From these, mature polyploid mega-karyocytes then develop through multiple DNA replications without nucleus and cell division (endomitosis). The thrombocytes (or platelets) arise through a "pinching off" of discrete portions of the megakaryocyte cytoplasm. Platelets are non-nucleated, 1–4 micrometers in size, and are made up of a delicate blue cytoplasm. Their life span its about 10 days. Approximately one-third of the total platelet population is temporarily (about 36 h) stored in the spleen (the reserve pool).

The measurement most relevant to laboratory diagnostics is the determination of the platelet count; additionally, the immature platelet fraction (IFP) can be used for the differentiation of thrombocytopenia.

4.5.1.3 Leukopoiesis – Generation of Myeloid Cell Lines

Under the influence of the cytokine GM-CSF, the CFU-GEMM hematopoietic stem cell forms the common precursor cell for monocytes and gran-ulocytes. Eos-CSF stimulates the formation of CFU-Eos (which develop into eosinophil granu-locytes), and Baso-CSF triggers the formation of CFU-Baso (from which differentiate the basophil granulocytes).

The neutrophil series is formed under the influence of G-CSF. Myeloblasts, which are the earliest recognizable precursor cells, develop via interme-diate cell types that are still capable of dividing, ultimately to give rise to mature forms that are no longer capable of dividing, the polymorpho-nuclear granulocytes (also known as segmented neutrophils). After being released from the bone marrow, they circulate for 10–20 hours in the blood, and then remain about five more days in the tissues.

The monocyte series is produced under the influence of M-CSF. The precursor cells mature through the monoblast and promonocyte stages into monocytes. These remain for about one day in the bloodstream before they enter the tissues and mature further.

4.5.1.4 Lymphopoiesis

Lymphocytes are immunocompetent cells. They are divided into subgroups: B cells, T cells, and NK cells. They differ in their immunologically detectable surface markers and their functions. Lymphocytes develop from lymphopoietic stem cells in the main formation sites, the bone mar-row for B-cells and the thymus for T-cells. The ma-ture cells remain capable of division, recirculate between the blood and lymph systems, and live in some cases for several years.

4.5.1.5 Hematopoiesis Disorders

Hematopoiesis disorders can result in an increase or decrease in one or more of the cell lineages. Re-active changes (due to infections, stress, trauma, etc.) are to be distinguished from pathological conditions.

Reductions can arise from defective produc-tion in the bone marrow, distribution disorders, or enhanced degradation can have their origin in the peripheral blood.

Examples of defective production of blood cells (or dyspoiesis) include:
- Infectious, toxic bone marrow damage
- Deficiency anemias
- Stem cell mutations with maturation and dif-ferentiation disorder (myelodysplastic syn-dromes)

Examples of distribution disorders include:
- Increased storage of cells in the spleen associ-ated with splenomegaly

Examples of enhanced degradation include:
- Immunologically based (autoantibodies against erythrocytes, platelets, or leukocytes)
- Mechanically based (hemolysis due to an arti-ficial heart valve)

In addition to reactive adaptation processes, causes of overproduction include hematologic neoplasms, which involve clonal propagation of a cell line. The affected (precursor) cells prolifer-ate uncontrollably, and supersede proper hema-topoiesis.

Examples of hematological diseases that give rise to clonal cell proliferation include:
- Acute leukemia
- Myeloproliferative neoplasia
- Lymphomas

4.5.2 Specialized Hematology – Pathologies, Disorders, Diagnosis, Differentiation

4.5.2.1 Anemia

Definition

Anemia is understood to mean a reduction in the hemoglobin concentration: below 13.0 g/dL in men, and below 12.5 g/dL in women. Age-related reference ranges are to be used with children.

The reduction in the hemoglobin concentration can be due to (a) a reduction in the total number of erythrocytes, (b) a decrease in the hemoglobin content of individual red blood cells, or (c) an increase in plasma volume with a resulting relative decrease in erythrocyte mass (= pseudo anemia).

Origins/pathogenesis

Pathogenetically, anemia can have two underlying origins:
- Defective production
  - Deficiency anemias (iron, vitamin B_{12}, or folic acid deficiencies)
  - Toxic damage (alcohol, medications, or poisons)
  - Infectious damage (parvovirus B19)
  - Iron metabolism disorders (anemia of chronic disease, ACD)
  - Erythropoietin deficiency (renal failure)
  - Inefficient erythropoiesis (MDS) and suppression of erythropoiesis (e.g., in leukemia)
- Increase cell destruction/loss
  - Hemolysis (autoantibodies, mechanical, membrane defects, etc. – see section on "Hemolysis")
  - Hemorrhage

Classification of anemias

The classification of anemia is based on the erythrocyte indices (MCV, MCH, MCHC), and the reticulocyte count.

The following two divisions facilitate drawing a rough conclusion on the cause of the anemia:

1. According to erythrocyte volume: The classification according to erythrocyte volume (mean corpuscular volume, MCV) distinguishes between microcytic anemias, normocytic anemias, and macrocytic anemias.

   a) Microcytic (MCV < 78 fL): iron deficiency anemia, anemia of chronic disease, thalassemia, and rare types of anemia (e.g., sideroblastic anemia)
   b) Normocytic: anemia of chronic disease, renal anemia, hepatic anemia, aplastic anemia, mixed deficiency anemia
   c) Macrocytic (MCV > 98 fL): vitamin B_{12}/folic acid deficiency, liver disease, MDS, myeloma, hypothyroidism, hemolytic anemias
2. According to the reticulocyte count:
   a) reduced or normal → hyporegenerative anemia; further differentiation is possible through classification according to MCV
   b) elevated → hyperregenerative anemia; hemolysis, acute hemorrhage, treatment of deficiency anemia

4.5.2.2 Eosinophilia

Definition

Eosinophilia is understood to mean an elevation of eosinophilic granulocytes in the peripheral blood. Eosinophilia measured at > 0.7 × 10^9/L requires clarification.

The eosinophilic granulocyte contains numerous granules in its cytoplasm. When activated, these release inflammatory mediators. They elicit inflammatory reactions, but also produce tissue damage. An eosinophil count of 10–20 × 10^9/L in the peripheral blood can already lead to organ dysfunction due to the tissue damage, especially in the presence of cardiac problems.

Origins

- Medications:
  - Antibiotics, neuroleptics, antidepressants, heparins, antidiabetics, chemotherapeutic agents, aspirin, and NSAIDs
  - DRESS syndrome" drug rash with eosinophilia and systemic symptoms; especially anticonvulsive drugs (phenytoin, carbamazepine), sulfonamides (cotrimoxazole), antiretroviral medications (abacavir), minocycline, allopurinol.
  - During a withdrawal attempt, normalization should occur within 10 days
- Allergies: allergy medical history
- Parasites: History of travel abroad

- Helminthic diseases (toxocariasis, filariasis, trichinellosis, schistosomiasis, hookworms, ascariasis, fascioliasis, taeniasis, echinococcosis)
- Immunological disorders
  - Check for the presence of indicative general symptoms
  - Churg-Strauss vasculitis, polyarteritis nodosa, SLE, sarcoidosis
- Malignant tumors:
  - Up to 60 % of neoplasms are associated with eosinophilia: solid tumors, hematological diseases
- Endocrinological origins
  - Adrenocortical insufficiency
- Chronic eosinophilic leukemia (CEL)/hypereosinophilic syndrome
  - In a non-reactive eosinophilia that persists longer than six months, a FIP1L1-PDGFRA rearrangement test should be performed.

The **most common** origins in the Western world are medication- and allergy-related eosinophilia, while world-wide it is parasitic eosinophilia.

A **thorough examination procedure** to clarify an eosinophilia, in addition to the medical history, current status, and laboratory tests, involves diagnostic imaging methods, especially echocardiography for detecting organ involvement and dysfunctions.

4.5.2.3 Hemolysis

Definition

Hemolysis refers to the release of intracellular components from blood cells (particularly red blood cells) into the extracellular space.

Shortening of the erythrocyte survival time results in an *in vivo* hemolysis, the magnitude of which depends on the capacity of the degradation sites (e.g., in the spleen) and the level of injury sustained by individual erythrocytes. This resulting free hemoglobin is rapidly bound by haptoglobin and eliminated from the circulation.

Erythropoiesis in the bone marrow increases to compensate for hemolysis. If the destruction of red blood cells outweighs their formation (usually this only occurs with a red blood cell survival time of < 20 days), anemia occurs with decreases in hemoglobin and hematocrit. Depending on the site of degradation, a distinction can be made between intravascular (within the blood vessels) and extravascular (outside the blood vessels, by macrophages of the reticuloendothelial system) forms.

This is different from the *in vitro* hemolysis that is a widespread preanalytical problem in laboratory analyses.

Origins

- Immune hemolysis (common cause of hemolysis)
  - Autoimmune hemolytic anemia: caused by autoantibodies to components of the red cell membrane (approximately 80 % warm autoantibodies, about 15 % cold autoantibodies, about 5 % Donath-Landsteiner hemolysin), primary are distinguished from secondary, e.g., through infections, autoimmune diseases, lymphomas or other malignancies, autoimmune hemolyses
  - Drug-induced hemolytic anemia
  - Alloantibody hemolytic anemia (transfusion reaction, hemolytic disease of the newborn)
  - Acute postinfectious hemolytic anemia
- Corpuscular defects
  - Hemoglobinopathies (quantitative abnormalities, such as in α- and β-thalassemias, and qualitative defects, for example, such as in sickle cell anemia, HbC, HbE); clarification is performed primarily through separation of the Hb fractions, and in some cases (e.g., α-thalassemia) a genetic analysis must be conducted.
  - Membrane defects (congenital: spherocytosis, elliptocytosis; and acquired: PNH = paroxysmal nocturnal hemoglobinuria); clarification in the case of spherocytosis focuses on the reduced osmotic resistance of erythrocytes (if necessary, genetic analysis), and in the case of PNH involves the flow cytometric analysis of GPI-anchored molecules.
  - Enzyme defects (most common: glucose-6-phosphate dehydrogenase deficiency and pyruvate kinase); clarification involves the measurement of enzyme activity (if necessary, genetic analysis)
- Vitamin B_{12}, folic acid deficiency
- Infectious origin
  - Viral, bacterial, parasitic

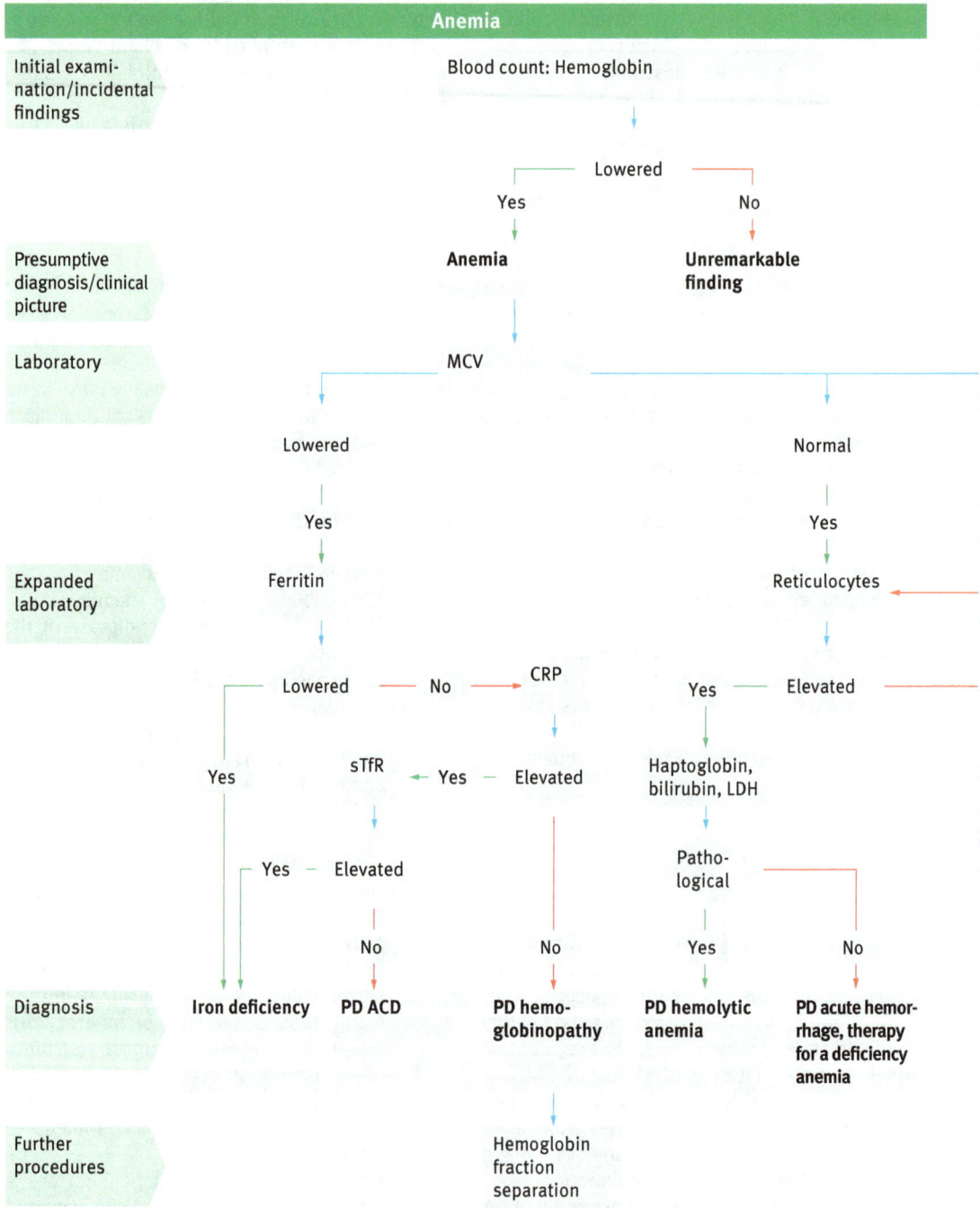

Anemia

| Initial examination/incidental findings | Blood count: Hemoglobin |

Lowered

Yes — No

| Presumptive diagnosis/clinical picture | **Anemia** — **Unremarkable finding** |

| Laboratory | MCV |

Lowered — Normal

Yes — Yes

| Expanded laboratory | Ferritin — Reticulocytes |

Lowered — No → CRP — Yes — Elevated

Yes — sTfR ← Yes — Elevated — Haptoglobin, bilirubin, LDH

Yes — Elevated — Patho-logical

No — No — Yes — No

| Diagnosis | **Iron deficiency** | **PD ACD** | **PD hemo-globinopathy** | **PD hemolytic anemia** | **PD acute hemorrhage, therapy for a deficiency anemia** |

| Further procedures | Hemoglobin fraction separation |

Figure 4.31 Note: these stepwise diagrams are kept relatively simple for reasons of clarity; they serve as an aid for making a diagnosis, and can be used as guidance for a majority of patients. However, in individual cases and especially when several concomitant diseases are present with complicated constellations of laboratory parameters or with laboratory parameters trending in opposite directions, deviations from this predetermined scheme must be considered.

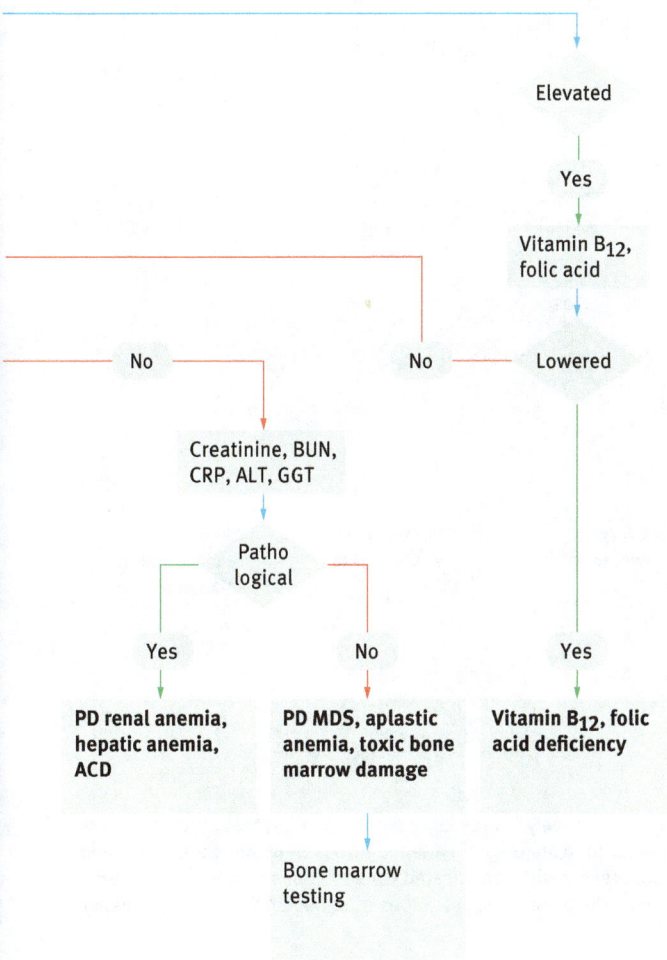

Elevated

Yes

Vitamin B$_{12}$, folic acid

No   No   Lowered

Creatinine, BUN, CRP, ALT, GGT

Patho logical

Yes   No   Yes

PD renal anemia, hepatic anemia, ACD

PD MDS, aplastic anemia, toxic bone marrow damage

Vitamin B$_{12}$, folic acid deficiency

Bone marrow testing

Eosinophilia		

Initial examination/incidental findings

Blood count: Eosinophils > 0.7 × 10⁹/L

No   Yes

Presumptive diagnosis/clinical picture

Unremarkable finding   **Eosinophilia**

Laboratory

Total IgE   Specific IgE   Stool examination
Serological examination
Autoantibody diagnostics

ANA, RF, pANCA, cANCA, C3, C4

Patho-logical   Patho-logical   Patho-logical

Expanded laboratory

Yes   Yes   Yes

Diagnosis

Allergic eosinophilia   **Parasitic eosinophilia**   **Systemic autoimmune disease**

Further procedures

Rule out medication-based origins

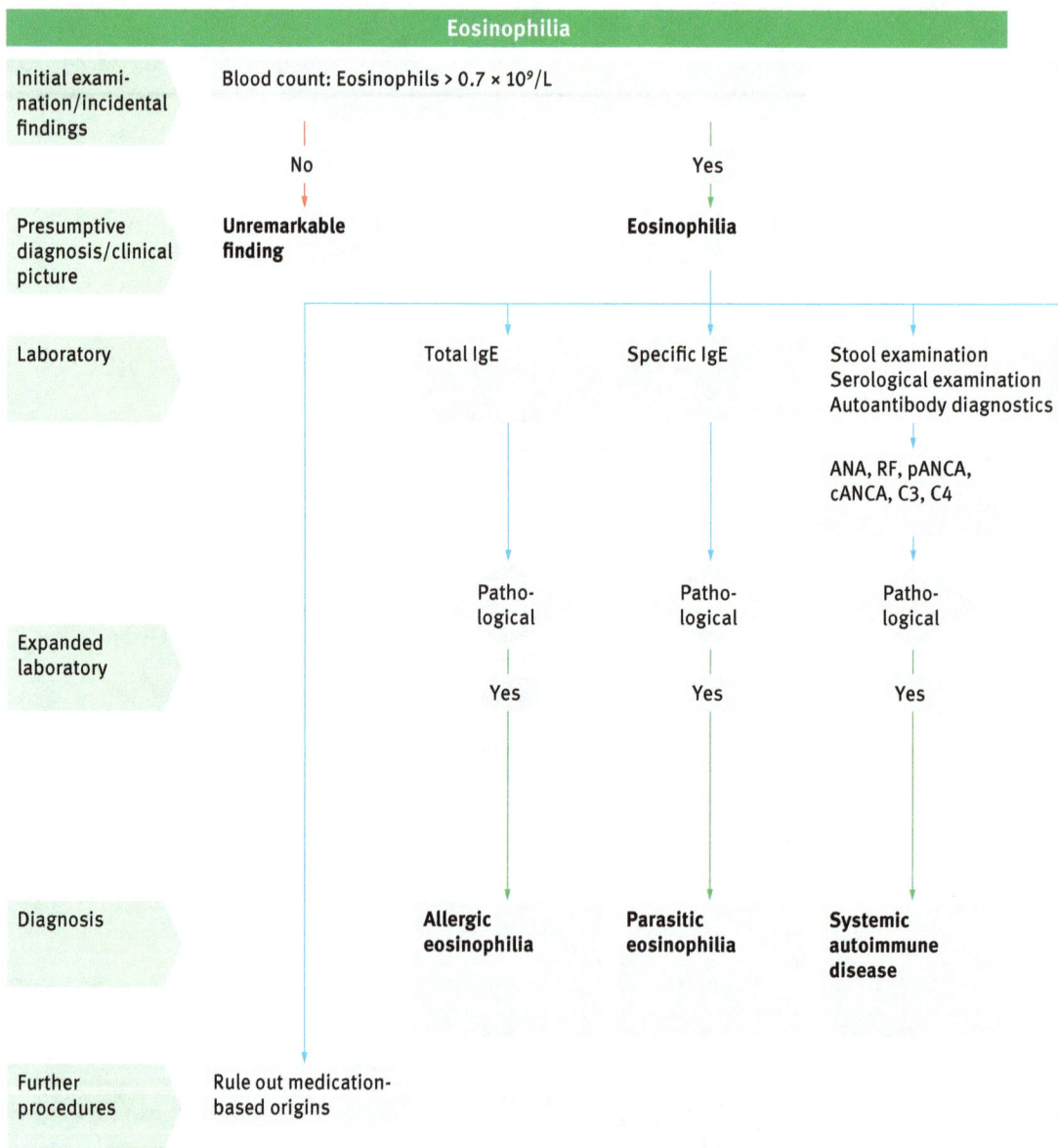

Figure 4.32 Note: these stepwise diagrams are kept relatively simple for reasons of clarity; they serve as an aid for making a diagnosis, and can be used as guidance for a majority of patients. However, in individual cases and especially when several concomitant diseases are present with complicated constellations of laboratory parameters or with laboratory parameters trending in opposite directions, deviations from this predetermined scheme must be considered.

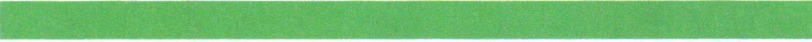

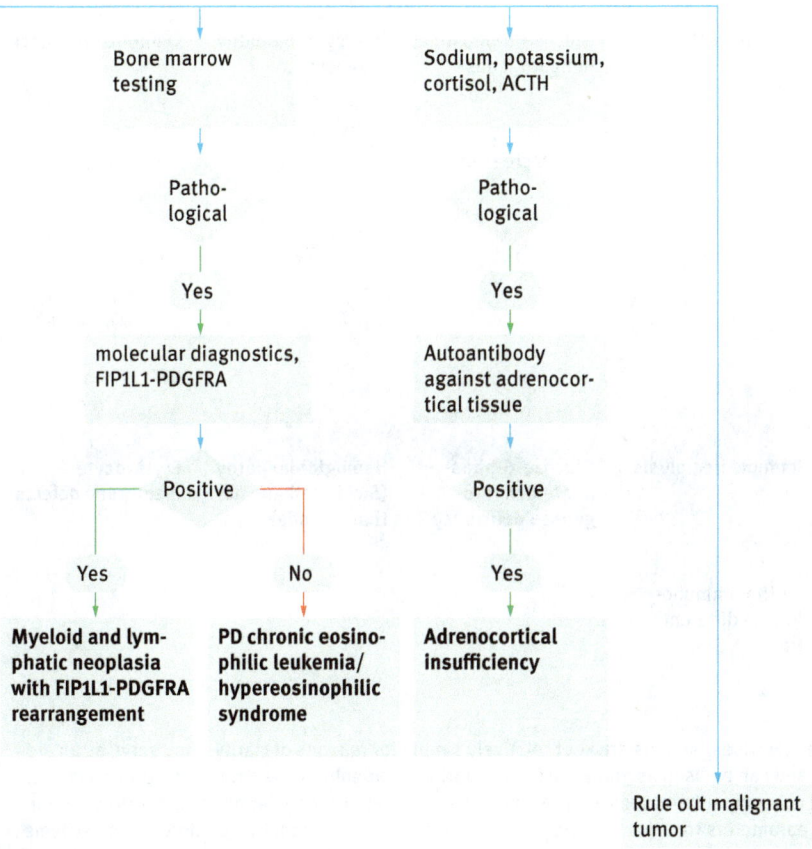

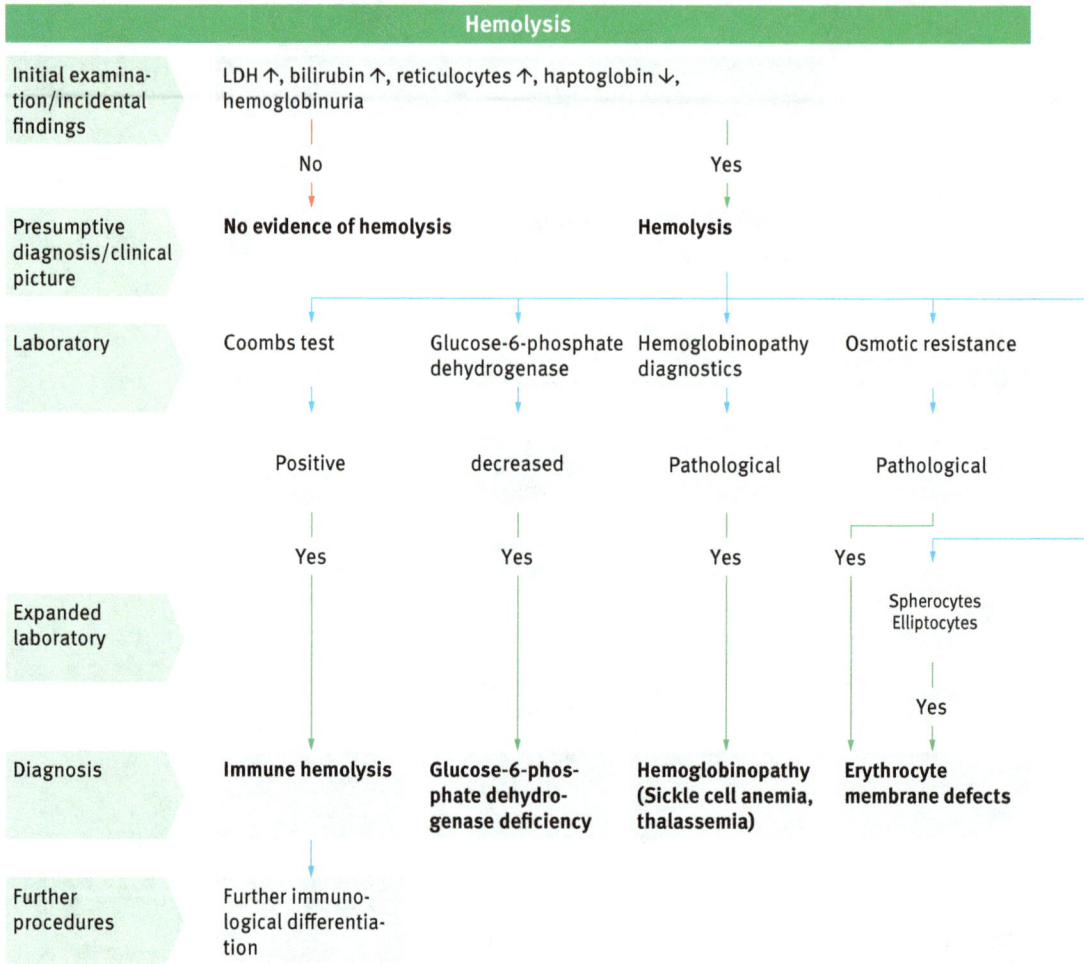

	Hemolysis			
Initial examination/incidental findings	LDH ↑, bilirubin ↑, reticulocytes ↑, haptoglobin ↓, hemoglobinuria			
	No		Yes	
Presumptive diagnosis/clinical picture	**No evidence of hemolysis**		**Hemolysis**	
Laboratory	Coombs test	Glucose-6-phosphate dehydrogenase	Hemoglobinopathy diagnostics	Osmotic resistance
	Positive	decreased	Pathological	Pathological
	Yes	Yes	Yes	Yes
Expanded laboratory				Spherocytes Elliptocytes
				Yes
Diagnosis	**Immune hemolysis**	**Glucose-6-phosphate dehydrogenase deficiency**	**Hemoglobinopathy (Sickle cell anemia, thalassemia)**	**Erythrocyte membrane defects**
Further procedures	Further immunological differentiation			

Figure 4.33 Note: these stepwise diagrams are kept relatively simple for reasons of clarity; they serve as an aid for making a diagnosis, and can be used as guidance for a majority of patients. However, in individual cases and especially when several concomitant diseases are present with complicated constellations of laboratory parameters or with laboratory parameters trending in opposite directions, deviations from this predetermined scheme must be considered.

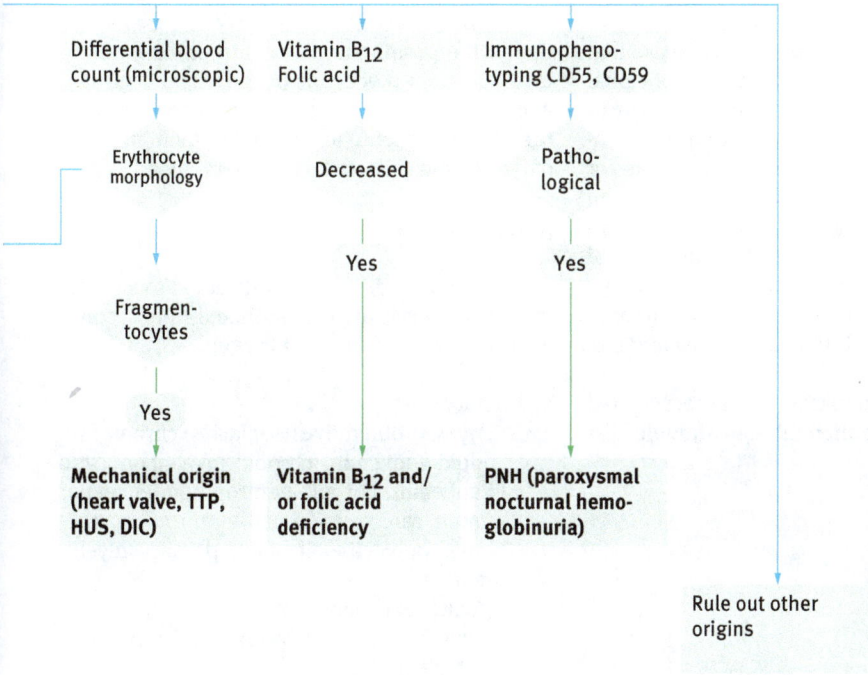

Differential blood count (microscopic)

Erythrocyte morphology

Fragmentocytes

Yes

Mechanical origin (heart valve, TTP, HUS, DIC)

Vitamin B_{12}
Folic acid

Decreased

Yes

Vitamin B_{12} and/ or folic acid deficiency

Immunophenotyping CD55, CD59

Pathological

Yes

PNH (paroxysmal nocturnal hemoglobinuria)

Rule out other origins

- Mechanical hemolysis
  - This involves mechanical intravascular destruction of red blood cells in the capillaries through microthrombi (e.g., TTP, HUS, DIC) or due to artificial structures (e.g., heart valves) in arterial vascular system.

4.5.2.4 Monoclonal Gammopathy

Definition

Monoclonal gammopathy refers to a disease that is accompanied by a proliferation of monoclonal immunoglobulins or fragments thereof (light or heavy chains). It is caused by uncontrolled proliferation of immunocompetent B lymphocytes or plasma cells. The proteins that are more common in the context of a monoclonal gammopathy include: complete immunoglobulin molecules of one class and one type, kappa- or lambda-type free light chains, and a combination of immunoglobulin molecules and free light chains and free heavy chains.

Monoclonal gammopathy can be associated with a number of malignant hematologic diseases:
- MGUS
- Multiple myeloma
- Amyloidosis
- Lymphoma

Clarification

The diagnostic pathway proceeds by carrying out a serum electrophoresis, if clinical symptoms (e.g. renal failure [RF], bone pain, osteolyses) or laboratory abnormalities (hypercalcemia, anemia, persistent ESR increase, or abnormal immunoglobulin level increase or decrease) are shown. With an unremarkable electrophoresis result but strong clinical suspicion of monoclonal gammopathy, an immunofixation in the serum and urine and the determination of free light chains in serum should nevertheless be carried out.

MGUS (monoclonal gammopathy of undetermined significance) is used to describe asymptomatic patients with a low M gradient (< 30 g/L), plasma cell count in the bone marrow < 10 %, and without end-organ involvement (CRAB: hypercalcemia, renal dysfunction, anemia, and lytic bone lesions); this clonal process is not deemed to be clearly neoplastic, since not all cases transform into neoplasia. In any case, these patients should be monitored continuously.

4.5.2.5 Leukocytosis

Definition

Leukocytosis is understood to mean an increase of leukocytes in the peripheral blood to $>10 \times 10^9/L$. The increased number of cells is frequently due to the proliferation of neutrophilic granulocytes and their precursors (reactive leukocytosis), and can also be caused by blast proliferation in the context of acute leukemias, or by high levels of lymphoma cells in the peripheral blood.

Origins

Primary origins that can be attributed to a defect in hematopoiesis are discriminated from secondary origins caused by other triggers.

- Primary origins:
  - Myeloproliferative neoplasias: chronic myeloid leukemia, chronic myelomonocytic leukemia, chronic neutrophilic leukemia; more rarely, in essential thrombocythemia, polycythemia vera, primary myelofibrosis
  - Acute leukemia
  - Lymphoma (see "Clarification of Lymphocytosis")
- Secondary (= reactive) origins:
  - Neutrophilia: acute infections, stress, trauma, noninfectious inflammation, acute hemorrhage, acute hemolysis, pregnancy, smoking, diabetes mellitus, renal failure, drugs (glucocorticoids, cortisone), Cushing syndrome
  - Lymphocytosis: (see section 4.5.2.6)
  - Monocytosis: certain infections, postinfection recovery period, rheumatic diseases, granulomatous diseases, drugs

Clarification

The diagnostic pathway always proceeds on the basis of an automated differential blood count, possibly with further microscopic differentiation. In most cases, secondary origins can be elucidated based on the medical and clinical history.

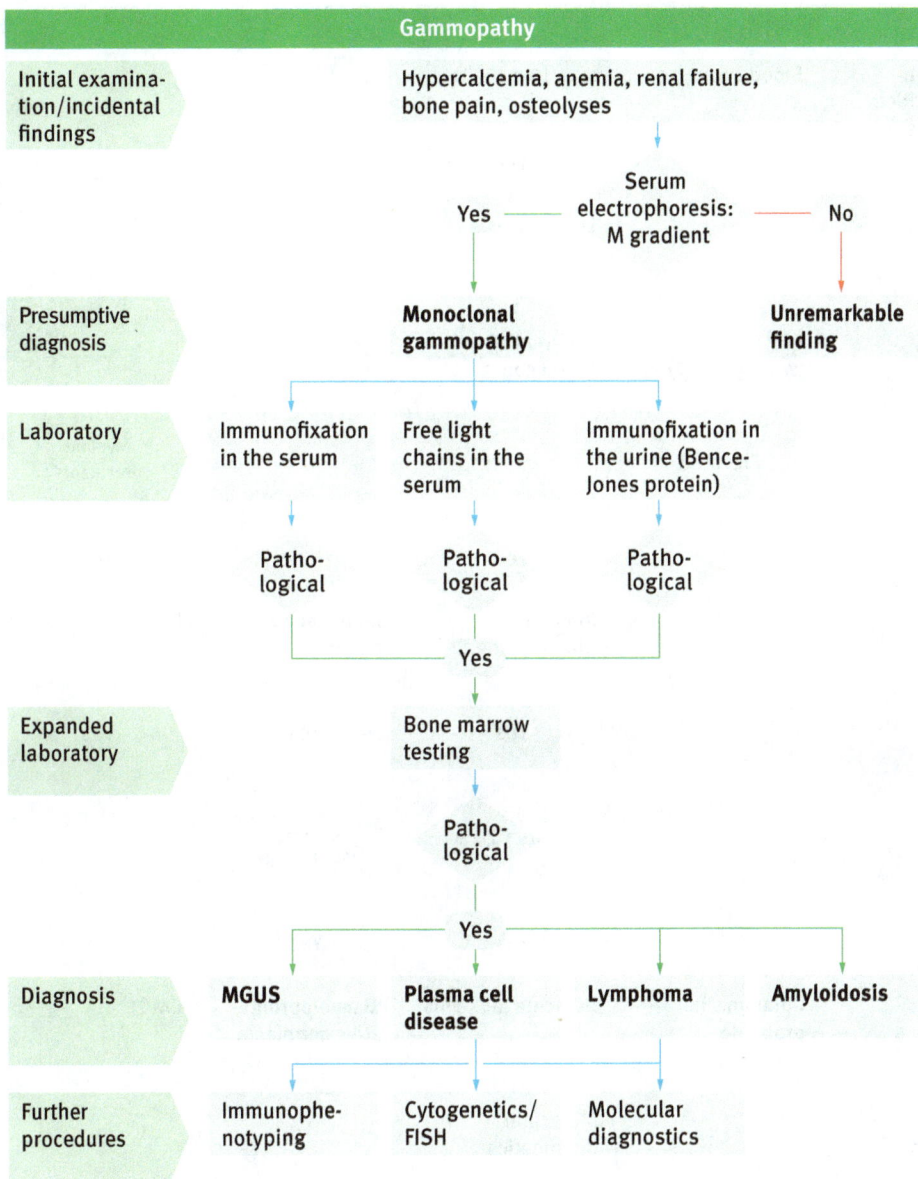

Figure 4.34 Note: these stepwise diagrams are kept relatively simple for reasons of clarity; they serve as an aid for making a diagnosis, and can be used as guidance for a majority of patients. However, in individual cases and especially when several concomitant diseases are present with complicated constellations of laboratory parameters or with laboratory parameters trending in opposite directions, deviations from this predetermined scheme must be considered.

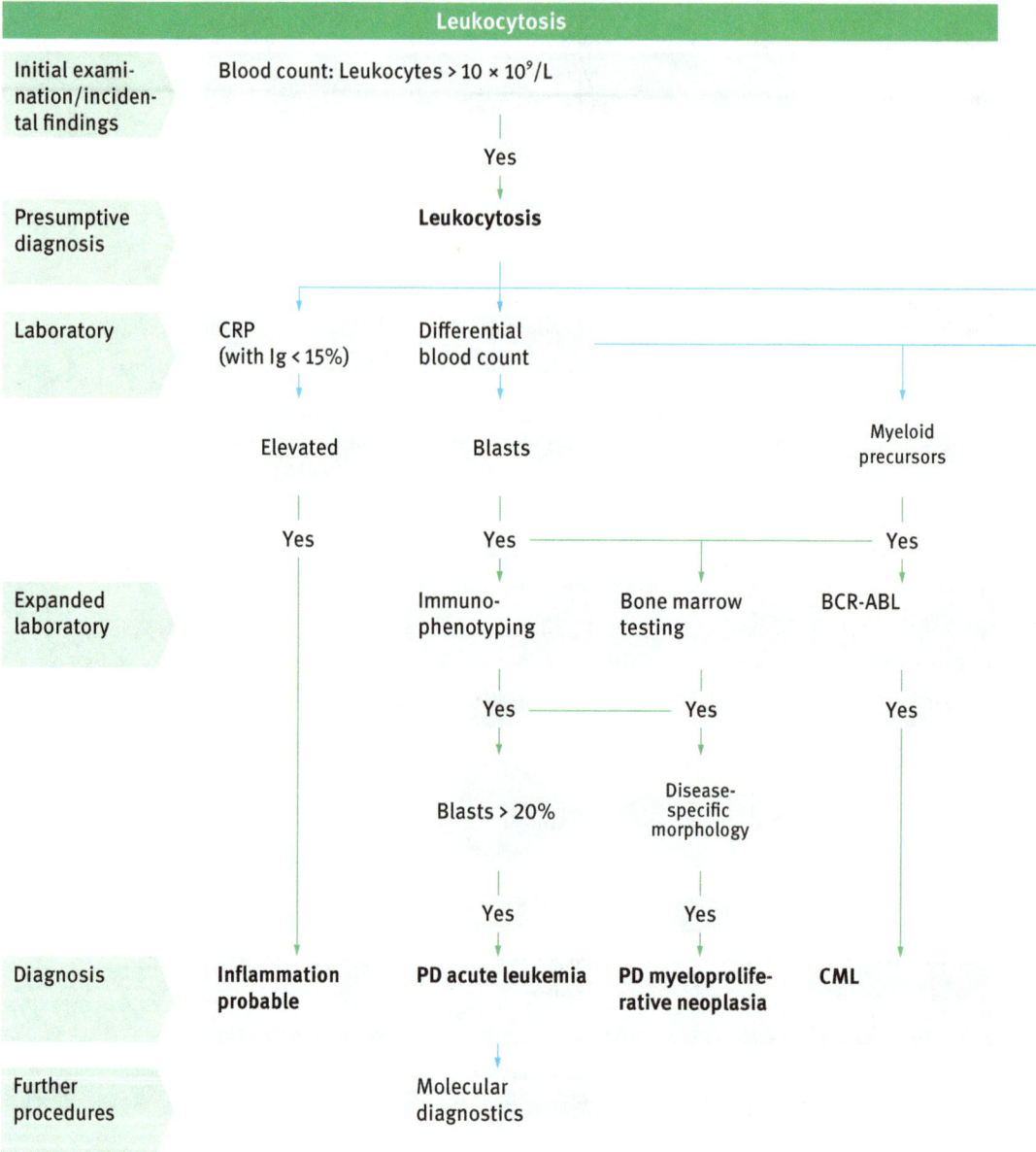

	Leukocytosis			
Initial exami-nation/inciden-tal findings	Blood count: Leukocytes > 10×10^9/L			
	Yes			
Presumptive diagnosis	**Leukocytosis**			
Laboratory	CRP (with Ig < 15%)	Differential blood count		Myeloid precursors
	Elevated	Blasts		
	Yes	Yes	Yes	Yes
Expanded laboratory		Immuno-phenotyping	Bone marrow testing	BCR-ABL
		Yes	Yes	Yes
		Blasts > 20%	Disease-specific morphology	
		Yes	Yes	
Diagnosis	**Inflammation probable**	**PD acute leukemia**	**PD myeloprolife-rative neoplasia**	**CML**
Further procedures		Molecular diagnostics		

Figure 4.35 Note: these stepwise diagrams are kept relatively simple for reasons of clarity; they serve as an aid for making a diagnosis, and can be used as guidance for a majority of patients. However, in individual cases and especially when several concomitant diseases are present with complicated constellations of laboratory parameters or with laboratory parameters trending in opposite directions, deviations from this predetermined scheme must be considered.

Primary origins are differentiated by means of flow cytometry immunophenotyping, molecular genetic detection of mutations, and through bone marrow tests.

4.5.2.6 Lymphocytosis

Definition

Absolute lymphocytosis means a proliferation in the absolute number of lymphocytes in the peripheral blood (age-dependent reference ranges).

In addition to the clinical history, the microscopic differential blood count supports the diagnosis.

The presence of reactive lymphocytes (microscopy: pleomorphic forms) indicates a secundary origin for the lymphocytosis, particularly caused by viral diseases, but also by drug-induced, endocrinological and autoimmune diseases.

The presence of many monomorphic lymphocytes (often in conjunction with smudge cells) suggests the presence of a monoclonal lymphocyte population, and thus a lymphoma. This can be detected by immunophenotyping using monoclonal antibodies (especially in the case of B-cell lymphoma). Lymphatic blasts that are mistakenly differentiated as lymphocytes in the automated differential blood count usually attract attention under microscopic examination, and raise a suspicion of acute leukemia.

Origins

- Infections:
  - Mononucleosis syndrome: EBV, CMV, *Toxoplasma gondii*, HIV, HSV, VZV, hepatitis virus, rubella virus, adenovirus
  - Chronic infections: brucellosis, tuberculosis, syphilis
- Hematological neoplasias
  - Lymphoma
  - Acute lymphatic leukemias
  - Special types: Persistent polyclonal B-lymphocytosis
- Medications
- Stress lymphocytosis:
  - e.g., cardiovascular collapse, post-traumatic, postoperative
- Autoimmune disorders
- Malignant tumors
- Endocrine disorders

Lymphocytes
↑

Yes

Rule out reactive origins

see section on "Lymphocytosis"

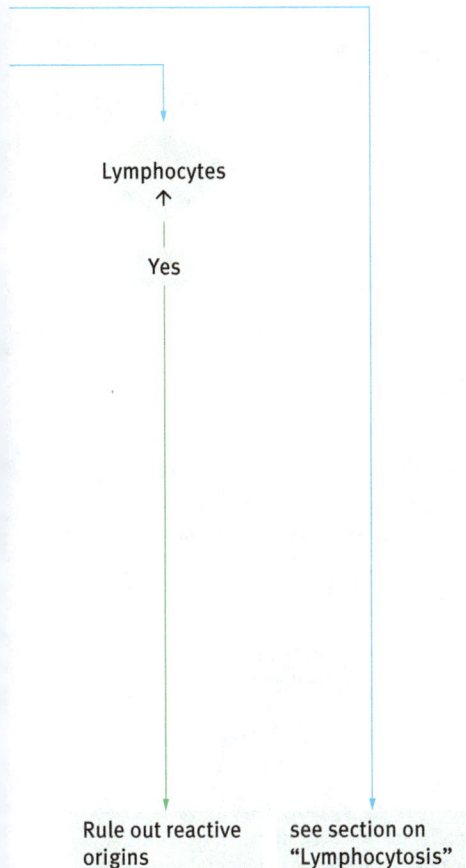

Lymphocytosis

Initial examination/incidental findings	Blood count: Lymphocytes > reference range [absolute]

Yes

Presumptive diagnosis	**Absolute lymphocytosis**

Laboratory	Differential blood count

	Lymphatic irritation patterns		Blasts	Monomorphic lymphocytes	Bilobed lymphocytes
Expanded laboratory	Serology (EBV, CMV, HIV, etc.)		Bone marrow testing	Immunophenotypingt	Immunophenotypingt
	Positive		Pathological	Pathological	Pathological
	Yes	No	Yes	Yes	Yes
Diagnosis	**Infectious lymphocytosis**	**Reactive lymphocytosis**	**Acute leukemia**	**Lymphoma**	**Benign polyclonal B-lymphocytosis**
Further procedures		Medication history		Rule out stress-related lymphocytosis	
				Rule out reactive origins	

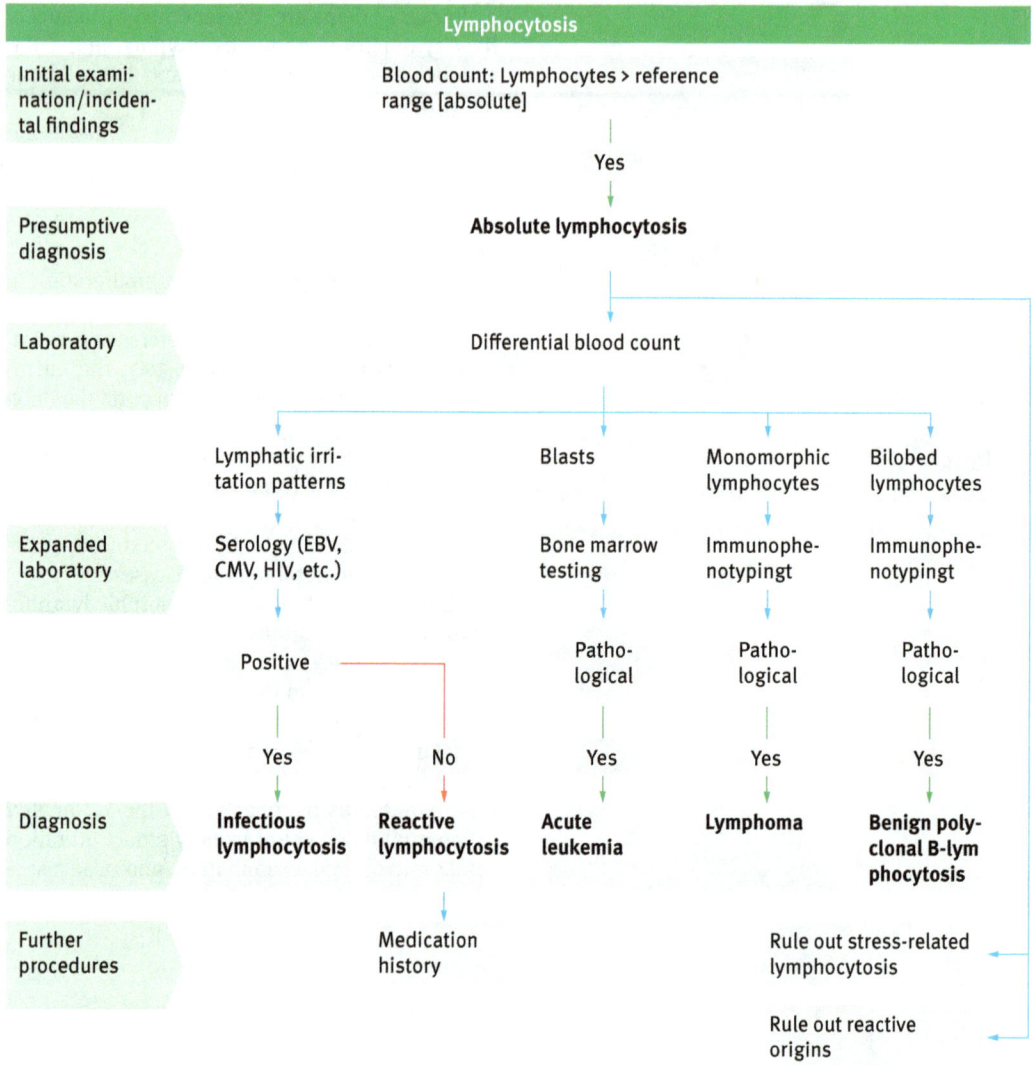

Figure 4.36 Note: these stepwise diagrams are kept relatively simple for reasons of clarity; they serve as an aid for making a diagnosis, and can be used as guidance for a majority of patients. However, in individual cases and especially when several concomitant diseases are present with complicated constellations of laboratory parameters or with laboratory parameters trending in opposite directions, deviations from this predetermined scheme must be considered.

4.5.2.7 Neutropenia

Definition

Neutropenia is defined as a reduction in neutrophils below 1500/μL. An increased tendency to infection usually only occurs at a neutropenia below 500/μL. **Agranulocytosis** is the almost complete absence of neutrophils in the blood, and occurs after the ingestion of certain medicines, after exposure to specific chemical substances, and also in cases of autoimmune disease (type I: autoimmune etiology with an acute course; type II: toxic origin with a slower course).

Origins

Neutropenia can be the result of reduced or insufficient granulopoiesis in the bone marrow, increased storage in the spleen, or increased destruction in the peripheral blood:
- Decreased production: bone marrow failure (acute leukemia, lymphoma, aplastic anemia, MDS, malignancy), congenital immunodeficiencies, drug-/toxin-related bone marrow damage, metabolic origins
- Increased pooling in the spleen: hypersplenism
- Increased destruction in the circulation; triggers: related to drug allergies, infectious, autoimmunological

The most common triggers of a drug-induced neutropenia are the drugs clozapine, antithyroid medications, and sulfasalazine. Additional drugs associated with neutropenia include metamizole, beta-lactam antibiotics, sulfamethoxazole, anticonvulsants, phenothiazines, antiarrhythmics, NSAIDs, ACE inhibitors, and others.

Viral infections often result in mild neutropenia, and are probably the most common cause of transient neutropenia. EBV and HIV infections result in prolonged neutropenia.

A number of bacterial and parasitic infections also are associated with neutropenia.

Primary autoimmune neutropenias are rare; more frequently, secondary neutropenias occur following other autoimmune diseases.

Congenital origins for neutropenia, i.e., congenital immunodeficiencies, should be considered, especially in pediatric patients.

Finally, a metabolic origin (nutritional or metabolic diseases) can be the underlying cause of neutropenia.

4.5.2.8 Pancytopenia

Definition

Pancytopenia is defined as a reduction in all 3 types of cellular components in the peripheral blood (tricytopenia), i.e., a combination of anemia, leukopenia and thrombocytopenia.

Based on the patient's medical/medication history, assumptions can be made relating to the contributions of toxins or drugs, and para-infectious/paratraumatic origins can be considered.

An imaging examination that shows splenomegaly will point to hypersplenism.

Origins

- Toxic bone marrow damage: drugs, radiation, chemotherapy, noxious substances (alcohol, benzene), malnutrition (megaloblastic anemias)
- Neoplastic bone marrow infiltration: acute leukemias, multiple myeloma, lymphoma, malignant tumor
- Aplastic anemia (toxic, immunological, related to medications or infections)
- Maturation disorders: myelodysplastic syndromes (MDS)
- Para-infectious/paratraumatic
- Paroxysmal nocturnal hemoglobinuria (PNH)
- Hypersplenism

Clarification

The clarification of pancytopenia requires a medication history, and the ruling out of contact with other toxic substances. Furthermore, suspicion of a para-infectious event indicates direct or serological examinations to detect the presence of pathogens.

A bone marrow puncture biopsy must be performed to rule out hematological disease (acute leukemia, MDS, aplastic anemia). In addition, splenomegaly can be ruled out using imaging.

4.5.2.9 Polycythemia

Definition

Polycythemia, a synonym for erythrocytosis, refers to erythrocyte proliferation, usually defined as an increase in hemoglobin and/or hematocrit (> two standard deviations beyond the age- and sex-specific reference ranges).

Origins

Polycythemia can be divided into congenital and acquired types:
1. The **congenital** forms are based on, for example, hemoglobinopathies, bisphosphoglycerate deficiencies, methemoglobinemia, and mutations of various signaling proteins (VHL, HIF, PHD, EpoR).

Neutropenia				
Initial examination/incidental findings		Blood count: neutrophilic granulocytes $< 1.6 \times 10^9/L$		
		Yes		
Presumptive diagnosis		**Neutropenia**		
Laboratory	Medical, clinical history	CRP	Differential blood count	Vitamin B$_{12}$, folic acid
		Elevated	Blasts	Lowered
		Yes	Yes — No	Yes
Expanded laboratory			Bone marrow testing	
Diagnosis		**Infection**	**PD acute leukemia** / **PD aplastic anemia, MDS, lymphoma**	**Vitamin B$_{12}$, folic acid deficiency**
Further procedures	Rule out drug-/toxin-induced neutropenia			

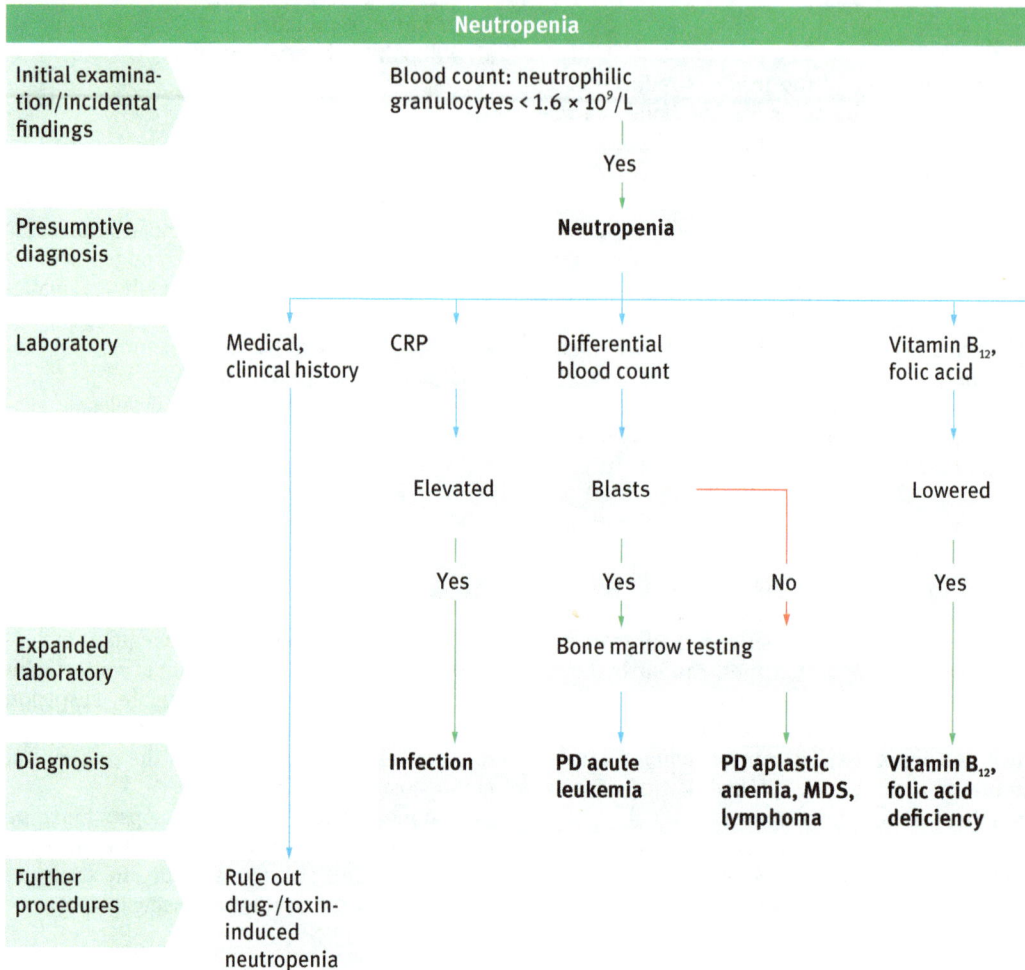

Figure 4.37 Note: these stepwise diagrams are kept relatively simple for reasons of clarity; they serve as an aid for making a diagnosis, and can be used as guidance for a majority of patients. However, in individual cases and especially when several concomitant diseases are present with complicated constellations of laboratory parameters or with laboratory parameters trending in opposite directions, deviations from this predetermined scheme must be considered.

2. The acquired forms are subdivided into the clonal and reactive varieties.

a) **Polycythemia vera** is a myeloproliferative neoplasm characterized by polycythemia. A specific mutation in Janus 2-tyrosine kinase (JAK2 V617F, or more rarely, a JAK2 mutation in exon 12) is detectable in almost all PV patients. The result is an erythropoietin-independent proliferation of red blood cell precursors.

b) **Non-clonal secondary** erythrocytosis can be further divided into hypoxia-dependent and hypoxia-independent types: The origins of the **hypoxia-dependent** type include chronic lung diseases, a cardiopulmonary shunt, residence at high altitude, smoking, CO poisoning, sleep apnea/hypoventilation, and renal artery stenosis.

The **hypoxia-independent** type occurs concomitant with the supply of EPO or androgens as well as with paraneoplastic EPO production.

```
          Autoantibody              Recheck blood
          diagnostics               count in 2–3 weeks


      ANA,           Anti-
     DNA Ab,      neutrophil           Normal
       Sm             Ab


      Yes            Yes               Yes


    PD SLE       PD auto-          PD cyclic
                 immune            neutropenia
                 neutropenia


                                   Rule out
                                   congenital
                                   immune
                                   defects
```

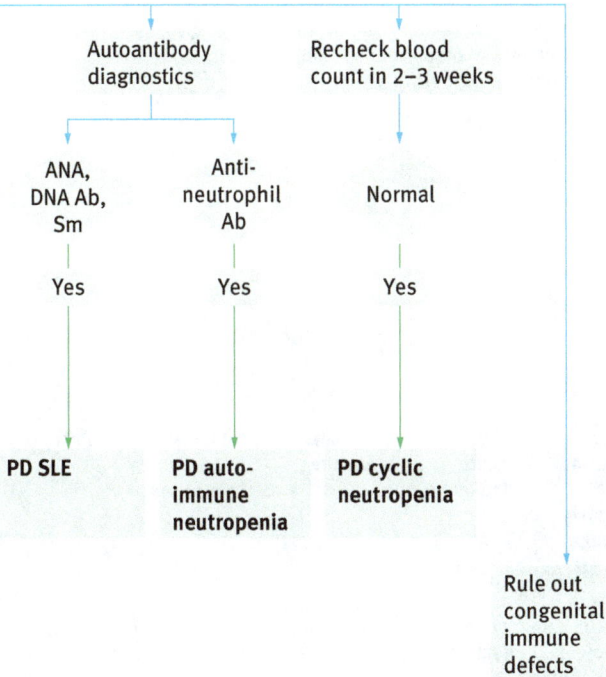

Clarification

The clarification of polycythemia using laboratory diagnostics proceeds with determination of the JAK2 mutation as well as the measurement of erythropoietin levels.

A bone marrow puncture biopsy can also contribute to the diagnostics. Suspicion of a congenital form of polycythemia indicates identification of the hemoglobin variants present by performing a hemoglobin fractionation, or obtaining evidence of mutation using PCR.

Polycythemia vera is diagnosed according to the 2010 WHO criteria.

If necessary, any secondary origins can be elucidated from the medical history, or by conducting additional physical or imaging examinations.

Literature

Thomas L, Labor und Diagnose, 7. Auflage, TH-Books Verlagsgesellschaft mbH, Frankfurt/Main, 2008.
Loffler H, Haferlach T, Hämatologische Erkrankungen, Springer-Verlag Berlin Heidelberg, 2010.

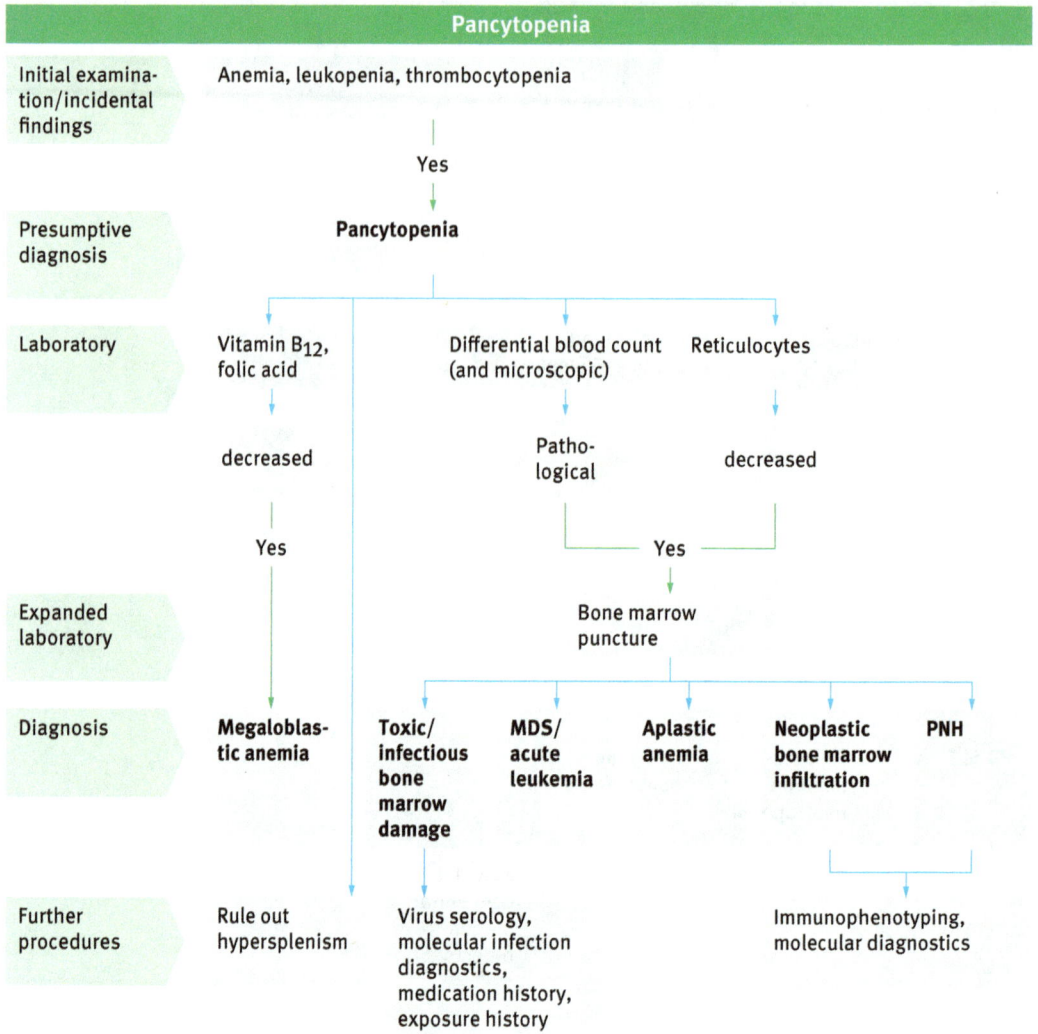

Figure 4.38 Note: these stepwise diagrams are kept relatively simple for reasons of clarity; they serve as an aid for making a diagnosis, and can be used as guidance for a majority of patients. However, in individual cases and especially when several concomitant diseases are present with complicated constellations of laboratory parameters or with laboratory parameters trending in opposite directions, deviations from this predetermined scheme must be considered.

Polycythemia				

Initial examination/incidental findings	Blood count: hemoglobin and/or hematocrit > reference range			

Yes ↓

Presumptive diagnosis	**Polycythemia**

↓

Laboratory	JAK2 mutation

↓

Positive — No

Yes

Expanded laboratory	JAK2 exon 12 mutation	Erythropoietin		Hemoglobin variants (HPLC, PCR)

	Positive	Normal/elevated		Positive

Yes   Yes   Yes

Diagnosis	**Polycythemia vera (according to WHO criteria)**	**Malignant tumor (paraneoplastic)**	**External EPO supply**	**Chronic hypoxia**	**Congenital erythrocytosis**

↓

Further procedures	Bone marrow testing

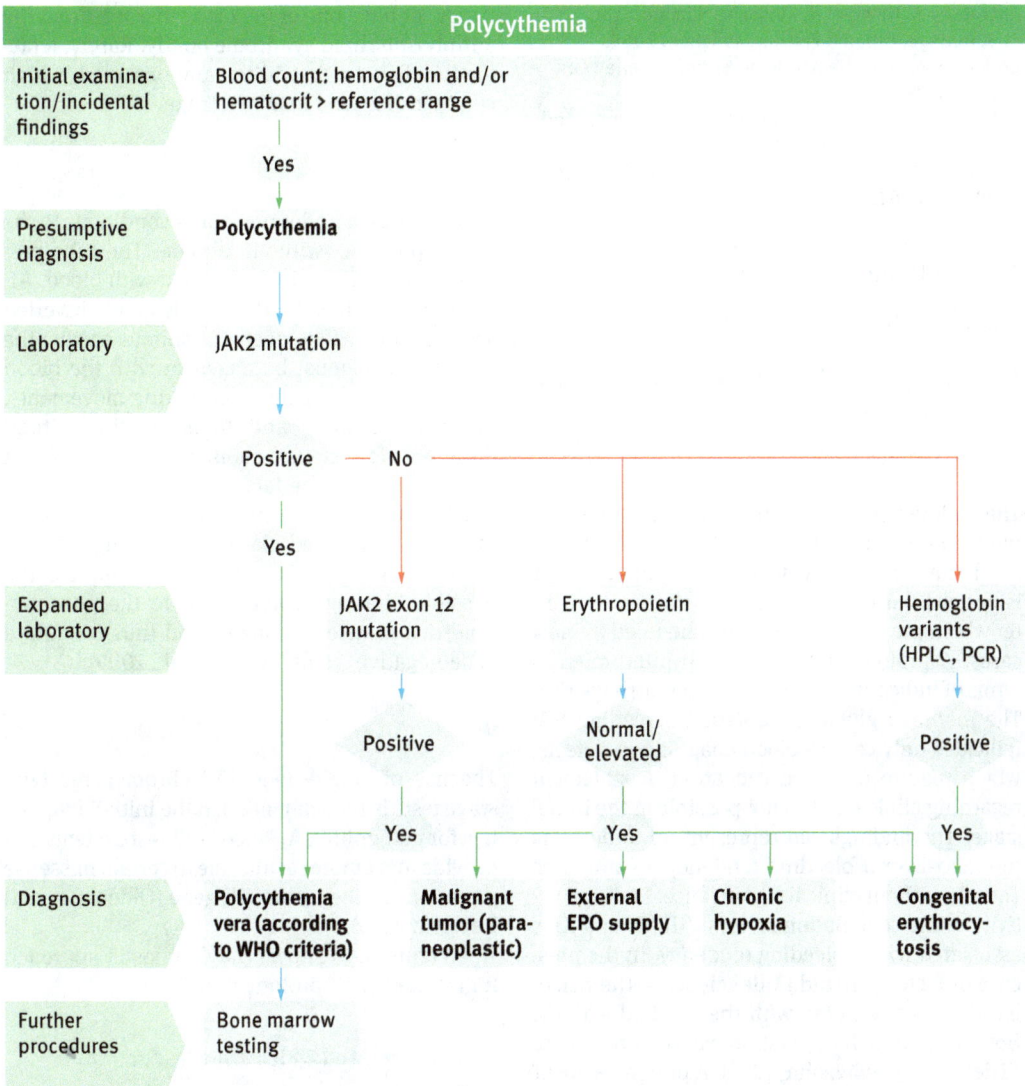

Figure 4.39 Note: these stepwise diagrams are kept relatively simple for reasons of clarity; they serve as an aid for making a diagnosis, and can be used as guidance for a majority of patients. However, in individual cases and especially when several concomitant diseases are present with complicated constellations of laboratory parameters or with laboratory parameters trending in opposite directions, deviations from this predetermined scheme must be considered.

Andreesen R, Heimpel H, Klinische Hämatologie, 3. Auflage, Urban & Fischer Munchen, 2009.

Beck N, Diagnostic Hematology, Springer Verlag London Limited, 2009.

WHO Classification of Tumours of Haematopoietic and Lymphoid Tissue (IARC WHO Classification of Tumours), World Health Organization, Fourth Edition edition, 2008.

Christian Martin Schambeck

4.6 Coagulation disorders

4.6.1 Diagnostic Pathways for Coagulation disorders

4.6.1.1 Isolated aPTT Prolongation

The isolated prolongation of the activated partial thromboplastin time (aPTT) is frequently an incidental finding. Typically, a prolonged aPTT is noticed during a preoperative clarification, after which the surgery date is rescheduled in most cases. A prolonged aPTT is often interpreted in terms of indicating an increased hemorrhage risk. The modified global coagulation screening test indicates only certain blood coagulation defects, which require further clarification. A statement regarding clinical risk is not possible at the initial stage. The findings can represent an underlying thrombosis or a bleeding tendency, or it can be entirely without clinical significance. Reduced activity of the coagulation factors VIII, IX and XI is associated with a bleeding tendency. In the presence of factor VIII and IX deficiencies, the risk of bleeding is associated with the residual activity. However, no such correlation exists with a factor XI deficiency (Seligsohn, 1993). A prolonged aPTT is induced by the reduction in factor VIII caused by von Willebrand disease. The common factor XII deficiency is not associated with either a spontaneous or intraoperative bleeding risk, even with the associated risk of thrombosis (Koster, et al., 1994; Girolami, et al., 2004). Apart from hereditary angioedema (Cichon, et al., 2006), a possible clinical significance of factor XII has been suggested so far only from work done in mouse models (Muller and Renne, 2008). A factor XII deficiency is not infrequently diagnosed together with von Willebrand disease. Antiphospholipid antibodies are often associated with a prolonged aPTT. These patients can be asymptomatic from the clinical perspective, exhibit either a prothrombotic ten-dency, or have one of the many diseases from the antiphospholipid syndrome family. Rarely, a factor II deficiency is additionally observed, which can then also lead to hemorrhage.

Preanalytical variables

Blood is drawn under non-stasis conditions to the extent possible, without jabbing. The tube pretreated with citrate is easily filled with blood. After filling completely, the tube is gently inverted several times. If it doesn't aspirate easily, the anticoagulant must be mixed in with the blood during the draw, using slight tilting movements. Protracted storage and transport times (total duration > four hours) should be avoided. An *in vitro* decrease in the labile factor VIII can mimic a deficiency. For detecting antiphospholipid antibodies, the citrated plasma is centrifuged twice, in accordance with guidelines, to suppress the possible binding of antibodies to the phospholipid-rich platelet fragments and thus rule out a false-negative result (Pengo, et al., 2009).

Decision Tree:

The use of single-stage and chromogenic two-stage tests is recommended in the initial diagnostics for hemophilia A, since both test systems can provide inaccurate results due to certain missense mutations in the factor VIII gene (Oldenburg and Pavlova, 2010).

▶ Figure 4.40 shows the diagnostic approach for isolated aPTT prolongation.

4.6.1.2 Isolated Quick Time Reduction

An isolated Quick value reduction that requires clarification is observed more rarely than an isolated aPTT prolongation. The finding often draws attention in advance of an operation. The perioperative hemorrhage risk cannot be predicted solely on the basis of the Quick value. If the clinical origin is not known in advance, the cause is often a congenital factor VII deficiency; this is the most common vitamin K-dependent factor deficiency, with an incidence of 1/1,500,000. Clinical bleeding diathesis ranges from mild all the way to severe forms, with hemarthrosis and cerebral hemorrhage. With a residual activity < 25 %, the genotype sometimes has more predictive power than the phenotype (Perry, 2002).

Isolated aPTT prolongation

Initial examination/incidental findings

Preliminary finding: aPTT prolongation

(Repeated) aPTT determination (without heparin or hirudin)

Prolonged — No → Preliminary finding: Heparin, long storage, longer transport, underfilled Monovette

Yes

Presumptive diagnosis/clinical picture

Asymptomatic   **Tendency to thrombosis**   **Bleeding diathesis**

Laboratory

Factor XII[1]   Antiphospholipid-antibody[1] (see section 4.6.1.6)   Factor VIII, IX, XI, von Willebrand factor[1]

[1] Only in the case that both other findings are negative.

decreased   Positive   decreased

No   Yes   No   Yes   No   Yes

Diagnosis

Factor XII deficiency   **Antiphospholipid Ab syndrome**   **PD fibrin polymerization disorder**   Confirmatory testing

Clarification of additional origins/additional procedures

Prekallikrein/high-molecular-weight kininogen

decreased   decreased

No   Yes   No   Yes

Coagulation factor deficiency of von Willebrand disease

"Normal variant"   **Prefactor deficiency**   **Thrombin time Reptilase time**   **"Transient" factor deficiency**   Plasma exchange, further von Willebrand diagnostics (see section 4.6.1.3)

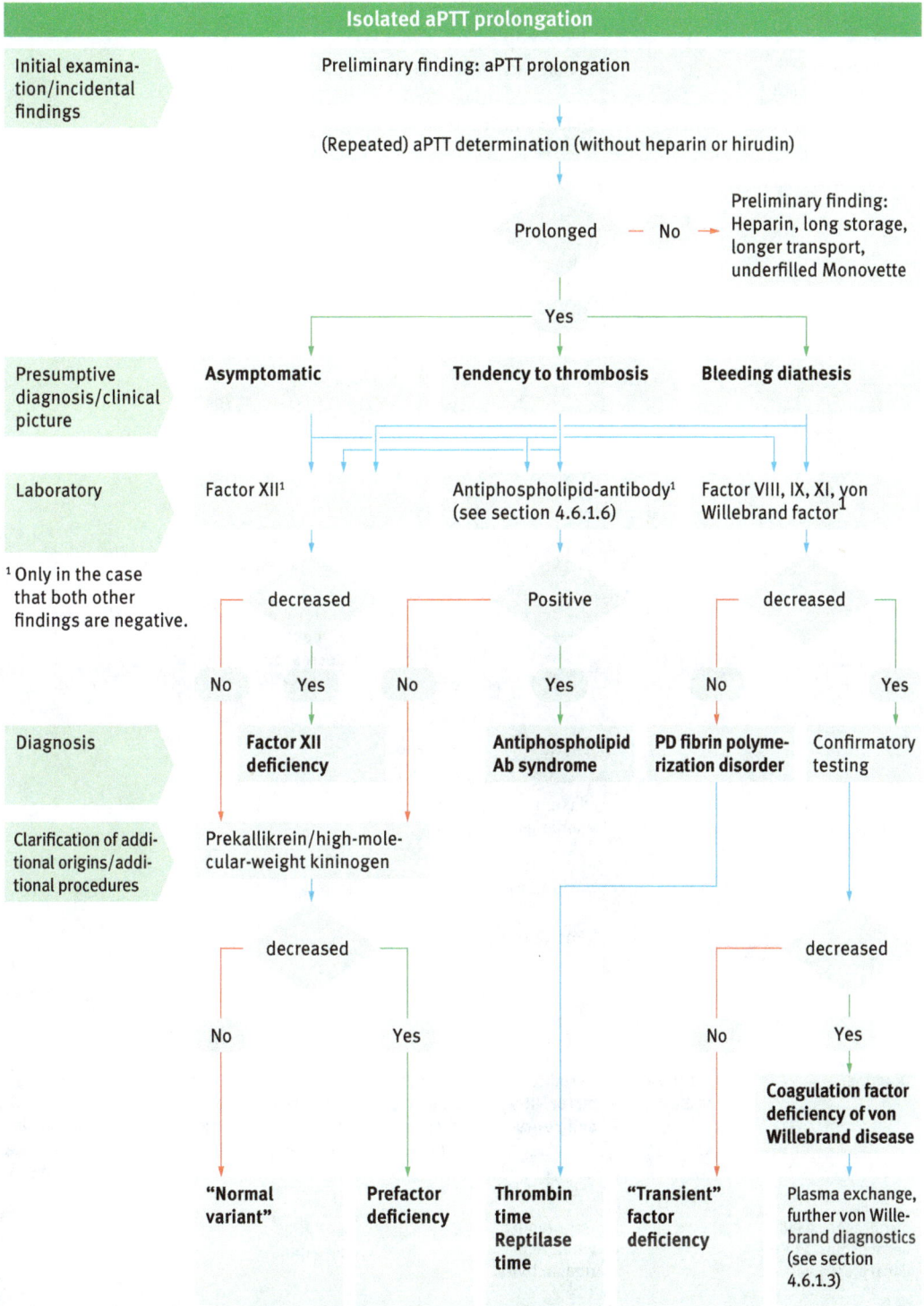

Figure 4.40 Diagnostic Pathway: Isolated aPTT prolongation.

Isolated Quick time reduction

Initial exami- nation/incidental findings	Preliminary finding: Quick value determination

Quick value redetermination

decreased —— No

Yes

Laboratory	Factor VII

No — Vitamin K
antagonists, pathological
liver parameters
(CHE) — Yes

decreased —— No

Yes

Factor X   Factor V or
X slightly
decreased

No — decreased

Expanded laboratory	Plasma exchange

Yes

Positive

Yes   No

Diagnosis	**Factor VII inhibitors**	**Hereditary factor VII deficiency**	**Vitamin K deficiency Other origins**	**Mild coagulation factor deficiency**	**Oral anticoa- gulation Liver disease**	**Preliminary finding: unfavorable preanalytical conditions**

Clarification of addi- tional origins/addi- tional procedures	Genotyping when resi- dual activity < 25%	Antiphos- pholipid Ab	

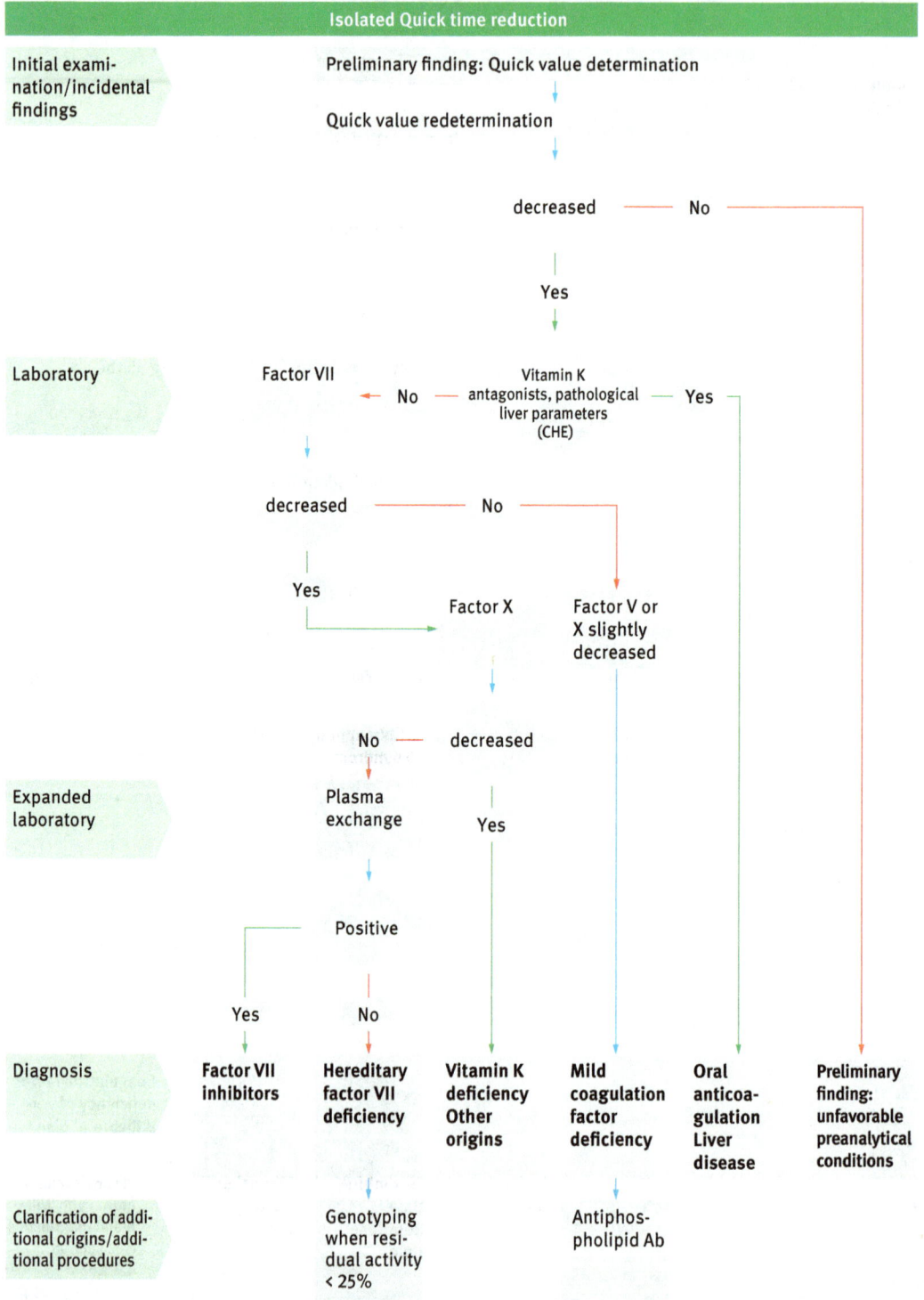

Figure 4.41 Diagnostic Pathway: Isolated Quick time reduction.

▶ Figure 4.41 shows the diagnostic approach for an isolated Quick time reduction.

Pre-analytical requirements

The guidelines to be observed during coagulation studies are also applicable here ▶ 4.6.1.1, section on "Pre-analytical requirements").

4.6.1.3 Bleeding diathesis

The medical history has not only the purpose of providing the indication for clarification of a hemorrhagic diathesis, but also to get a "feel" for the clinical pretest probability. If the laboratory diagnostic clarification remains unsuccessful with a high probability for a coagulation disorder, therapeutic recommendations should still be made. At a low clinical pretest probability, further diagnostics can probably be omitted following a negative result, and prophylactic measures are to be recommended with restraint.

One should not be limited to general questions in taking the medical history, but rather try to quantify the clinical information as much as possible. Thus, for example, most women feel that the amount of their menstrual bleeding is "normal" for them, but interindividual differences become apparent only after a more precise inquiry in terms of days ("Do you need to change the napkin/tampon more than six times/day? Even at night?"). A standardized medical history form is helpful here. "Bleeding diaries" to quantify the menstrual bleeding are tedious to manage. Outlining the timeframe of the clinical bleeding characteristics is crucial to distinguishing congenital from acquired disorders (heavy menstrual bleeding since menarche, since the pregnancy, or in the years before menopause?).

Signs of bleeding include:
1. A predisposition to developing petechiae, ecchymoses and hematomas (frequency, circumstances, location, and extent),
2. Epistaxis (frequency, duration, circumstances, one or both nostrils affected),
3. Blood in stool/urine (following illness),
4. Menstrual bleeding (duration and intensity, mitigation under contraception), and
5. Postoperative hemorrhage (Immediate or delayed posthemorrhage? Corrective measures required? Transfusion required?)

The bleeding duration after accidental cuts is often included. This bleeding characteristic is rather difficult to quantify, though, because the depth of the cut can vary greatly. Extensive bleeding and hemarthrosis are typical of coagulopathies, while petechiae and mucosal bleeding point to von Willebrand disease and platelet functional defects.

In addition to characterizing the type of bleeding, three other important elements are recognized:
1. Comorbidities,
2. Medication history, and
3. Family medical history

Special importance is attached to the patient's medication history. Here it is important not only to record the current medications, but to do the detective work to identify the medications taken in the past (frequency, "occasional" use of aggregation-inhibiting drugs, and interactions with other substances).

Pre-analytical requirements

Sensitive preanalytics are essential for laboratory diagnostics in the area of blood coagulation, and this is particularly true in platelet function testing. Platelets can become activated through improper sampling. A maximum of three minutes stasis is permissible only to facilitate performing the puncture. The blood draw begins only after releasing the stasis. The sample is aspirated gently using a wide-lumen puncture needle (18–20 gauge). The filled tube is immediately inverted several times gently so that the applied anticoagulant can mix thoroughly with the blood. The appropriate anticoagulant in platelet diagnostics is 0.109 M sodium citrate for use in Born aggregometry, release testing, and flow cytometry. Exposure to cold or transport on ice must be strictly avoided. Pneumatic tube delivery should be considered carefully, since the forces that occur can activate platelets. The aggregometry measurement process should begin as early as 45 minutes after the blood draw. After centrifugation, platelet-rich plasma requires a rest period of 15 minutes at room temperature. Ideally, the measurement should be completed in two hours. For these reasons, blood samples should be drawn near the analysis laboratories. If this is not possible, special attention should be paid when transporting by the usual means. Thus, for example, the exact time of the blood drawn should be documented.

Decision Tree

The diagnosis of von Willebrand disease is sometimes difficult. The precision of the ristocetin cofactor assay is unsatisfactory, and so an "antibody-binding activity assay" was developed as an alternative to the traditional assay. In this assay, the epitope of the antibody targets the GPIbα chain at the von Willebrand factor binding site. Type 2 von Willebrand disease is not enough recognized with sufficient reliability, so that in this case the ristocetin cofactor assay cannot be replaced. A newly developed activity assay could prove to be a viable alternative to the ristocetin cofactor assay within the next few years. This newer method employs a recombinant GPIbα fragment instead of stabilized human platelets (Patzke and Schneppenheim, 2010; Schneppenheim and Budde, 2006).

The classic bleeding time screening test is easy to use, but lacks sensitivity and specificity (Witt and Patscheke, 1997). Another screening method is the PFA-100, which is very sensitive to large von Willebrand factor multimers, detects rare severe platelet defects well, but mild platelet defects are often insufficiently recognized (Harrison, 2005). The test is subject to numerous interfering parameters. In certain individual cases, no cause can be assigned to an observed positive test result, even after thorough clarification. A diagnostic algorithm that incorporates these screening tests has been proposed (DGKL, 2004).

The gold standard in the diagnostics of platelet function is Born aggregometry, also referred to as light transmission aggregometry (Budde, 2002), although there is hardly any standardization and the results are strongly laboratory- and examiner-dependent. Other limitations of this analysis technique are the time-consuming (and platelet activating) procedure for working up the sample material, and measurement in an artificial matrix. The citrate employed as anticoagulant binds calcium, an important activator of platelet function. A more suitable analysis technique is impedance aggregometry (McGlasson and Fritsma, 2009). In this method, whole blood is used, matrix mimics physiological conditions far more closely, and importantly the hirudin anticoagulant does not deprive the platelets of calcium. Neither system can produce shear stress conditions. As a result of the calcium depletion, Born aggregometry can detect release abnormalities, while in this case special supplementary techniques are required in imped-

ance aggregometry. However, Born aggregometry exhibits low sensitivity for the common secretion abnormalities, so that it is prudent to follow-up with complementary diagnostics, for example, luminometric detection of the delta granules (also referred to as dense granules) (Cattaneo, 2009).

▶ Figures 4.42a and b illustrate the diagnostic procedures for bleeding diathesis.

4.6.1.4 Acute Venous Thromboembolism

Most mobile patients with deep vein thrombosis present at a hospital or private medical practice with complaints of a swollen leg, a feeling of tension or even bursting pain in the foot and calf. In order of frequency, the symptoms that occur include edema, pain, and cyanosis. By contrast, however, a deep vein thrombosis often causes no symptoms in bedridden patient. Pelvic vein thrombosis sometimes manifests itself as tearing pains in the lumbar region. In mobile patients, the classic compression and stretching pain signs (e.g., Homans' sign, Payr's sign, etc.) are of highly variable sensitivity with insufficient specificity, while these signs are frequently unsuitable in bedridden patients. By contrast, an acute pulmonary embolism manifests itself in sudden dyspnea, chest pain, syncope, or hemoptysis.

The interdisciplinary AWMF S2 guidelines (DGA, 2010) for the diagnosis of venous thromboembolism are based on the assessment of clinical probability derived from the medical history and clinical results. The best evaluation tool is the clinical scoring scheme developed by Wells (Wells, et al., 2000; Wells, et al., 2003; ▶ Tables 4.24 and ▶ 4.25.). Once the clinical probability has been established, a D-dimer determination should made. In practice, and contrary to the Guidelines, the process is streamlined by performing the D-dimer determination and diagnostic imaging in tandem. A high D-dimer value might then be mistakenly interpreted as confirmation of the presumptive diagnosis. D-dimers arise as the final product in the proteolysis of fibrin that has been cross-linked by factor XIII. An increased D-dimer concentration is not specific for a venous thromboembolism, and can also be observed following operations, etc., secondary to hematomas, trauma, and during pregnancy. Due to the high sensitivity but relatively low specificity, the D-dimer determination is more suitable for ruling out a diagnosis. Evidence of D-dimers is used for clarification in an ambulatory patient, while the lack of specificity had a substantial effect with bedridden patients. Various assays exhibit different levels of specificity. Upon suspicion of a massive pulmonary embolism, the algorithm should be disregarded and a transthoracic echocardiogram performed immediately.

Table 4.24 Wells score to assess the clinical probability of deep vein thrombosis (DVT).

Parameter	Wells score
Active cancer	1
Paralysis or recent immobilization of the legs	1
Bed rest (> 3 days), major surgery (< 12 weeks)	1
Pain without induration along deep veins	1
Swelling of the entire leg	1
Swelling of the lower leg > 3 cm compared with the contralateral leg	1
Compressible edema on the symptomatic leg	1
Collateral veins	1
Earlier document DVT	1
Alternative diagnosis at least as probable as DVT	–2

Table 4.25 Wells score to determine the clinical probability of pulmonary embolism.

Clinical symptom	Score
Signs of venous thrombosis	3
Pulmonary embolism more probable than other diagnoses (medical and clinical history, ECG, chest X-ray, blood gases)	3
Heart rate > 100/min	1.5
Immobilization/operation < 4 weeks	1.5
Earlier venous thromboembolism	1.5
Hemoptysis	1
Tumor	1

Pre-analytical requirements

The D-dimer determination is sufficiently robust. The basic recommendations for the proper blood drawing procedures also apply here. A lack of thorough mixing of the blood with the anticoagulant submitted can lead to plasma activation and thus to fibrin production, leading to falsely high results.

Decision Tree

▶ Figure 4.43 shows the diagnostic procedures for acute venous thromboembolism.

4.6.1.5 Heparin-induced Thrombocytopenia (Type 2 HIT)

The algorithm for the diagnosis of HIT is similar to that for a suspected venous thromboembolism. Here too, the determination of clinical probability forms the beginning of the diagnostic workflow. The 4T score has been proven suitable for this purpose (Lo, et al., 2006; ▶ Table 4.26.). And here too, the role of the laboratory diagnostics is to rule out the presumptive diagnosis. A positive test does not confirm the diagnosis. The specificity of the test vs. the heparin-PF4 antibody procedure is increased through use of assays that only detect the pathogenetically significant IgG antibodies (Greinacher, et al., 2007). The next few years will see the availability of IgG-specific tests with a short turnaround time, so that the assays against all three antibodies (IgG, IgM and IgA) will be increasingly obsolete. High titers, as measured by quantitative IgG-specific tests, will even be able to confirm a presumptive diagnosis. Only anti-PF4/heparin antibodies are detected in the conventional tests. However, antibodies against other antigens can also be causative, such as anti-NAP2/heparin or anti-IL8/heparin antibodies, etc. When a clinical suspicion still persists, and at the latest following a negative PF4/heparin Ab test result, a functional test (e.g., HIPA or serotonin release assay) should be performed.

Pre-analytical conditions

In contrast to conventional coagulation diagnostics, the pre-analytics for clinical laboratory evidence of HIT are not critical. Citrated plasma or serum is used in the antigen test, and serum for the functional tests. Antibody detection is still possible up to three days after the blood draw.

Decision Tree

▶ Figure 4.44 shows the procedures for HIT diagnosis.

4.6.1.6 Thrombophilia

Indications

The medical benefits of thrombophilia screenings has sometimes been considered controversial. The opinion follows a rhythmic flow from

Bleeding diathesis 1

Initial examination/incidental findings
postoperative bleeding, hematoma, epistaxis, hypermenorrhea, internal joint or muscle hemorrhage, possibly positive family medical history

Presumptive diagnosis/clinical picture

One-time sudden bleeding event — Yes → Drug-induced (Marcumar, heparin, antiaggregatory medications)? Surgery related? Specialty clinic: liver cirrhosis, amyloidosis, etc.

No → Bleeding diathesis

Laboratory

Platelet dysfunction   **Plasmatic coagulation disord**   **Hyperfibrinolysis**

aPTT and TPZ Quick tests

No

Normal value — No → aPTT and TPZ Quick tests are pathological

Yes

Yes

von Willebrand factor: (Ristocetin cofactor) activity and antigen   Factor VIII

Acute phase ← No — decreased ──────── decreased

No   Yes   Yes   Yes

Both pathological → → →

No   Yes

Activity/ antigen ratio is pathological

Expanded laboratory

von Willebrand factor ↓

No   Yes

Possibly plasma exchange

CBAs or multimer differentiation

No

Diagnosis

Substantially rule out factor VIII deficiency and/or von Willebrand disease   **Doubtful von Willebrand disease**   **von Willebrand disease**

Clarification of additional origins/additional procedures

Repeat testing (during an inflammation-free interval)   RIPA

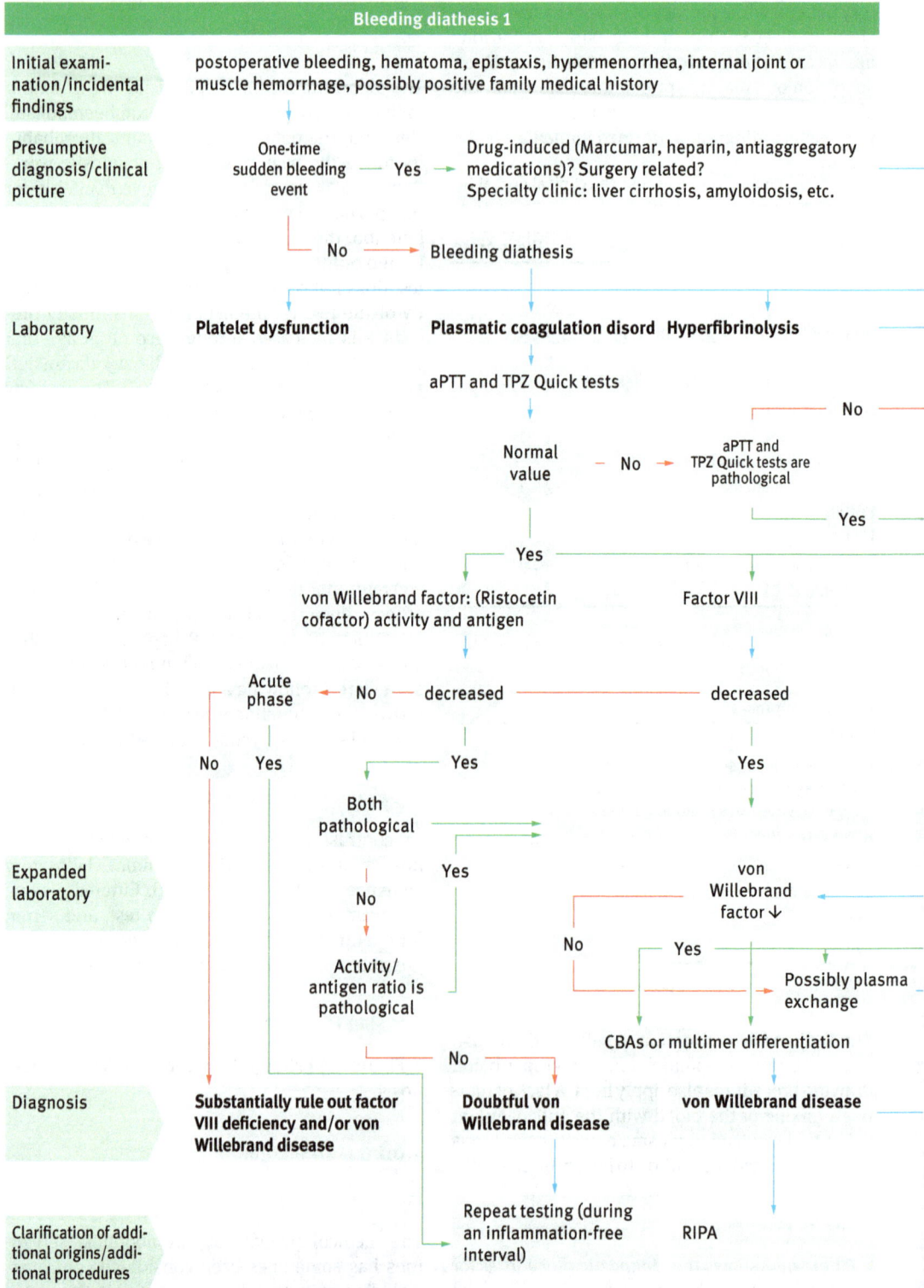

Figure 4.42a Diagnostic Pathway: Bleeding diathesis 1.

Still suspicion of coagulation disorder:
Suspected inhibitors, acquired von
Willebrand disease

Fibrin polymerization disorders

see the sections on "Isolated Quick time
reduction" or "Isolated aPTT prolongation"

e.g., chronic DIC

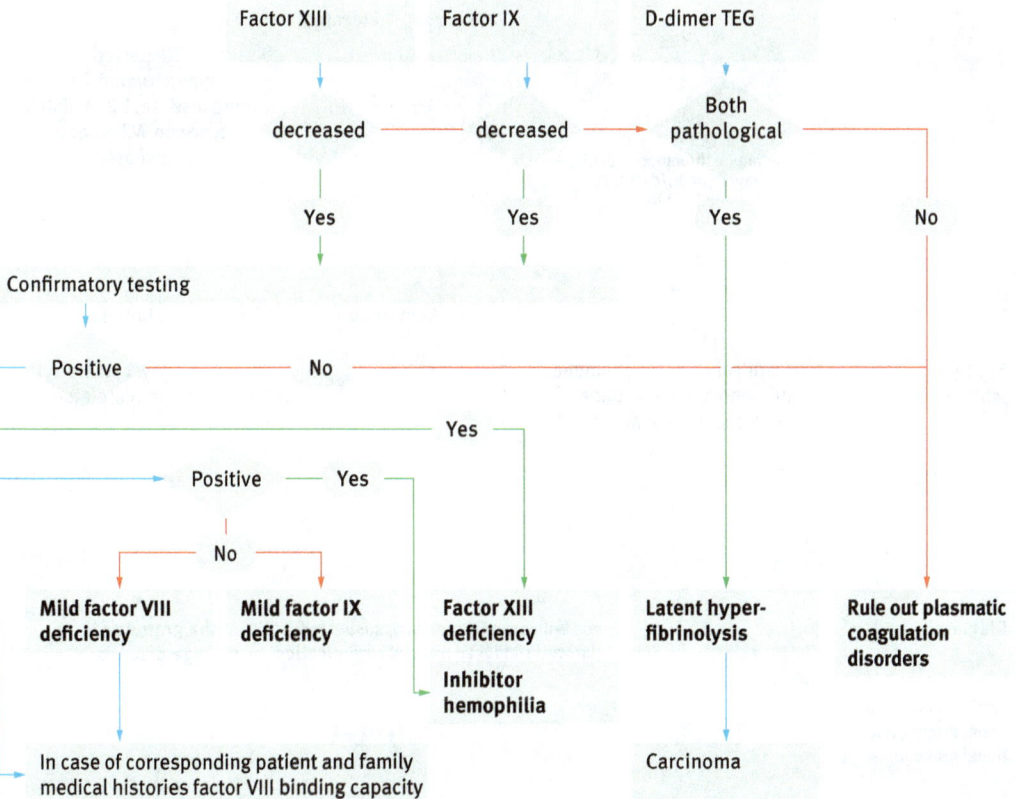

Factor XIII   Factor IX   D-dimer TEG

decreased   decreased   Both
                                    pathological

Yes   Yes   Yes   No

Confirmatory testing

Positive   No

                              Yes

          Positive   Yes

                No

Mild factor VIII   **Mild factor IX**   **Factor XIII**   **Latent hyper-**   **Rule out plasmatic**
deficiency   **deficiency**   **deficiency**   **fibrinolysis**   **coagulation**
                                                                                  disorders

                                             Inhibitor
                                             hemophilia

In case of corresponding patient and family   Carcinoma
medical histories factor VIII binding capacity

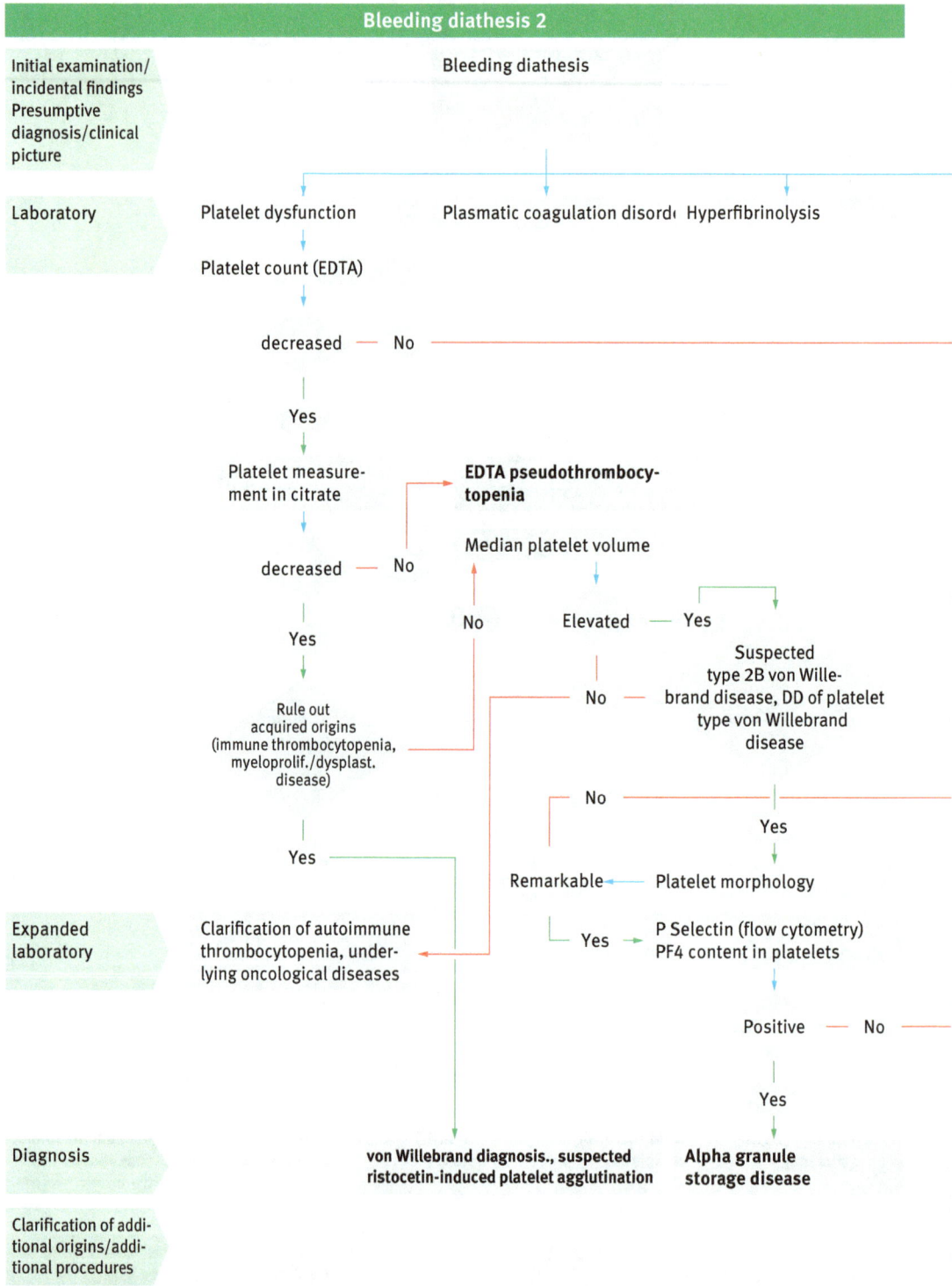

Bleeding diathesis 2

Initial examination/ incidental findings Presumptive diagnosis/clinical picture

Bleeding diathesis

Laboratory

Platelet dysfunction   Plasmatic coagulation disord   Hyperfibrinolysis

Platelet count (EDTA)

decreased — No

Yes

Platelet measurement in citrate → **EDTA pseudothrombocytopenia**

Median platelet volume

decreased — No

Yes   No   Elevated — Yes

Rule out acquired origins (immune thrombocytopenia, myeloprolif./dysplast. disease)   No — Suspected type 2B von Willebrand disease, DD of platelet type von Willebrand disease

No   Yes

Yes   Remarkable ← Platelet morphology

Expanded laboratory   Clarification of autoimmune thrombocytopenia, underlying oncological diseases   Yes → P Selectin (flow cytometry) PF4 content in platelets

Positive — No

Yes

Diagnosis   **von Willebrand diagnosis., suspected ristocetin-induced platelet agglutination**   **Alpha granule storage disease**

Clarification of additional origins/additional procedures

Figure 4.42b Diagnostic Pathway: Bleeding diathesis 2.

Fibrin polymerization disorders

Aggregometry

Release tests (ATP, PF4)

Positive — No — Positive

Yes   Yes

Confirmatory   Confirmatory
testing   testing

Positive — No — Positive

Yes   Yes

Aggregometry

After
ristocetin is
decreased or absent — No
compared to other
activators

Yes

GPIb/V/IX
(flow cytometry)

e.g., GPIIb/IIIa,   P-Selectin, mepacrine,
(flow cytometry)   (flow cytometry), intra-
                                cellular ATP/PF4,
                                electron microscopy

Positive — No

Yes

Bernard-Soulier disease   **MYH9-associated
diseases**

Receptor defects   **Secretion disorder,
pool disorder**

molecular genetic   Thrombocytopathy
clarification   unidentifiable

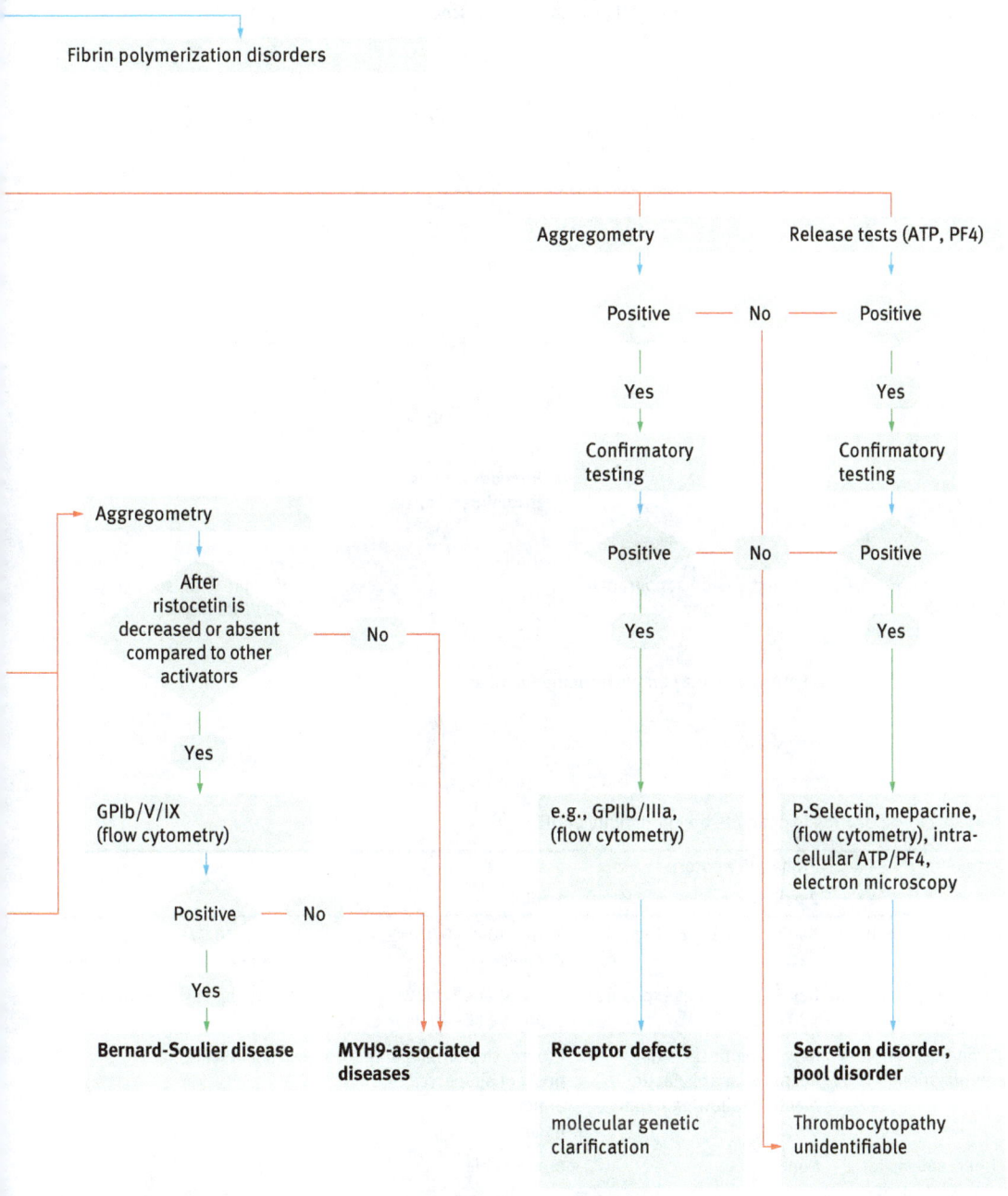

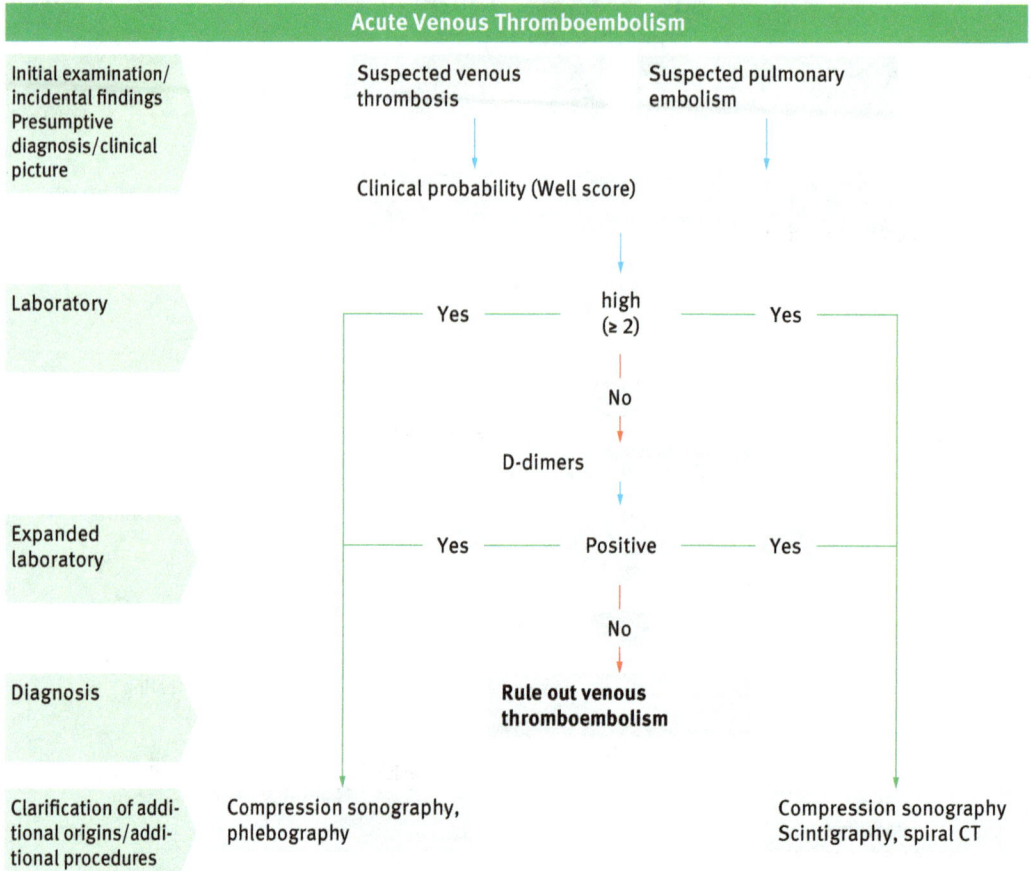

Figure 4.43 Diagnostic Pathway: acute venous thromboembolism.

Table 4.26 4-T-scoring to estimate the probability of HIT.

Parameter	Probability criteria		
	2 points	**1 point**	**0 points**
Thrombocytopenia	Nadir* ≥ 20 G/L and > 50 % decrease	Nadir* 10–19 G/L or 30–50 % decrease	Nadir* < 10 G/L or < 30 % decrease
Timeframe for the platelet decrease	Day 5–10 or ≤ 1 at exposure < 30 days	> Day 10 or ≤ 1 day at exposure 30–90 days earlier	Day < 5 (no earlier exposure)
Thrombosis or other complications	New thrombosis, skin necrosis, anaphylactic reaction following heparin bolus	Progressive or relapsing thrombosis or suspected thrombosis, or non-necrotizing skin lesions	No complications
Other reasons for platelet decrease	None	Conceivable	Definitive

* Nadir = means the lowest value measured

non-critical recommendations (such as in the mid-90s) and complete rejection (as a few years ago). The current S2 Guideline for the treatment of venous thromboembolism has been rather reticent regarding thrombophilia screening, and provides only a very rough framework – such as for the duration of oral anticoagulation (DGA, 2010).

The classical indication is the assessment of the **risk of recurrence of a first or repeated venous thromboembolism**. From this is derived a recommendation on how long after an event to begin anticoagulation. Immediately after an event, the risk of recurrence is particularly high. However, with an increasing interval since the acute event, the risk of recurrence is always higher than the risk for a first venous thromboembolism (Lindhoff-Last, 2011). An estimated incidence of > 5 %/year favors prolonged anticoagulation therapy. The cumulative recurrence rate after five years is 40 % for antithrombin deficiency, protein C deficiency, and protein S deficiency, but only 10 % with factor V disorders, prothrombin 20210 polymorphism, and elevated factor VIII (Lijfering, et al., 2009; Brouwer, et al., 2009). The recurrence risk is particularly high with triple positivity for antiphospholipid antibodies (Pengo, et al., 2010).

Thrombophilia screening is an important step in a multimodal approach. The therapy recommendation rests on a detailed medical history, examination findings at the time of the acute event, family medical history, and a possible residual thrombosis several months later. Aspects to consider include compliance or a possible risk of bleeding. The duration of oral anticoagulation therapy depends crucially on the precise treatment history. An idiopathic event is perceived differently than a secondary event. The exact circumstances in run-up to venous thromboembolism must be investigated. Only after repeated inquiries does it often turn out that a thrombosis event was actually provoked due to an exogenous factor. Trauma, immobilization, or surgery are typical contributing factors, but also any unusual exertion, an abrupt increase in exercise intensity, or excessive, unusual physical activity (par effort) all favor venous thrombosis. The family medical history is important in its own right. Laboratory diagnostics often provide the physiological coagulation correlate to a positive family history. However, the laboratory findings can be negative with a positive family history, and even so a hidden hereditary thrombophilia must be assumed in some individual cases. If several first-degree relatives are affected at an early age, and also when distant relatives have experienced a thrombosis, negative laboratory results must not be considered to rule out a congenital risk.

The family medical history is subject to strong subjective influences. Patients frequently do not distinguish between a superficial and a deep vein thrombosis. In such cases, targeted questions (did the relatives need to take a vitamin-K-antagonist?) can increase the specificity of the family medical history. Also the effect of a residual thrombosis was investigated in several studies for the probability of recurrence. Another key element is also the sex of the patient: men have a higher risk of recurrence following idiopathic venous thrombosis. Thrombophilia screening should be carried out in younger patients (< 50 years), regardless of whether the complaint concerned spontaneous or secondary venous thrombosis. An early age of onset is characteristic of hereditary thrombophilia. Antiphospholipid syndrome has a first peak age between 20 and 30 years. Thrombosis with an atypical localization (sinus, mesenteric, and subclavian thrombosis) are suggestive of thrombophilia. A laboratory diagnostic clarification of thrombosis in advanced age is not recommended, because the basal risk of thrombosis increases continuously with age, especially after the age of 55 years. This recommendation should not be considered absolute, since the antiphospholipid syndrome has a late peak age.

A **positive family medical history** can be an indication if previously asymptomatic relatives of an affected person with a positive laboratory finding will in all likelihood display high compliance. The relatives should be willing to guard against thrombosis in particular risk situations (long plane or car trips, being bedridden), and to internalize a multi-level approach – from simple gymnastic exercises through the wearing of effective compression tights up to undergoing temporary anticoagulation treatment. Hereditary thrombophilia is usually ruled out, but the occurrence of antiphospholipid antibodies can also exhibit a familial predisposition.

Fertility treatments are becoming increasingly significant in the clarification of thrombophilic conditions. Fibrin deposits impair not only the perfusion at the maternal-fetal boundary, but also trophoblast differentiation and proliferation. The placenta matures up to the 24th week of gestation, and disturbed placentation can result in mis-

HIT diagnostics

Initial examination/ incidental findings Presumptive diagnosis/clinical picture

Suspected heparin-induced thrombocytopenia (HIT)

4T score

> 3 points — No

Yes

Laboratory

IgG-specific assay for anti-PF4/heparin antibodies

High optical density (e.g., > 1) — Yes — Positive — No — Strong suspicion of HIT — No

Yes No Yes

Expanded laboratory

Function test (to detect heparin-dependent Ab against Ag other than PF4/heparin)

Yes — Positive

No

Diagnosis

Heparin-induced thrombocytopenia (HIT)   **HIT doubtful**   **HIT ruled out**

Clarification of additional origins/additional procedures

Repeat Ag test if still at the beginning of the timeframe

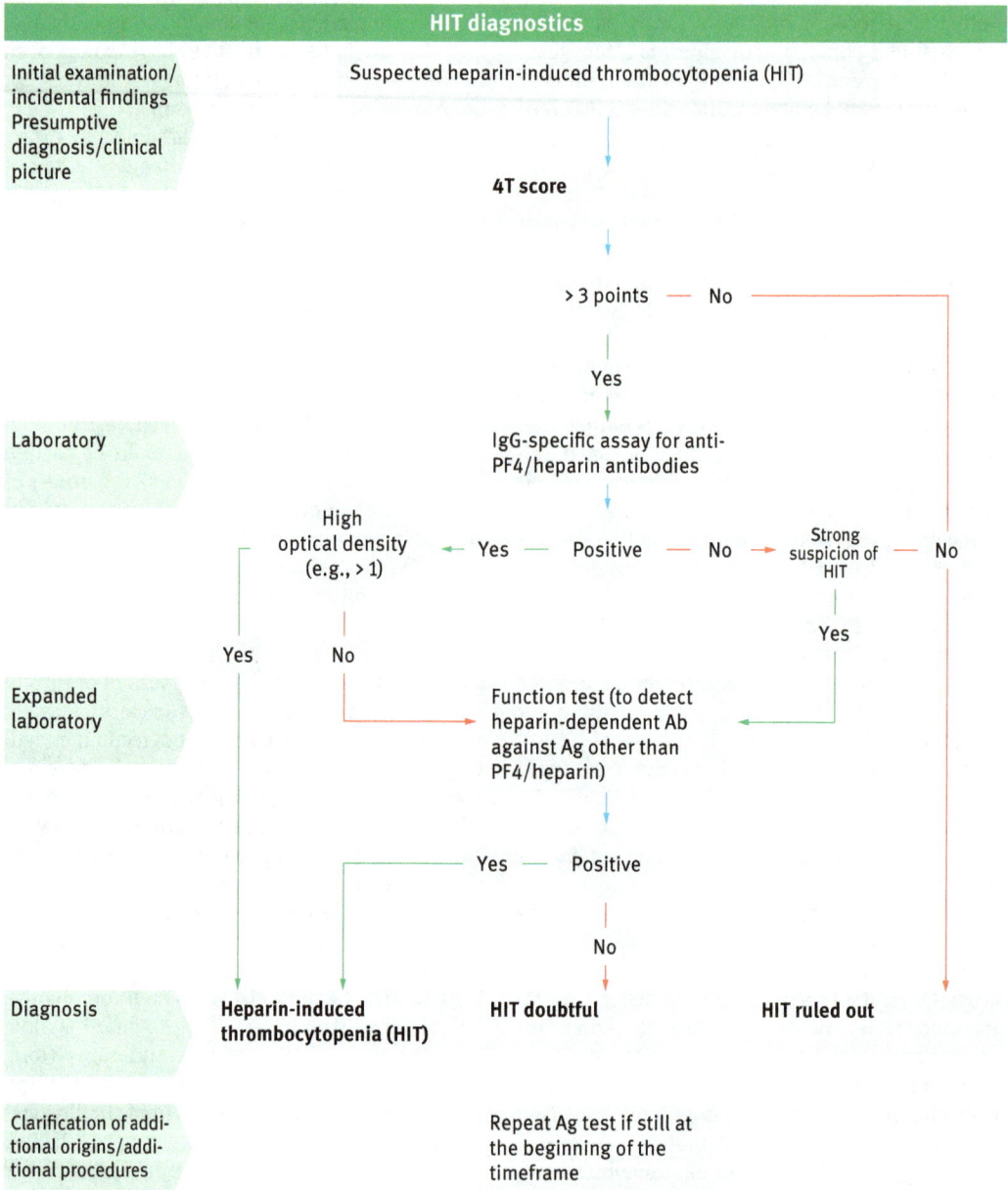

Figure 4.44 Diagnostic Pathway: heparin-induced thrombocytopenia (Type 2 HIT).

carriage and other pregnancy complications such as intrauterine growth retardation. In addition to numerous other factors, habitual miscarriage (three or more miscarriages in a row) can be caused by antiphospholipid syndrome. The combination of acetylsalicylic acid and heparin reduces the abortion rate. Clarification of the antiphospho-lipid antibodies is therefore recommended by the ACCP, while the importance of hereditary thrombophilia is still viewed with reservations (Bates, et al., 2008). According to a meta-analysis, the risk of both early and late miscarriage increases by about two times due to a factor V disorder or the prothrombin 20210 polymorphism (Robertson, et al., 2005). Whether an affected patient benefits from heparin cannot yet be judged reliably. The recently published randomized controlled ALIFE and SPIN trials included only 13 % and 4 % patients (respectively) with a thrombophilic defect (Clark, et al., 2010; Kaandorp, et al., 2010). The available data on pregnancy complications, such as preeclampsia, placental detachment, or intrauterine growth retardation, exhibit no clear patterns. Repeated implantation failure in assisted reproduction warrants clarification (Nelson, 2011). Performing diagnostics prior to beginning a fertility treatment is not without controversy, but could be justifiable given the psychological and socioeconomic dimensions of this type of therapy. No sufficiently powered intervention studies are available, and the costs/benefits of anticoagulation therapy must be weighed carefully. The incidence of serious adverse events with the use of heparin in prophylactic doses is low, so that this risk might be outweighed by the possible benefits. However, the bleeding rate is significantly increased by concomitantly administered aspirin.

Pre- and Post-analytical Principles

The optimal time for drawing a blood sample is four weeks after oral vitamin-K-dependent anticoagulation therapy has been completed. The normalization of the protein S activity in plasma takes several weeks to achieve. Clarification is advisable while oral anticoagulation treatment is still underway so that a deficiency in protein S or protein C can be validly ruled out after the vitamin-K-antagonist is discontinued. The presence of antiphospholipid antibodies can support a decision not to terminate anticoagulation therapy prematurely. Two months since the thrombosis event should have elapsed if thrombophilia is to be investigated during vitamin-K-antagonist treatment. This timing is optimal for anticoagulation with the newer oral antithrombotics, such as rivaroxaban. To this end, blood should be drawn before the morning dose (i.e., 24 hours since the previous administration), since many clotting parameter results are falsified after absorption of the drug. Avoid drawing a blood sample at the time of an acute event, regardless of whether before or during heparinization, or while already under oral anticoagulation treatment, since the protein C will be falsely negative, protein S falsely positive, and factor VIII will exhibit an

Table 4.27 Temporary (acquired) causes of selected thrombophilia risk factors.

Laboratory parameters	Influencing variables
Antithrombin	Heparin, hepatopathy, protein loss
Protein C	Anticoagulation treatment, acute thrombotic events, hepatopathy, vitamin K deficiency
Protein S	Acute phase reaction (CRP), hepatopathy, pregnancy, anticoagulation, vitamin K deficiency, female sex hormones
Factor VIII	Acute phase reaction (CRP), postoperative condition, acute thromboembolism, vascular disorders, hepatopathy, malignant tumor, pregnancy, stress, medications (steroids, DDAVP, adrenalin)
Homocysteine	Folic acid, vitamin B_6, or vitamin B_{12} deficiencies; renal failure, hypothyroidism, malignant tumor, hepatopathy, zinc deficiency, medications (methotrexate, theophylline, carbamazepine, phenytoin, oral contraceptives, steroids, CyA, L-dopa, cholestyramine, niacin)

acute-phase-dependent elevation. A clarification at such an early stage has no therapeutic implications. Subsequent to a thromboembolism, the guidelines specify vitamin-K-antagonist treatment aimed at a target INR of between 2.0 and 3.0 or administration of a proven dosage of one of the newer oral antithrombotics.

Blood is drawn under non-stasis conditions to the extent possible, without jabbing. Inducing stasis for several minutes causes factor VIII levels to rise by up to 20 %. The transport of blood samples should be completed within four hours. Protein S levels can drop *in vitro*. Homocysteine should only be determined when the sample material is processed immediately after the blood draw, or when the blood is stored and transported in a special Monovette. The patient must be fasting in this case. For detecting antiphospholipid antibodies, the citrated plasma is centrifuged twice, in accordance with guidelines, to suppress the possible binding of antibodies to the phospholipid-rich platelet fragments and thus rule out a false-negative result .

The post-analytical phase is viewed as just as critical as the pre-analytics. Some laboratory parameters can be affected to a considerable degree by variables that must be known to correctly assess the findings (▶ Table 4.27). The most significant source of interference is antiphospholipid antibodies, which can falsify all coagulation findings.

Decision Tree

A classical, stepwise approach is always suggested, roughly corresponding to the prevalence of the defects. Accordingly, only after obtaining a negative result for the common factor V disorder mutation and for the prothrombin 20210 polymorphism should the rarer inhibitor defects be investigated. This proposal ignores the fact that, not infrequently, a combination of defects can be detected. Such a finding can be the grounds on which to recommend prolonged oral anticoagulation treatment.

Stepwise diagnostics for APC resistance makes sense if the downstream genotyping is more expensive than the functional tests. The falling cost of genotyping prompts the omission of the functional test, which today – in contrast to the first assay – is specifically designed for the factor V mutation. The table provides an overview of the temporary causes for decreased inhibitors and higher levels of factor VIII and homocysteine. According to the guidelines, a positive antiphospholipid antibody finding should be confirmed after 12 weeks. A finding is positive if a medium- or high-grade titer is observed for anticardiolipin or anti-β2-glycoprotein 1 antibodies and/or a lupus anticoagulant can be detected. The complex diagnostics are explained in more detail elsewhere (Pengo, et al., 2009; Miyakis, et al., 2006).

▶ Figure 4.45 shows the diagnostic procedures for thrombophilia.

Further Diagnostics

Screening for mutations in the antithrombin gene is justified with a type 2 deficiency. A type 2b carries a lower thrombosis risk than do other forms of antithrombin deficiency. Genotyping of a protein S deficiency is usually not helpful with borderline findings from the clotting tests. In individual cases, screening for mutations in the protein S and protein C genes is indicated if, for example, coumarin derivatives are not to be discontinued. There are a number of parameters with little evidence basis that lack therapeutic implications, and these are not worth pursuing if the findings are negative. The MTHFR 677 and 1298 polymorphisms do not represent independent risk factors, but rather have a moderate effect on plasma homocysteine levels. Here, the phenotype is more decisive than the genotype, an observation that also applies to PAI1-4G/5G polymorphism. These genotypes can also increase the thrombosis risk due to a factor V disorder or other defect.

Literature

Seligsohn U. Factor XI deficiency. Thromb Haemost 1993; 70: 68–71.

Koster T, Rosendaal FR, Briet E, Vandenbroucke JP. John Hageman's factor and deep-vein thrombosis: Leiden Thrombophilia Study. Br J Haematol 1994; 87: 422–4.

Girolami A, Randi ML, Gavasso S, Lombardi AM, Spiezia F. The occasional venous thromboses seen in patients with severe (homozygous) FXII deficiency are probably due to associated risk factors: a study of prevalence in 21 patients and review of the literature. J Thromb Thrombolyis 2004; 17: 139–43.

Cichon S, Martin L, Hennies HC, Muller F, Van Driessche K, Karpushova A, Stevens W, Colombo R, Renne T, Drouet C, Bork K, Nothen MM. Increased activity of coagulation factor XII (Hageman factor) causes hereditary angioedema type III. Am J Hum Genet 2006; 79: 1098–104.

Muller F, Renne T. Novel roles for factor XII-driven plasma contact activation system. Curr Opin Hematol 2008; 15: 516–21.

Pengo V, Tripodi A, Reber G, Rand JH, Ortel TL, Galli M, de Groot PG. update of the guidelines for lupus anticoagulant detection. J Thromb Haemost 2009; 7: 1737–40.

Oldenburg J, Pavlova A. Discrepancy between onestage and chromogenic factor VIII activity assay results can lead to misdiagnosis of haemophilia A phenotype. Hämostaseologie 2010; 30: 207–11.

Perry DJ. Factor VII deficiency. Br J Haematol 2002; 118: 689–700.

Patzke J, Schneppenheim R. Laboratory diagnosis of von Willebrand disease. Hämostaseologie 2010; 30: 203–6.

Schneppenheim R, Budde U. Von Willebrand-Syndrom und von Willebrand-Faktor. Aktuelle Aspekte der Diagnostik und Therapie. 2. Auflage. UNI-MED Verlag AG Bremen, London, Boston 2006.

Witt P, Patscheke H. Blutungszeit – Standortbestimmung. J Lab Med 1997; 21: 299–301.

Harrison P. The role of PFA-100 testing in the investigation and management of haemostatic defects in children and adults. Br J Haemtol 2005; 130: 3–10.

Consensus Papier der DGKL-Arbeitsgruppe „Hämostaseologische Labordiagnostik". Blutungsneigung: Diagnostische Strategie zur Abklärung einer Thrombozytendysfunktion. J Lab Med 2004; 28: 453–62.

Budde U. Diagnose von Funktionsstörungen der Thrombozyten mit Hilfe der Aggregometrie. J Lab Med 2002; 26: 564–71.

McGlasson DL, Fritsma GA. Whole blood platelet aggregometry and platelet function testing. Semin Thromb Hemost 2009; 35: 168–80.

Cattaneo M. Light transmission aggregometry and ATP release for the diagnostic assessment of platelet function. Semin Thromb Hemost 2009; 35: 158–67.

DGA. Interdisziplinare S2-Leitlinie zur Diagnostik und Therapie der Venenthrombose und der Lungenembolie. VASA 2010; 39: S/78.

Wells PS, Anderson DR, Rodger M, Ginsberg JS, Kearon C, Gent M, Turpie AG, Bormanis J, Weitz J, Chamberlain M, Bowie D, Barnes D, Hirsh J. Derivation of a simple clinical model to categorize patients probability of pulmonary embolism: increasing the models utility with the SimpliRED D-dimer. Thromb Haemost 2000; 83: 416–20.

Wells PS, Anderson DR, Rodger M, Forgie M, Kearon C, Dreyer J, Kovacs G, Mitchell M, Lewandowski B, Kovacs MJ. Evaluation of D-dimer in the diagnosis of suspected deep-vein thrombosis. N Engl J Med 2003; 349: 1227–35.

Lo GK, Juhl D, Warkentin TE, Sigouin CS, Eichler P, Greinacher A. Evaluation of pretest clinical score (4T's) for the diagnosis of heparin-induced thrombocytopenia in two clinical settings. J Thromb Haemost 2006; 4: 759–65.

Greinacher A, Juhl D, Strobel U, Wessel A, Lubenow N, Selleng K, Eichler P, Warkentin TE. Heparin-induced thrombocytopenia: a prospective study on the incidence, platelet-activating capacity and clinical significance of anti-PF4/heparin antibodies of the IgG, IgM, and IgA class. J Thromb Haemost 2007; 5: 235–41.

Lindhoff-Last E. Bewertung des Rezidivthromboserisikos venoser Thromboembolien. Hämostaseologie 2011; 31: 7–12.

Lijfering WM, Brouwer J-L P, Veeger NJGM, Bank I, Coppens M, Middeldorp S, Hamulyak K, Prins MH, Buller HR, van der Meer J. Selective testing for thrombophilia in patients with first venous thrombosis: results from a retrospective family cohort study on absolute thrombotic risk for currently known thrombophilic defects in 2479 relatives. Blood 2009; 113: 5314–22.

Brouwer JL, Lijfering WM, ten Kate MK, Kluin-Nelemans HC, Veeger NJGM, van der Meer J. High long-term absolute risk of recurrent venous thromboembolism in patients with hereditary deficiences of protein S, protein C and antithrombin. Thromb Haemost 2009; 101: 93–9.

Pengo V, Ruffatti A, Legnani C, Gresele P, Barcellona D, Erba N, Testa S, Marongiu F, Bison E, Denas G, Banzato A, Padayattil Jose S, Iliceto S. Clinical course of high-risk patients diagnosed with antiphospholipid syndrome. JTH 2010; 8: 237–42.

Bates SM, Greer IA, Pabinger I, Sofaer S, Hirsch J. Venous thromboembolism, thrombophilia, antithrombotic therapy, and pregnancy. Chest 2008; 133: 844S–886 S.

Robertson L, Wu O, Langhorne P, et al. The Thrombosis Risk and Economic Assessment of Thrombophilia Screening (Treats) Study: thrombophilia in pregnancy; a systematic review. Br J Haematol 2005; 132: 171–96.

Clark P, Walke I, Laghorne P, Crichton L, Thompson A, Greaves M, et al. SPIN (Scottish Pregnancy intervention) study: a multicenter, randomized controlled trial of low-molecular weight heparin and low-dose aspirin in women with recurrent miscarriage. Blood 2010; 115: 4162–7.

Kaandorp SP, Goffijn M, van der Post JAM, Hutten BA, Verhöve HR, Hamulyak K, et al. Aspirin plus heparin or aspirin alone in women with recurrent miscarriage. N Engl J Med 2010; 362: 1586–96.

Nelson SM. Is placental haemostasis relevant to recurrent implantation failure? Thromb Res 127 Suppl. 3 (2011) S93–S95.

Miyakis S, Lockshin MD, Atsumi T, Branch DW, Brey RL, Cervera R, Derksen RHWM, de Groot PG, Koike T, Meroni PL, Reber G, Shoenfeld Y, Tincani A, Vlachoyiannopoulos PG, Krilis SA. International consensus statement on an update of the classification criteria for definite antiphospholipid syndrome (APS). J Thromb Haemost 2006; 4: 295–306.

Thrombophilia

Presumptive diagnosis/clinical picture

Deep venous thromboembolism: positive patient or family medical history; miscarriage predisposition (pregnancy complications)

Laboratory

Hereditary factors

APC resistance	Genotyping factor II	Antithrombin chromogen	Protein S activity	Protein C activity	Fibrinogen (Clauss)

hetero- or homo-zygote

decreased — decreased — decreased — decreased

APC ratio decreased

Yes — Yes — Yes — Yes

Yes — Yes

Rule out temporary origins — No

Expanded laboratory

Genotyping

Confirmatory testing

hetero- or homo-zygote — No

Positive — Yes

No

Yes

Rule out antiphos-pholipid antibodies

Yes

Yes

Antithrom-bin Ag	Protein S free	Protein C Ag	Fibrinogen Ag

Normal value or Clauss ratio: Ag ~0.5

Diagnosis

Factor V Leiden | **Prothrombin 20210 poly-morphism** | **Congenital inhibitor deficiency** | **Dysfibrino-genemia**

Clarification of additional origins/additional procedures

Genotyping if necessary

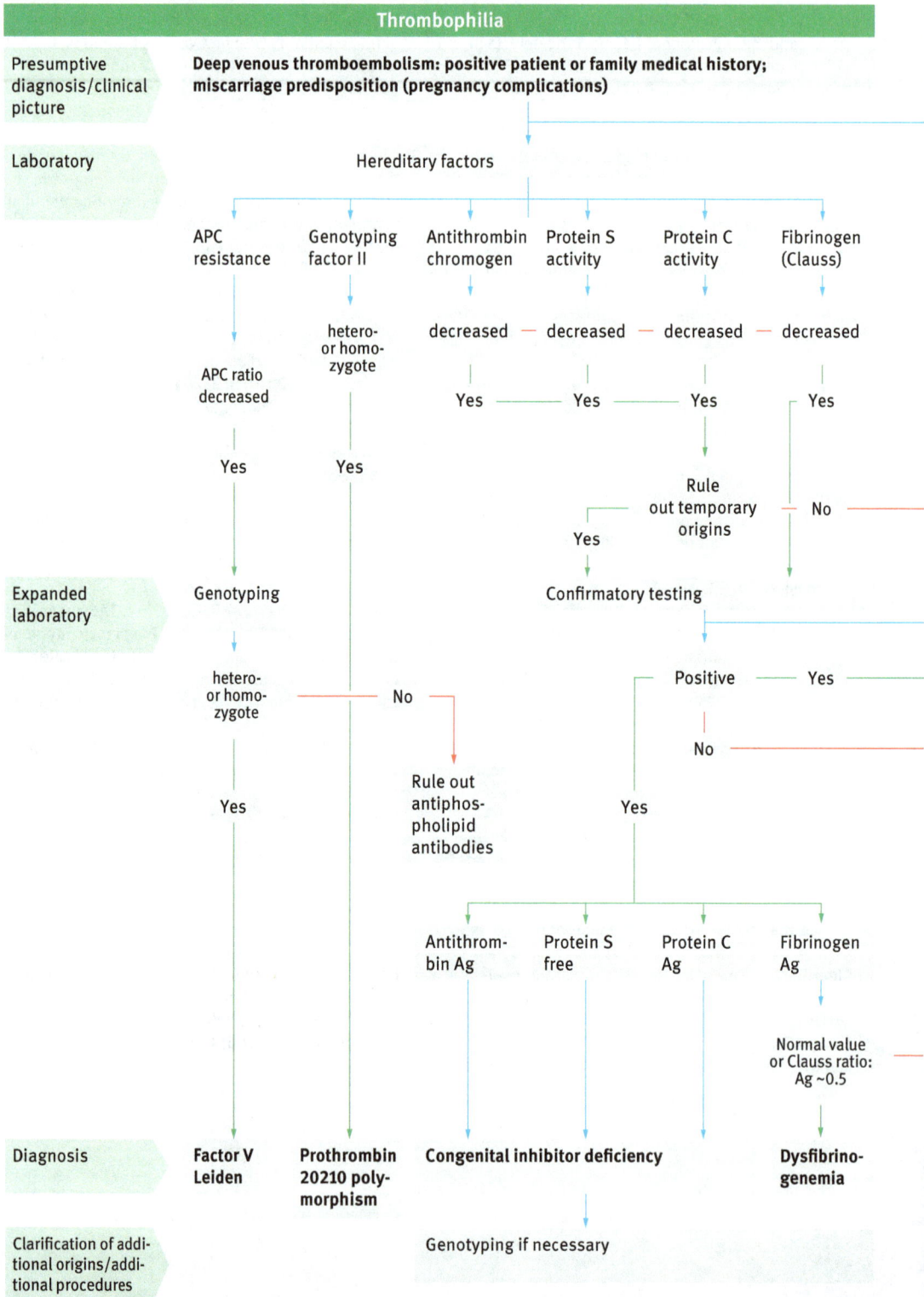

Figure 4.45 Diagnostic Pathway: Thrombophilia.

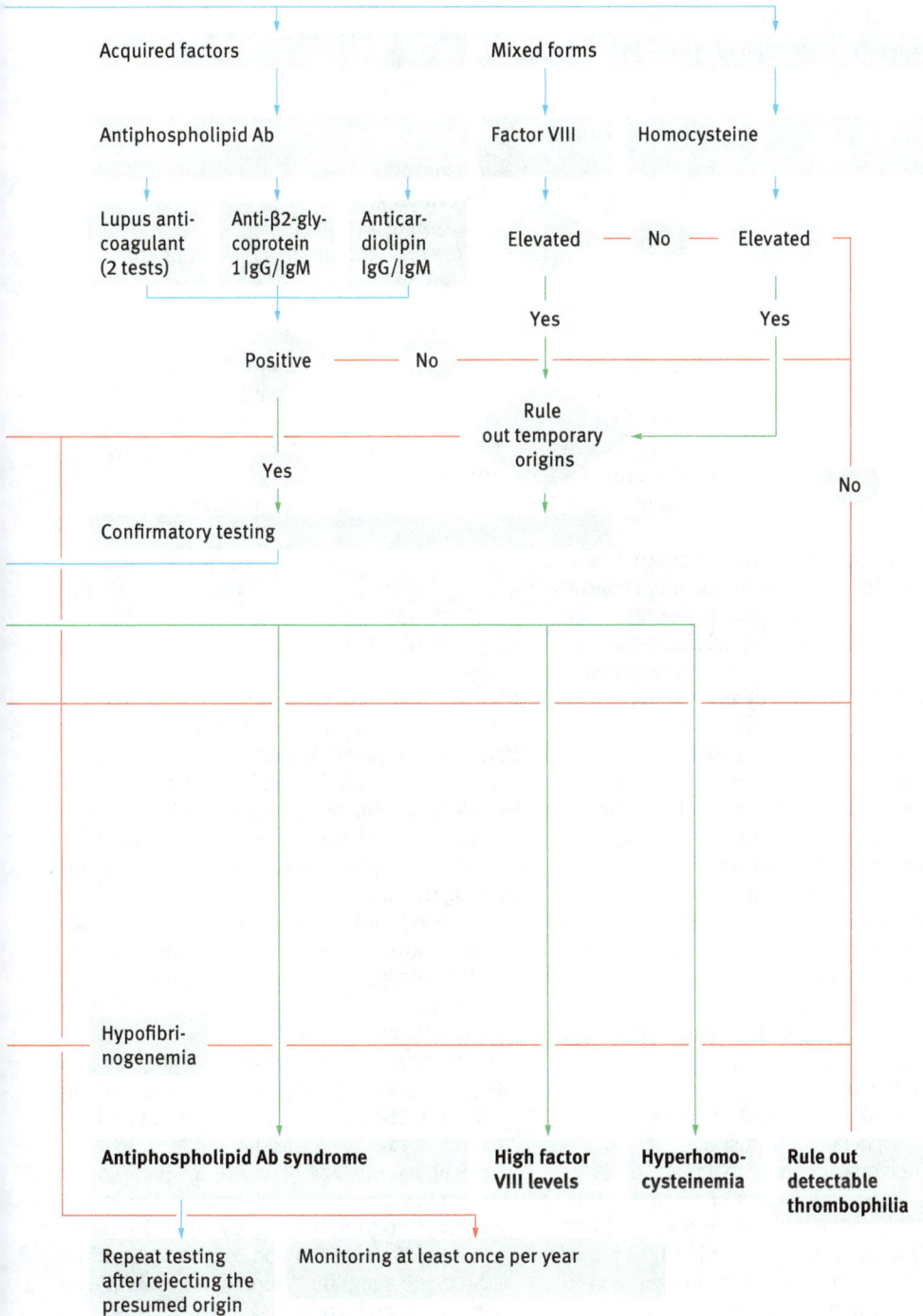

Acquired factors   Mixed forms

Antiphospholipid Ab   Factor VIII   Homocysteine

Lupus anti-   Anti-β2-gly-   Anticar-   Elevated — No — Elevated
coagulant   coprotein   diolipin
(2 tests)   1 IgG/IgM   IgG/IgM

                                            Yes   Yes

            Positive ——— No

                                            Rule
                                          out temporary
                                            origins

                                                           No

            Yes

Confirmatory testing

Hypofibri-
nogenemia

Antiphospholipid Ab syndrome   **High factor**   **Hyperhomo-**   **Rule out**
                                          VIII levels   **cysteinemia** **detectable**
                                                                             thrombophilia

Repeat testing   Monitoring at least once per year
after rejecting the
presumed origin

Manfred Wolfgang Wick, Hans Jurgen Kuhn,
Markus Otto, Hela-Felicitas Petereit,
Hayrettin Tumani, Manfred Uhr und
Brigitte Wildemann

In cooperation with the German Society
for Cerebrospinal Fluid Diagnostics and
Clinical Neurochemistry (DGLN).

4.7 Neurological Disorders

4.7.1 Neurological Laboratory Diagnostics

4.7.1.1 Characteristics of Neurological Laboratory Di agnostics

1. Categorically ruling out a CNS disorder with a few simple laboratory methods is not possible. Cerebrospinal fluid (CSF) diagnostics are not screening tests, but are often indicated in the first place for the diagnosis of inflammatory diseases and additionally for hemorrhage, tumor involvement, and dementia syndromes.
2. If deemed necessary, a lumbar puncture must be preceded by a CT scan to rule out a contraindication (e.g., intracranial pressure); additional blood tests might be helpful to rule out severe coagulopathy, to identify any systemic inflammations, and to detect pathogens by blood culture.
3. Lumbar puncture is carried out as an emergency diagnostic procedure comprising cell and erythrocyte counts, glucose or lactate and total protein, or, more often, as a basic test program comprising cytology, CSF/serum albumin and immunoglobulin ratios and oligoclonal bands supplemented by targeted specialized examinations depending on the medical indication.
4. Many CSF parameters, especially protein concentrations, depend on the blood/CSF barrier function and must therefore be interpreted as a CSF/serum quotient.
5. In addition, blood or urine analyses are also required, especially for diseases of the peripheral nervous system or metabolic diseases (e.g. autoantbody detection in serum for PNP work-up, copper metabolism in the blood and urine in Wilson's disease, vitamin B12 in serum and possibly methylmalonic acid excretion in the urine, in vitamin B_{12} deficiency).

4.7.1.2 Cerebrospinal Fluid Diagnostic Parameters

Emergency program:
- Cell and erythrocyte count (chamber counts)
- Preliminary cell differentiation
- Total protein
- Glucose or lactate
- Rapid pathogen test (Gram stain, latex antigen test)

Basic program:
- CSF cytology
- Pathogen detection culture
- CSF/serum quotient for albumin, IgG, possibly also IgA and IgM
- Oligoclonal IgG

Special diagnostics:
- Pathogen-specific antibody indices
- PCR for detecting the pathogen genome (primarily for viruses)
- Immunocytology or immunophenotyping
- Tumor markers
- Destruction and dementia markers
- Ferritin

4.7.1.3 Pre-analytics in Cerebrospinal Fluid Diagnostics

Only the essential pre-analytical requirements for CSF diagnostics are specified here; extensive treatments of preanalytical laboratory medical principles and analyte stability can be found in the relevant clinical chemistry and microbiology textbooks as well as in the recommendations of the DGKL Pre-analytics Working Group (www.dgkl.de).

1. At lumbar puncture, avoid artificial contamination with blood, cartilage or bone marrow cells, and skin flora as much as possible; this is not always possible under demanding anatomical circumstances. If this is not possible or not assessable in a repeat lumbar puncture (e.g., following iatrogenic, traumatic, spinal SAH),the CSF should still be analyzed and the degree of falsification estimated by a post-analytical assessment of multiple quantitative determinations: e.g. by comparing the leukocyte/erythrocyte ratios in blood and CSF; in the case of artificial blood contamination, the "three-vial sampling" approach is useful (see the section on "bloody CSF").

2. CSF samples for emergency diagnosis should be processed immediately (within one hour), and temperature fluctuations and excessive agitation during transport should be avoided. Otherwise, a significant decrease in cell count might occur along with effects on the cell profile (granulocytes and siderophages in the CSF matrix are especially unstable, whereas T lymphocytes can survive for one day). Glucose and lactate levels depend on the cell content, particularly at room temperature in the absence of enzyme inhibitors, and can be unstable.
3. CSF and serum should be obtained in parallel for protein and antibody analyses, since otherwise the basic assumptions regarding the diffusion equilibrium between the blood and CSF compartments (a prerequisite for evaluating the quotient) are not reliable.
4. Most of the proteins and antibodies in the CSF and serum are stable for at least one week at refrigerator temperatures, but immunoglobulins should not be frozen.
5. Some proteins, e.g., ß-amyloid, tend to adhere to certain plastic surfaces such as polystyrene; for this reason, polypropylene tubes should be used for diagnostic procedures related to dementia.

4.7.2 Diagnostic Pathways and Procedures

4.7.2.1 Clinical Spectrum and Underlying Guidelines from Clinical Professional Associations

Starting from different clinical syndromes or CSF analysis results, the following diagnostic pathways have been developed by various working group members. Descriptions of procedures and typical findings for virtually all the issues discussed in the group are now available:

- Acute meningitis/encephalitis, including opportunistic CNS infections
- Bloody CSF/suspected SAH
- Radicular syndromes including meningeal carcinomatosis
- Chronic inflammatory CNS diseases including MS
- Inflammatory CSF syndrome of unknown origin
- Dementia syndromes
- Wilson's disease

Strict implementation in decision trees and their graphical representation proved to be difficult in some cases, such as chronic inflammation, inflammation of unknown origin, and dementias.

The work is based on the DGLN guidelines and methods catalog (Petereit, Sindern, Wick (Ed.) 2007; update available at: www.dgln.de) – where necessary taking into account the guidelines of the German Neurological Society (DGN: www.dgn.org) as far as references are made to laboratory findings found there. It can reasonably be concluded that the requirement for participation of the appropriate clinical professional associations is met because the CSF diagnostics experts from the DGN and DGKL are generally also affiliated with the DGLN. Furthermore, the source material includes several recent standard CSF diagnostics textbooks, along with contributions from many authors affiliated with the DGLN, DGN and DGKL (Felgenhauer and Beuche, 1999; Zettl, Lehmitz, and Mix (ed.), 2005; Kluge, Wiezcorek, Linke, Zimmermann and Witte, 2005; Wildemann, Oschmann, and Reiber, 2010).

4.7.2.2 Acute Meningitis

Although meningitis is a rare disease with an incidence of 10 per 100,000, due to its potentially lethal course and the availability of treatment options with curative potential, no diagnosable case should be missed. Acute meningitis thus represents the archetypal case for emergency CSF diagnostics. In the absence of contraindications to lumbar puncture, from the medical and preanalytical perspective, the emergency analysis and consequent decisions for further diagnosis and treatment must proceed within two hours. At a minimum, the presence of bacterial meningitis must be confirmed or confidently excluded within this time frame, and if necessary an initial pathogen identification made via microscopy or latex test.

The flow diagram shows the process starting from a clinical suspicion (▶ Figure 4.46).

Further differentiation is carried out as in ▶ Table 4.28.

Finally, it should be noted that at a very early stage, the lymphocytic meningitis cell profile can initially appear granulocytic or mixed.

A low or normal cell count can indicate a meningeal irritation, such as in a systemic infection.

Acute Meningitis	
Initial examination	Headache , fever, and neck stiffness; rule out intracranial pressure, CT
Presumptive diagnosis	**Acute Meningitis**
	Lumbar puncture
Laboratory	Appearance, cell counts, cell differentiation, glucose, lactate, total protein

No —— Patholo- gical (primarily cell findings)

Normal findings   Yes

Diagnosis	**Differential diagnosis, see table 4.28**
Further tests	Gram preparation/antigen detection (Differentiation, see table 4.29) Imaging methods

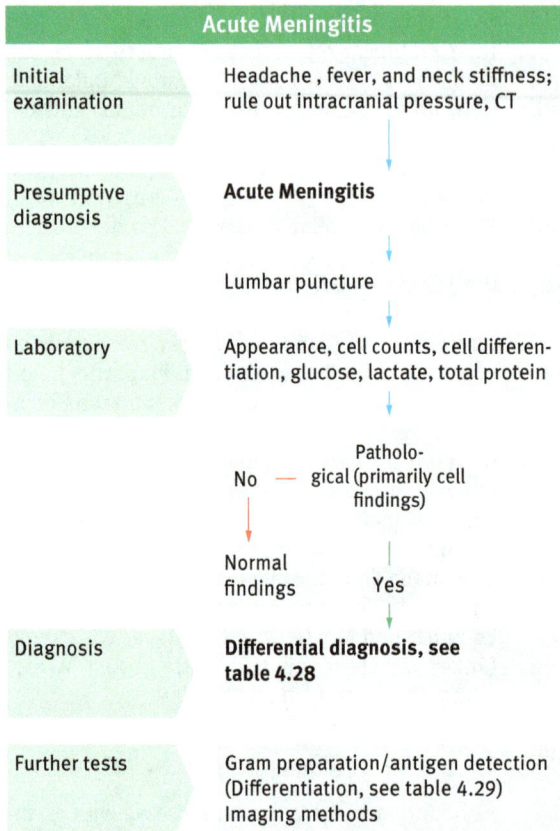

Figure 4.46 Diagnostic Pathway: acute Meningitis.

Table 4.28 Differential diagnosis of meningitis (DGLN Guidelines, 2007; modified from Felgenbauer und Beuche, 1999).

CSF parameter	Purulent meningitis	Lymphocytic (primarily viral) meningitis	Tuberculous meningitis
Cell count/µL	>1000	<1000	<1000
Cytology	Granulocytic	Lymphocytic	Mixed cellular
Glucose quotient	Lowered	Normal	Lowered
Lactate, mmol/L	>5	<5	>5
Total protein, mg/L	>1000	<1000	>1000
Blood/CSF barrier	Seriously disrupted	Normal to moderately disrupted	Seriously disrupted

Note: In an "apurulent" meningitis, the cell count might be only slightly increased, while the bacterial density is substantial. This special form of bacterial meningitis is associated with a poor prognosis, and is often found in immunocompromised patients. Also in the early stages of bacterial meningitis, a still low cell count can lead to an erroneous assessment. When in doubt, a repeat puncture must be done after 24 hours.

The pathogen diagnosis is made based on the preliminary results:

Purulent meningitis:
- Blood culture, CSF culture, Gram stain from the CSF, possibly a rapid test for suspected cryptococcal meningitis using an India ink preparation.

Table 4.29 Microscopic identification of the most common meningitis pathogens: + = positive, – = negative.

Pathogen	Gram reaction	Localization	Form
Staphylococci	+	Intra- or extracellular	Clusters of cocci
Meningococci	–	Intracellular	Roll-shaped diplococci
Pneumococci	+	Extracellular	Lancet-shaped diplococci
Haemophilus influenzae	–	Extracellular	Fine rods in a "school of fish" arrangement
E. coli and other Enterobacteria	–	Predominantly extracellular	Plump rods
Listeria	+	Intra- or extracellular	Few plump rods

Table 4.30 Diagnostic work-up of lymphocytic meningitis.

Basic tests:

HSV AI, VZV AI, Borrelia AI, HSV PCR, VZV PCR

In patients with concomitant HIV or other immune deficiencies

CMV AI, EBV AI, TPHA AI, toxoplasmosis AI, CMV PCR, EBV PCR, JCV PCR

In cases of relevant exposure:

TBE AI

Other viruses:

Depends on the therapeutic relevance (e.g., mumps); possibly no specific diagnostics

Tuberculous meningitis (with a clinical suspicion of tuberculous meningitis, initiate a four-fold treatment regimen):

- TB PCR, also repeatedly (if enough material, send at least 5 mL), cultures, also from urine, BAL, Ziehl-Neelsen stain or modified Kinyoun stain

If the patient had not yet been pretreated with antibiotics in a case of purulent meningitis, microscopic identification of the likely pathogen will usually be possible as shown in ▶ Table 4.29 below. However, the microscopic detection of tuberculosis bacteria from CSF, e.g., with Ziehl-Neelsen staining, gives low sensitivity.

Otherwise, if necessary, a latex agglutination test for antigen detection, then culturing for resistance testing and multiplex PCR is essential. Overall, the pathogen is detected in approx. 80 % of purulent meningitis cases, while in only about 50 % TB cases.

The diagnostic procedure for lymphocytic meningitis is shown in ▶ Table 4.30.

It should be noted here that PCR is the most sensitive method for viral genome detection in the early phase. After a few days in immunocompetent patients, the humoral immune response starts and detection be accomplished via the pathogen-specific antibody index (AI); by contrast, AI is the only practicable method for Borrelia and toxoplasmosis.

4.7.2.3 Opportunistic CNS Infections

Opportunistic infections and atypical or weak reactions must be considered in patients with immune deficiencies, as shown in ▶ Table 4.31 and

Table 4.31 Opportunistic CNS infections – bacteria, fungi, protozoa.

Neurotuberculosis: meningitis or granuloma: CSF: mixed pleocytosis, serious barrier disruption with IgA production, increased glucose consumption; DD also neurosarcoidosis

Septic embolic encephalitis (hematogenic):
CSF: Similar to TB, somewhat higher cell counts, pathogen: Blood culture, if necessary,

Cryptococcal meningoencephalitis (most often secondary to HIV):
CSF: pathogen by microscopy > 80 %, antigen and culture, barrier disruption with weak cell response and pathological glucose consumption

CNS aspergillosis (often secondary to leukemia or bone marrow transplantation [BMT]): aspergillosis in imaging procedures; pathogens usually not in the CSF; barrier disruption possibly with weakened cell response, and pathological glucose consumption

CNS toxoplasmosis (most often secondary to HIV):
MRI: DD CNS tuberculosis and NHL; few CSF changes, rarely tachyzoites; if necessary, toxoplasma AI

Table 4.32 Viruses of the herpes group – frequently as opportunistic pathogens.

HSV 1	Hemorrhagic necrotizing meningoencephalitis
HSV 2	Mollaret meningitis (recurring)
VZV	Zoster ganglionitis, facial nerve paresis; with immunodeficiency: meningoencephalitis
CMV	Encephalitis, retinitis, possibly radiculitis (most often secondary to HIV and immunosuppression)
EBV	B cell involvement; note in presence of immunodeficiency: transformation into B cell NHL

Table 4.32. This includes reactivation of latent pathogens, such as tuberculosis, toxoplasmosis, and herpes group viruses, or infections by pathogens that do not normally cause encephalitis. Basically, atypical patterns of findings are to be expected, for example, only mild cellular reactions, particularly weak pathogen-specific antibody production; under these conditions, serological findings can be unreliable (possible false negatives). Thus, the direct detection of pathogens is of particular importance here.

4.7.2.4 Suspected SAH/Bloody Cerebrospinal Fluid

- With a clinical suspicion of subarachnoid hemorrhage (SAH), first a CT scan to confirm the diagnosis – even simply to rule out contraindications to lumbar puncture. Note: approximately 10–20 % of SAH are CT-negative. With an unclear diagnosis and absence of contraindications: perform lumbar puncture. If there is any uncertainty about the uniformity of blood-tinged CSF, the three-vial sampling protocol should first be carried out, with subsequent verification in the laboratory; first, emergency diagnostics with cell and erythrocyte counts, assessment for xanthochromia, if necessary, after centrifugation while taking the total protein concentration into account.
- With a xanthochromia at a total protein of < 1000 mg/L: actual hemorrhage is quite probable; look for the source of the bleeding. Otherwise, assess the cytology, and if necessary, make a ferritin determination from the CSF; assess the cell and erythrocyte counts, and cell profile, if necessary with comparison to peripheral blood. Evidence of a scavenger reaction with significant erythrophagocytosis or even siderophages: actual hemorrhage is confirmed.
- By contrast, with a CSF composition resembling diluted blood: artificial hemorrhage is likely; DD fresh bleeding < 12 h. If uncertainty persists, or with a clear, cell-poor CSF to rule out previous SAH: ferritin determination. If ferritin > 15 ng/mL, an actual hemorrhage is quite probable if bacterial meningitis can be ruled out.
- The procedure for a clinically suspected SAH is shown in Figure 4.47, and an algorithm for work-up of bloody CSF is shown in ▶ Figure 4.48.

4.7.2.5 Radicular Syndromes

Clinical definition

Radicular syndrome refers to sensory, motor and/or vegetative-trophic disorders in the dermatomes, which can be associated with a distribution area of the spinal nerve root. It can affect individual nerve roots (monoradiculopathy) or multiple nerve roots (polyradiculopathy). The procedure for suspected radicular syndrome is shown in ▶ Figure 4.49.

Differential diagnosis

In addition to mechanical origins, such as disc herniation, inflammatory (pathogen- or autoimmune-related) and neoplastic diseases are also considered.

The most common inflammatory origins are autoimmune inflammatory (Guillain-Barré syndrome [GBS], Miller-Fisher syndrome, sarcoidosis, vasculitis) or infectious diseases (Borrelia, mycobacteria, VZV, HSV1/HSV2, EBV, Leptospira, CMV) and lymphomatous or carcinomatous meningitis.

Since the clinical picture alone often cannot distinguish between the various etiologies, spinal imaging should be performed first. Once a mechanical origin has been ruled out, proceed to clarify an inflammatory or neoplastic etiology.

Steps in laboratory diagnostics

Even in the absence of signs of systemic infection, the indication for lumbar puncture is given since an isolated intrathecal inflammation can often be present.

Thunderclap headache – suspected SAH

Initial exami-
nation/incidental
findings

Thunderclap headache

Imaging
procedures

No — Hemor-
rhage — Yes

Clinic

Intra-
cranial pressure
or coagulation
disorder

— No → Lumbar puncture, if necessary using
the three-vial sampling protocol

Yes

Laboratory

Yes — CSF bloody
test strip — No

Ferri-
tin > 15 µg/L
or positive for erythro-
phages/sidero-
phages

Xantho-
chromia, ferritin
> 15 µg/L or positive for ery-
throphages/sidero
phages

No   Yes   Yes   No

Expanded
laboratory

Rule out meningitis

If neces-
sary, repeat lumbar
puncture after 12 h
with hemorrhage
detection

Yes

Diagnosis

Artificially bloody CSF
With persistent clinical
suspicion

**Hemorrhage
detected**

No

Yes

Clarification of addi-
tional origins/addi-
tional procedures

MRI: actual hemorrhage
or other disease

Search for hemorrhage
source (e.g., angiography)

MRI: actual hemorrhage
or other disease

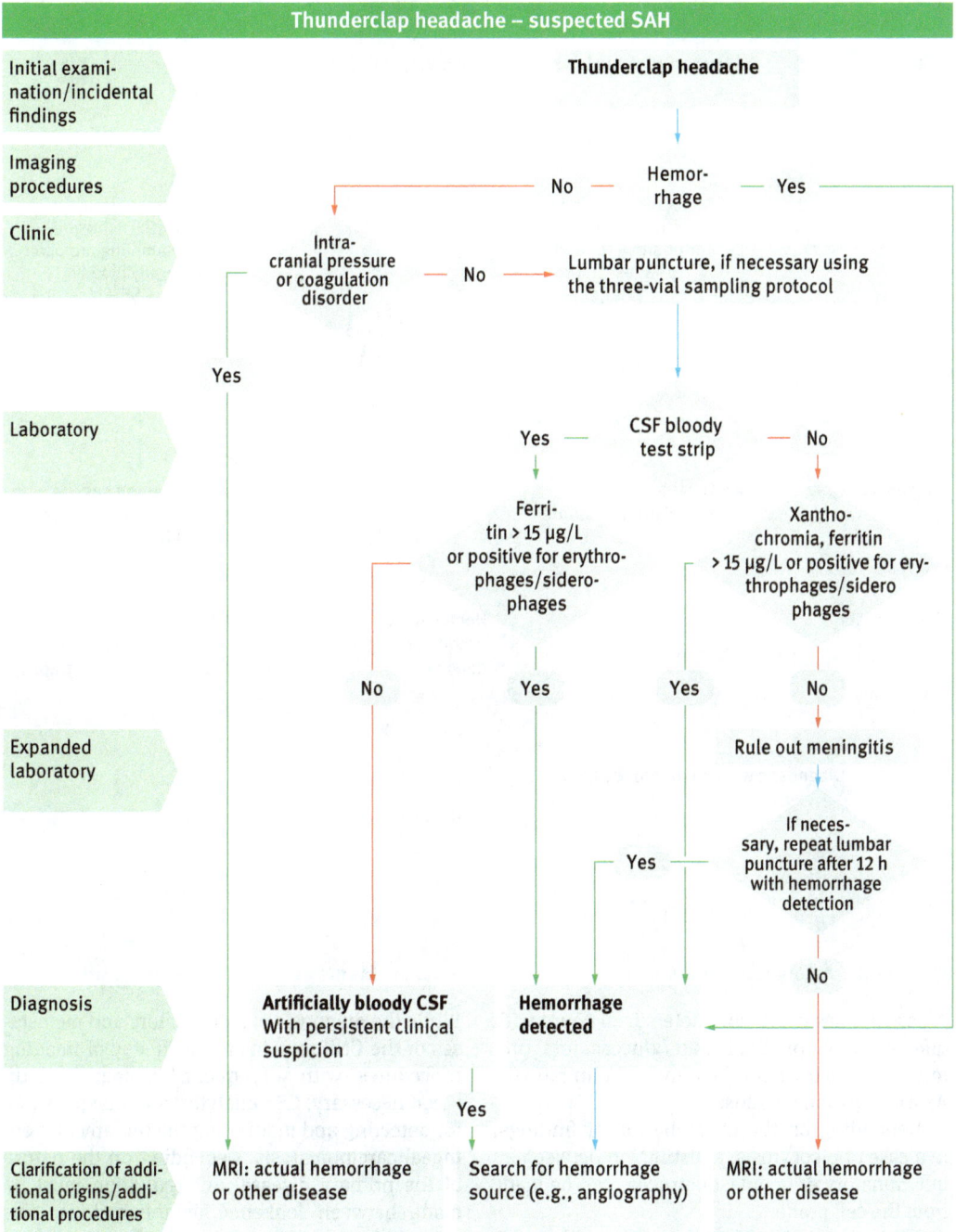

Figure 4.47 Diagnostic procedure of a thunderclap headache – clinical suspicion of SAH.

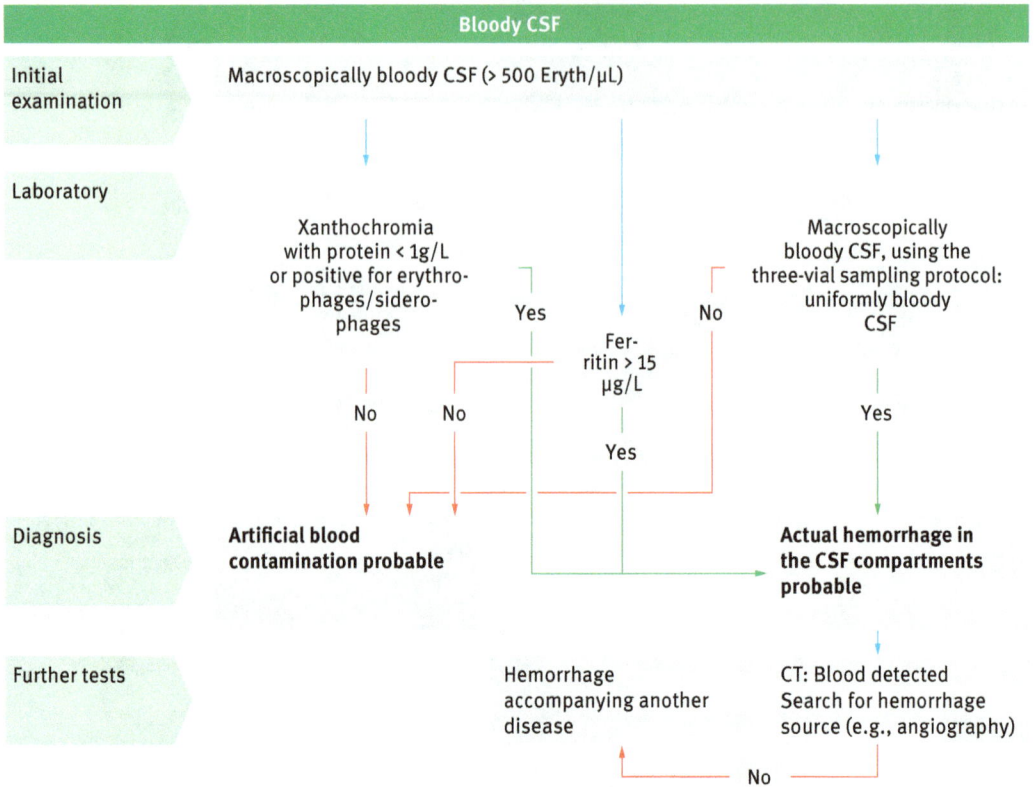

Figure 4.48 Diagnostic work-up of bloody CSF.

Is an inflammatory CSF syndrome present?

Assess the basic CSF parameters (cell count with differential cell profile, lactate/glucose, total protein, albumin quotient, immunoglobulin ratio (G, A, M), oligoclonal bands.

Depending on the constellation of findings, in a case of pleocytosis, a distinction between an inflammatory or neoplastic process can be made from the cell profile.

The constellation of findings from cell counts with the other protein parameters can provide indications of possible pathogenic origins, such as Borrelia infection (pleocytosis, normal lactate, three-class Ig synthesis with IgM predominant), so that a targeted PCR or pathogen-specific serological diagnosis can be carried out.

4.7.2.6 Meningeal tumor involvement

While the diagnosis of solid tumors and metastases of the CNS remains the mainstay of imaging procedures, with subsequent histology work-up when necessary, CSF analytics are indispensable for detecting and monitoring the therapy of meningeal carcinomatosis. Depending on the nature of the primary disease, differentiation must be made between leukemic, lymphomatous, carcinomatous, melanomatous, and sarcomatous meningitis, and also the relatively rare meningitis of primary brain tumors. Apart from the always indispensable cytomorphology, further procedures depend critically on this differentiation. Occasionally, extensive diagnostics are required if the meningitis is the first manifestation of an as

Radicular Syndrome

Initial examination	Sensory, motor and/or vegetative disorders in the spinal nerve root area

Presumptive diagnosis — Radicular Syndrome

Laboratory — Lumbar puncture ← No — Spinal cord imaging procedures: mechanical origin

Appearance, cell counts, cell differentiation, glucose, lactate, total protein, CSF protein differentiation, oligoclonal bands

Yes

Pathological — No → Normal findings

Yes

Inflammatory

Yes   No →   High CSF Protein or Albumin Ratio

Further tests — PCR, pathogen-specific serological diagnosis, autoantibodies: positive result?   Malignant cells in CSF

Yes   No   No   Yes   No   Yes

If necessary, repeat the lumbar puncture

Diagnosis — **Depending on the results, *inter alia*, GBS or infectious radiculitis**   **Meningeal carcinomatosis**   **e.g., Tumor-herniated disc**   **GBS**

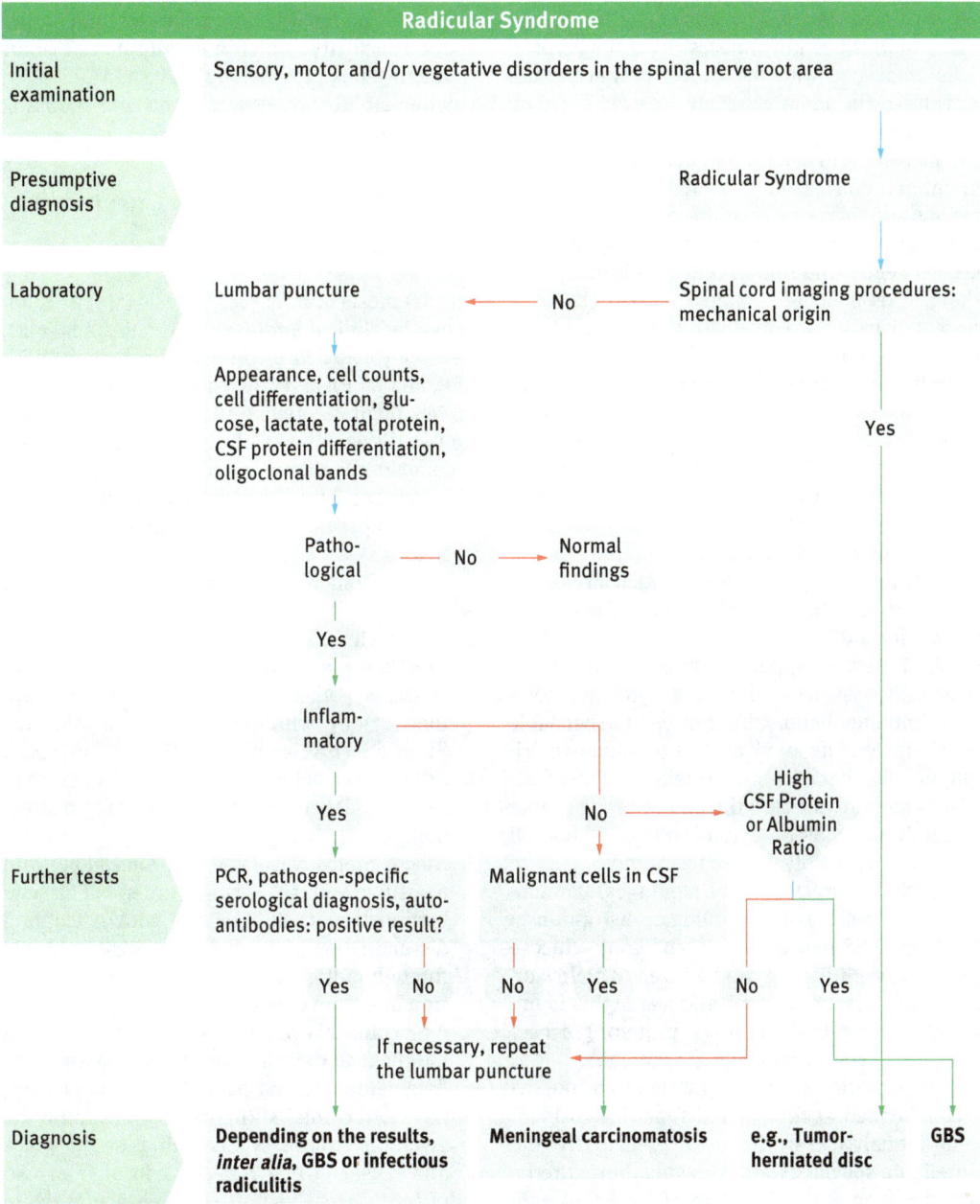

Figure 4.49 Diagnostic work-up of Radicular syndrome.

yet unknown neoplasia. Conversely, further investigation is usually unnecessary if the atypical cells associated with the known primary tumor can already be unambiguously detected based on cytomorphology.

The cell count determination is required as basic information for producing the cytologic preparations and follow-up over the course of disease, although it cannot confirm or rule out the diagnosis. Between 0 and 10,000 cells/μl, basically anything is possible; CSF samples in cases of hematological disease have about 10- to 100-fold higher cell counts than in solid tumors.

In the first lumbar puncture, with a sufficient cell recovery and provided the examiner is experienced, a cytologic sensitivity of approximately 70–80 % is possible with solid tumors; a sensitivity of over 90 % can be expected in acute leukemias and highly malignant lymphomas (although not in primary CNS lymphomas!). In principle, it remains problematic to differentiate lymphocytic CSF pleocytosis in a case of low-malignancy lymphoma for a differential diagnosis of neoplastic meningitis versus opportunistic infections; this is often only possible with immunocytology. Moreover, immunophenotyping can be indispensable for characterizing atypical cells of unknown origin, or cells that constitute a relatively low fraction in individual cases; the choice of the proper antibody depends on cytomorphology and cell counts, and possibly the primary tumor.

Another characteristic of meningeal carcinomatosis is a somewhat significant disruption in the blood/CSF barrier and an anaerobic glucose metabolism. Still, both can be absent with low tumor load. However, neoplastic meningitis is unlikely if all the basic findings (protein, glucose/lactate, cell count, cytology) are normal.

The majority of tumor markers cannot be recommended at the present time due to inadequate analytical or diagnostic sensitivity and unreliable specificity and/or evaluation criteria. An exception is the detection of local CEA synthesis with sensitive analytical methods; this has been shown to be a viable supplementary method to cytology for use in carcinomas with proven high specificity. Due to a lack of specificity, however, elevated beta-2-microglobulin cannot be regarded as an indicator for leukemia or lymphoma involvement, although if an inflammatory process has been ruled out, it can have a value in differential diagnosis and in ruling out a

neoplastic meningitis. Other markers with higher tissue specificity, which normally do not occur in the CNS (e.g., thyroglobulin, PSA, AFP, sHCG) can be helpful with respect to the corresponding primary tumor.

4.7.2.7 Chronic Inflammatory CNS Disorders

Multiple sclerosis

The diagnosis of multiple sclerosis (MS) is established by clinical findings and craniospinal MRI. Neurophysiological tests (evoked potentials: VEP, SEP, and MEP), and CSF results are supportive of an MS diagnosis. Definite MS requires the detection of dissemination of disease symptoms and inflammatory lesions (as detected by cranial MRI) in space and time. The presence of MS is additionally supported by typical inflammatory CSF changes.

The McDonald diagnostic criteria are fulfilled when:
1. A first clinical event (clinically isolated syndrome, e.g. optic neuritis, myelitis, brainstem syndrome, other focal or multifocal CNS symptoms) along with positive cranial MRI (i.e. Swanton criteria of dissemination in space fulfilled, see below), is followed by a new neurological deficit (as above) (clinically definite MS), or
2. After a clinically isolated syndrome along with a positive MRI (i.e. Swanton criteria of dissemination in space fulfilled, see below), temporal dissemination of the disease process is proven through radiological detection of a new T2 lesion in a repeat cranial MRI .
3. A first clinical event (see above) coincides with radiological detection of dissemination of inflammatory lesions in both space and time, i.e. when cranial MRI abnormalities fulfill the Swanton criteria of dissemination in space and reveals ≥ one T2-lesions in at least two of four typical regions (periventricular white matter, juxtacortical white matter, infratentorial white matter, spinal cord, and ≥ one clinically asymptomatic contrast-enhancing T1-lesion(s)
4. Continous neurologic deterioration (over at least one year) coincides with two of the following conditions: positive cranial MRI (at least one T2-lesion in at least one of the following regions: periventricular, juxtacortical, in-

fratentorial), positive spinal MRI (at least two focal T2-lesions, positive CSF (i.e. intrtahecal IgG synthesis as detected by CSF-restricted oligoclonal bands or an elevated IgG-index) (Primary progressive MS)

Typical CSF findings support the diagnosis and can be expected in 95 % of MS cases, independent of the clinical diseases course (relapsing, secondary, or primary chronic progressive).

First stage of diagnostics: the cell profile (cell count and CSF cell cytomorphology) are pathological in 60 % of patients. Typical abnormalities include a lymphocytic pleocytosis up to 30/µL and cytological evidence of few transformed lymphocytes and plasma cells (2–5 %). However, a normal cell count and cytology do not rule out MS. With higher sensitivity (75 %), quantitative alterations in the protein profile findings are detectable. Total protein is normal or only slightly elevated (< 800 mg/L), while the albumin quotient (QAlb) is normal and in only 10 % of cases might show a slight ($8–10 \times 10^{-3}$) or moderate ($10–20 \times 10^{-3}$) blood/CSF barrier disruption. A characteristic finding is local IgG synthesis (82 %), or, more rarely, local synthesis of IgM or IgA, as revealed by illustration of CSF/serum quotients for albumin and immunoglobulins (QAlb, QIgG, IgM, QIgA) in quotient diagrams. Qualitative proof of intrathecal IgG synthesis is obtained with highest sensitivity by detection of oligoclonal IgG bands (OCB) using isoelectric focusing (> 95 %: type 2 OCB = 2 or more CSF-restricted bands, or type 3 OCB = 2 or more CSF-restricted bands in addition to identical bands in the CSF and serum).

Second stage of diagnostics: In 90 % of MS cases, the MRZ reaction (polyspecific intrathecal IgG synthesis against viral antigens with detection of a positive AI (> 1.4; measured by ELISA, or > 4; measured in titer steps) such as measles, rubella, HSV, and zoster in multiple combinations) is positive. As compared to OCB, the MRZ reaction is thought to more specifically reflect the underlying chronic autoimmune process in the central nervous system (CNS). Glucose and especially lactate are normal (< 2.1 mmol/L). If neuromyelitis optica (NMO, Devic's syndrome) or an NMO spectrum disorder (NMOSD) is considered in the differential diagnosis in patients with opticospinal

symptoms, serological screening for aquaporin-4 antibody (AQP4-IgG, highly specific for NMO) or, myelin-oligodendrocyte-glycoprotein (MOG)-IgG) is required. Serological screening for ANA (positive in 20–40 % of MS cases, but only exceptionally > 1:320), and, when positive, for ANA-profile (negative in MS) might help to differentiate MS from neurological manifestations of connective tissue diseases.

Diagnoses other than MS should be taken into consideration with:

- Cell counts > 40–50/µL;
- Marked blood/CSF barrier disruption;
- Negative OCB;
- Pronounced local IgM synthesis;
- A positive serology for AQP4-IgG oder MOG-IgG;
- Important differential diagnoses include:
- Isolated pleocytosis in the absence of an abnormal humoral immune reaction:
  - Neuromyelitis optica (Devic's syndrome);
  - Neurosarcoidosis;
  - Neurological manifestations of systemic vasculitides and collagenoses;
  - Neurological manifestations of Behcet's disease;
- Isolated blood/CSF barrier disruption:
  - Space-occupying processes;
  - Neurodegenerative diseases;
- Isolated IgA synthesis with or without pleocytosis:
  - Tuberculous meningitis and tuberculoma
  - Embolic focal encephalitis;
  - Brain abscess;
  - Whipple's disease;
  - Leprosy;
  - Adrenoleukodystrophy;
- Isolated IgM synthesis with or without pleocytosis:
  - Neuroborreliosis
  - Mumps meningoencephalitis;
  - Neurological manifestations of non-Hodgkin's lymphoma.

The main differential diagnoses for MS that may mimick clinical symptoms and CSF findings are shown in ▶ Table 4.33.

The procedure for differentiating between chronic inflammatory CNS diseases, multiple sclerosis, and other demyelinating diseases is presented in ▶ Figure 4.50.

Table 4.33 Differential diagnosis of multiple sclerosis.

Clinically isolated syndrome (CIS), e.g., optic neuritis: the subsequent transition into definite MS is depicted with higher sensitivity by the presence of CSF-restricted OCB, and with higher specificity by a positive MRZ reaction

Devic's syndrome (neuromyelitis optica, NMO) and NMOSD: CSF-restricted OCB detectable in only 20–30 % of cases, MRZ reaction usually negative, antibodies against AQP4, and, in some AQP4-IgG seronegative cases, against MOG in the serum

Acute disseminated encephalomyelitis (ADEM): postinfectious, monophasic; acute course, OCB detectable in only 20–60 % of cases, MRZ reaction usually negative

Chronic neuroborreliosis: local Borrelia-specific Ab production and inflammatory pleocytosis

Collagen vascular disorders and systemic vasculitides with CNS involvement (SLE, Sjögren's syndrome, mixed connective tissue disease, Wegener's granulomatosis): blood/CSF or barrier disruption, elevated cell count in many cases, rarely CSF-restricted OCB, confirmation by detection of specific autoantibodies in the serum

Other demyelinating diseases

1. Acute demyelinating encephalomyelitis (ADEM) and Weston-Hurst syndrome

ADEM and and its maximum variant, acute hemorrhagic leukoencephalitis (AHLE, or Weston-Hurst syndrome) are prototype monophasic inflammatory CNS diseases, and frequently occur as para-infectious disorders.

First stage of diagnostics: In contrast to MS, ADEM and AHLE significantly more often produce pleocytosis of > 50 cells/µL; lymphocytes and monocytes predominate, however, cytology may also reveal some neutrophilic and eosinophilic granulocytes. Similar findings are also obtained in the acute form of MS (Marburg type), and inconcentric sclerosis of Baló type. Unlike MS, the total protein is elevated in ADEM and AHLE (> 800–900 mg/L) and the blood/CSF barrier dysfunction can be significantly more pronounced (8–10×10^{-3} or > 10×10^{-3}). CSF-restricted OCB are only detectable in 20–60 % % of cases, most often only transiently. Thus, a follow-up lumbar puncture within 4–6 weeks after the onset of symptoms might be useful to support the diagnosis.

Second stage of diagnostics: Current and only partially published studies indicate that a positive MRZ reaction is absent or rarely found in ADEM and AHL. No changes in glucose or lactate are expected.

2. Neuromyelitis optica (NMO, Devic's syndrome);

NMO is characterized by the repeated or, more rarely monophasic, occurrence of transverse myelitis (on spinal MRI extension of lesions over ≥ three vertebral segments) and optic neuritis (ON) and, mostly absent cerebral involvement at onset (note: brain lesions develop in up to 80 % of cases during the course of disease). NMO spectrum disorders (NMOSD) include isolated or recurrent longitudinally extensive transverse myelitis (LETM), and recurrent ON and brainstem encephalitis. NMOSD are mediated by dominant humoral autoimmune mechanisms and respond to antibody- and B-cell-depleting therapies such as plasma exchange and B cell-depletion by monoclonal antibodies.

First stage of diagnostics: A highly specific serum marker for NMO is directed against the water channel protein aquaporin-4 (originally called NMO-IgG). NMO-IgG/AQP4-IgG, by using immunohistochemistry or recombinant cell-based assays, is detectable in the serum of up to 80 % of patients with NMOSD, and is not found in other inflammatory or non-inflammatory neurological or rheumatologic disorders. Of note, NMO-IgG/AQP4 Ab is not detectable in MS sera, thus discriminationg the two disorders with extremely high specificity.NMO-IgG/AQP4-IgG are present in the serum of patients with systemic lupus erythematosus (SLE) and Sjögren's syndrome (SS), presenting with but not in those without opticospinal symptoms suggesting that NMOSD and connective tissue disease concur in these individuals and are not caused by the connective tissue disorder.

Unlike MS, pleocytosis of > 50 cells/µL and a predominance of granulocytes are often found during phases of acute disease activity. The total protein concentration is increased (> 800–900 mg/L), and the blood/CSF barrier disruption is more pronounced (8–10×10^{-3} or > 10×10^{-3}). CSF-restricted OCB are only detectable in 20–30 % of cases, most often only transiently. Thus, a follow-up lumbar puncture 4–6 weeks after the onset of symptoms

Chronic inflammatory CNS disorders, MS, and other demyelinating diseases

At onset — Clinical symptoms: optic neuritis, myelitis, brainstem syndrome, MRI: inflammatory foci disseminated in space and time

Presumptive diagnosis — Differential diagnosis of multiple sclerosis.

Laboratory analysis — Lumbar puncture

Appearance, cell count, cytology, glucose, lactate, total protein, oligoclonal bands, quotient diagram

No — Pathological (particularly oligoclonal bands)

Normal findings — Yes

Diagnosis
- **Multiple sclerosis probable**
- Other diagnoses to be taken into consideration, such as: **neuromyelitis optica, borreliosis, collagenoses, ADEM, vasculitides**, etc., see Table 4.33.

Further tests
- **MRZ reaction** — Yes → **MS**
- neurophysiological measuring methods (evoked potentials: VEP, SEP MEP)
- autoantibodies (aquaporin-4, ANA, ANA profile, ANCA, cardiolipin in serum)
- Paraneoplasias
- *Borrellia* AI

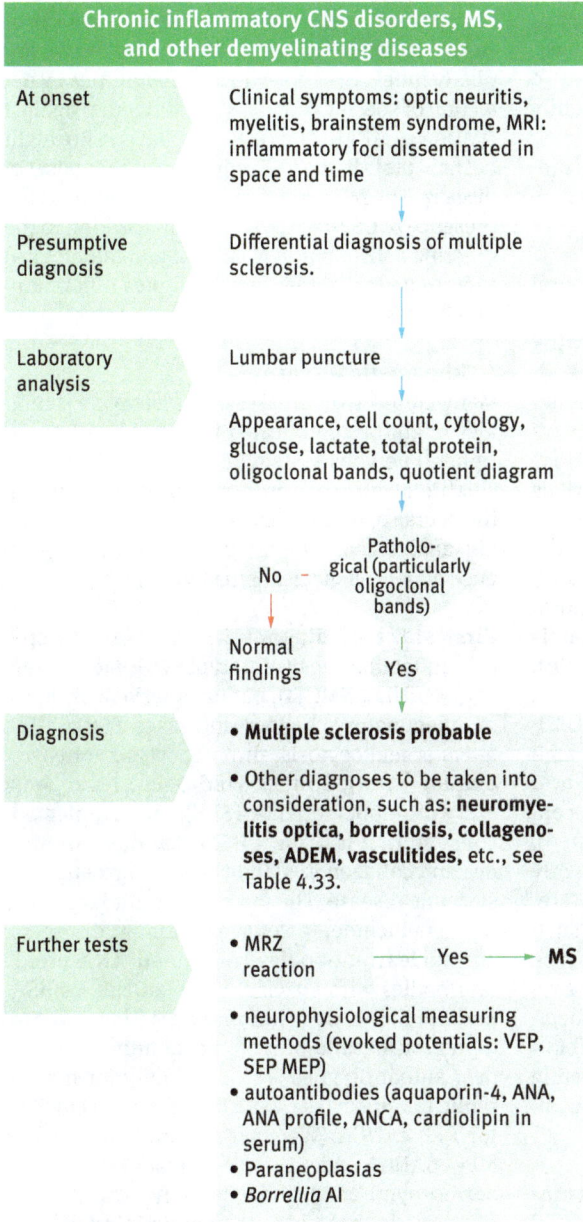

Figure 4.50 Procedure for differentiating chronic inflammatory CNS diseases, multiple sclerosis and other demyelinating diseases.

might be useful NMOSD from from MS when ON and myelitis are presenting manifestations.

Second stage of diagnostics: In contrast to MS, the MRZ reaction is negative or only exceptionally positive in patients with NMOSD. The glucose and lactate are normal.

3. Paraneoplasias of the CNS and autoimmune encephalitis

Paraneoplasias of the CNS (limbic encephalitis, rhombencephalitis, paraneoplastic cerebellar degeneration, opsoclonus myoclonus syndrome, stiff person syndrome) are caused by an autoimmune reaction against onconeural antigens. The serum and CSF of about 60 % of patients comprise high titers of onconeural antibodies, and, when directed against intracellular epitopes, point to the presence of underlying tumor. The recently identified autoimmune encephalitides associated with serum antibodies against neural surface proteins, more often emerge as non-tumour –associated disorders

First stage of diagnostics: Distinct onconeural immune responses (tumor-associated in > 90 % of cases) are antibodies against the following target antigens (index tumor in parentheses): Hu (small-cell lung cancer), Yo (breast, ovarian cancer), Ri (breast cancer), Ma2 (testicular tumor), amphiphysin (small-cell lung cancer), Tr/ DNER (Hodgkin's disease), CV2/CRMP5 (various tumors), Amphiphysin (small-cell lung cancer, breast cancer), SOX1 (small-cell lung cancer) . According to recent findings, autoantibodies with specificity for neuronal surface proteins occur in patients with limbic or more diffuse encephalitis (LGI1 (leucine-rich glioma inactivated 1 protein), CASPR2 (contactin-associated protein-like 2), $GABA_AR$ (γ-amino-butyric acid-A receptor), $GABA_BR$ (γ-amino-butyric-B receptor), AMPAR (α-amino-3-hydroxy-5-methyl-4-isoxazolepropionic-acid receptor], NMDAR (N-Methyl-D-Aspartat receptor), DPPX (dipeptidyl-peptidase-like protein 6). Seropositivity for NMDAR occurs predominantly in females and is associated with ovarian teratoma in up to 50 % cases. The detection of such antibodies indicates a relatively good response to immunotherapy. The onconeural immune response can be detected with immunohistochemistry, and is confirmed by immunoblot or ELISA using recombinant antigens. Antibodies targeting neuronal surface proteins are detected by recombinant cell-based assays..

Second stage of diagnostics (highly recommended): The cell and protein profiles in CSF are frequently abnormal in patients with CNS paraneoplasias and autoimmune encephalitis, however, normal CSF findings do not rule out these diseases. Characteristic changes include pleocytosis of up to 30–40 cells/μL, the detection of transformed lymphocytes and/or plasma cells in CSF smears, slightly increased total protein (500–1000 mg/L), as well as intrathecal IgG synthesis as measured quantitatively or qualitatively. Onconeural antibodies targeting intracellular

epitopes are synthesized intrathecally in 88 % of cases (detection by calculating the respective antibody index, or in specialized laboratories by detection of specific OCBs), as are antibodies against NMDAR, AMPAR, and $GABA_BR$. NMDAR-Ab might be detectable in the CSF only shortly after onset of disease. The MRZ reaction is negative even in the presence of CSF-restricted OCB. In addition to the differing constellation of clinical and radiological symptoms and signs, this facilitates differentiation from MS.

4. Rheumatic Diseases

Many connective diseases and systemic vasculitides might be complicated by central and/or peripheral nervous system involvement. Neuropsychiatric symptoms can occur initially or during the course of disease. Laboratory diagnostics and CSF analysis can support, but not prove, the presence of neurological manifestations.

First stage of diagnostics: Unlike CNS specific inflammations (prototype: MS; more rarely ADEM/AHLE, NMOSD, paraneoplasias), evidence of inflammatory changes (increased ESR or CRP, anemia, leukocytosis, thrombocytosis) or eosinophilia (Churg-Strauss syndrome); leukopenia and thrombocytopenia (SLE), or complement consumption (C3, C4, CH50) (various vasculitides and collagenoses) indicates the presence of a systemic disease. The most important laboratory markers include, in collagen vascular disorders: antinuclear antibodies (ANA) and ANA profile (antibodies with specificity for dsDNA, Ro/SSA, La/SSB, Scl70, U1-RNP, centromere histone, Sm, alpha-fodrin, and others); in immune vasculitides: autoantibodies with specificity for neutrophilic granulocytes (ANCA) with fine specificities for PR3 cANCA (Wegener's granulomatosis) or MPO pANCA (microscopic polyangiitis, Churg-Strauss syndrome), and, optionally, other autoantibodies (rheumatoid factor, cardiolipin Ab, lupus anticoagulant, and others). The significance of antibodies directed against ribosomal P protein and NMDAR (subtype differing from those detectable in autoimmune NMDAR-encephalitis) in SLE-associated psychoses remains controversial. When neuropsychiatric involvement is suspected, the presence of pleocytosis and/or intrathecal Ig-synthesis with or withoutblood/CSF barrier disruption, or of CSF-restricted OCB, can be diagnostically decisive. CSF analysis is of enormous importance in ruling out secondary consequences of treatment (mainly infections).

Second stage of diagnostics: Unlike in NMOSD and CNS paraneoplasias/autoimmune encephalitis, theMRZ reaction is positive in many cases. The diagnostic significance of intrathecal synthesis of complement factors and/or ANA/ANCA remains uncertain.

4.7.2.8 Inflammatory Cerebrospinal Fluid Syndrome of Unknown Origin

Definition

When will inflammatory CSF be present?
- The following CSF findings are considered "inflammatory":
  - Pleocytosis (leukocytes > 4/µL);
  - Intrathecal synthesis of the immunoglobulins IgG, IgA or IgM (> 10 % intrathecal fraction in the quotient diagram);
  - Oligoclonal IgG bands (pattern 2 and pattern 3, according to Andersson, et al., 1994);
  - Direct detection or cultivation of disease pathogens;
  - Local synthesis of antibodies (pathogen-specific or autoimmune), detected for example as an elevated antibody index (AI).

Differential diagnoses of "inflammatory CSF syndrome"

Are the above-named CSF changes associated with an inflammatory nervous system disorder?
- An increased cell count can also occur in malignant diseases, and as epiphenomena in other conditions (reactive pleocytosis; e.g., repeated lumbar puncture (LP), ischemia, hemorrhage, neurosurgical procedures, spinal catheter, intrathecal or systemic administration of certain drugs, such as steroids, immunoglobulins, and antibiotics).

Is it caused by a pathogen-related or autoimmune-mediated disease?
- The distinction between these groups of diseases is difficult, especially in chronic disorders. For example, CSF-restricted OCB are usually detectable in both types of disease. Specific analyses, such as intrathecally-produced pathogen-specific antibodies (MRZ reaction) or autoantibodies, can be helpful here.

4.7.2.9 Dementia syndromes

Depending on the medical history and symptomatology, the diagnostic work-up of dementias requires a complex interplay of neuropsychological, radiological, and CSF diagnostic testing procedures, and does not readily enable a simple scheme of yes/no decisions. Since no single laboratory result can be taken by itself as specific for a particular disease, the detection of dementia and destruction markers only makes sense in the context of a relevant clinical question, and not as a screening procedure. The benefit for a patient only develops slowly after initial therapeutic approaches become apparent at an early stage. The representations in the following ▶ Tables 4.34 and 4.35 are thus very tentative. However, there is widespread agreement that after ruling out various other diseases with secondary dementia (e.g., ischemia, encephalitis, or NPH) following findings are helpful:

Table 4.34 Diagnostic procedure of dementia syndromes.

- **Imaging methods:** ruling out vascular dementia as well as normal pressure hydrocephalus
- **CSF:** Ruling out chronic encephalitis

Rapidly progressive prion diseases, such as Creutzfeldt-Jakob:
- Initially often unclear;
- *In vivo* detection of prion aggregates in the CSF is not possible by routine methods
- Surrogate markers such as NSE and S-100 in the CSF show acute tissue destruction;
- Specific: tau strongly increased in the CSF, as well as detection of protein 14-3-3

Table 4.35 Chronic primary dementias.

- Most common forms: Alzheimer's disease and Lewy body dementia (associated with Parkinson's disease) as well as frontotemporal dementia
- Early detection in the stage of "mild cognitive deficit" possible; however, no reliable differentiation of different forms
- Characteristic pattern of findings: increased release of tau and phospho-tau, and increased consumption and tissue deposition of the β-amyloid 1-42 fragment of β-APP (or a reduced Aβ1-42/Aβ1-40 quotient)

1. Significant release of the surrogate markers tau protein and protein 14-3-3 into the CSF supports a diagnosis of Creutzfeldt-Jakob disease;
2. Chronic primary dementia (including Alzheimer's disease, Lewy body and frontotemporal dementia), which can be detected early by a typical pattern of findings (increased release of tau and phospho-tau, increased consumption of the β-amyloid fragment 1-42, and/or possibly a reduced Aβ1-42/Aβ1-40 ratio);
3. Distinguishing between various subtypes of chronic primary dementia based on a marker profile is currently not possible with confidence;
4. For valid findings, compliance with the pre-analytical requirements (polypropylene tube) is essential.

4.7.2.10 Wilson's disease

In any inexplicable liver disease in childhood, adolescence, or early adulthood, Wilson's disease should be ruled out as in neurological psychiatric symptoms (tremor, dysarthria, hypersalivation,

dystonia, personality changes, etc.), with or without a liver involvement.

The diagnostics process for Wilson's disease is shown in the Figure ▶ 4.51.

First stage of diagnosis – preliminary diagnostics: Serum ceruloplasmin and copper determinations are made, and both parameters will generally be decreased (90 %). In the hemolytic stage of the disease, the copper level might be normal or slightly increased.

The basal copper excretion in 24-hour urine will be increased, and the value will be greater than 1 µmol/d. If borderline findings are obtained, a D-penicillamine loading test (2 × 500 mg D-penicillamine) can be performed with subsequent determination of urinary copper; however, this test is not standardized.

An ophthalmological evaluation with evidence of a Kayser-Fleischer corneal ring from the slit lamp examination is required only from the age of 10. Assessment:
• If all parameters are normal, develop alternative diagnoses.

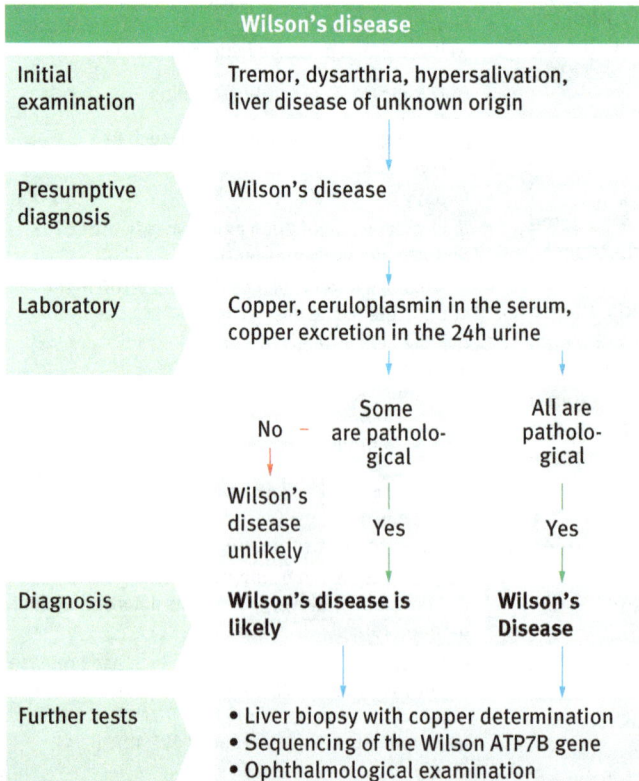

Figure 4.51 Diagnostics process for Wilson's disease.

- If all the parameters are pathological, the diagnosis can be considered reliable.
- With discrepancies in the results, further studies are necessary.

Second stage of diagnostics – confirmatory tests:

Confirmatory tests that can be used include:
- Liver biopsy with quantitative copper determination (increased more than 250 µg/g dry weight). Histology and histochemistry are not mandatory;
- Sequencing of the Wilson **ATP7B** gene;
- Intravenous radiocopper test: at the moment not available.

Literature

Felgenhauer K., Beuche W. Labordiagnostik neurologischer Erkrankungen. Stuttgart: Thieme 1999

Kluge H., Wieczorek V., Linke E., Zimmermann K., Witte O. Atlas of CSF Cytology. Stuttgart: Thieme 2007

Petereit H.-F., Sindern E., Wick M., editors. Liquordiagnostik. Leitlinien und Methodenkatalog der Deutschen Gesellschaft für Liquordiagnostik und Klinische Neurochemie. Heidelberg: Springer 2007

Wildemann B., Oschmann P., Reiber H. Laboratory Diagnosis in Neurology. Stuttgart, New York: Thieme 2010)

Zettl U., Lehmitz R., Mix E., editors. Klinische Liquordiagnostik, 2nd ed., Berlin: de Gruyter 2005

Zettl UK, Tumani H. Cerebrospinal fluid and multiple sclerosis. Blackwell Publishing, Oxford 2005

4.7.3 Authors and Working Group

4.7.3.1 Spokesperson for the Working Group

- Dr. med. M. Wick, Laboratoriumsmedizin, Klinikum der LMU, Campus Großhadern, Marchionini-strasse 15, 81377 Munchen, E-Mail: manfred.wick@med.uni-muenchen.de

4.7.3.2 Members of the Working Group

The task of reviewing and editing the basic (laboratory) diagnostic procedures in neurology in compliance with the requirements of DGKL was initially undertaken by an interdisciplinary working group assembled from the board of the German Society for Cerebrospinal Fluid Diagnostics and Clinical Neurochemistry (DGLN), enabling cooperation between clinicians and clinical chemists, although all of the involved neurologists themselves also have laboratory experience:

- Dr. H.-J. Kühn, formerly Clinical Chemistry, University of Leipzig
- Prof. Dr. M. Otto, Neurology, University of Ulm
- PD Dr. Dr. M. Uhr, MPI for Psychiatry, Munich
- Dr. M. Wick, Laboratory Medicine, LMU Munich, Campus Großhadern
- PD Dr. H.-F. Petereit, Neurology, Praxis rechts vom Rhein, Cologne
- Prof. B. Wildemann, Neurology, University of Heidelberg
- Prof. Dr. H. Tumani, Neurology, University of Ulm and Director Fachklinik für Neurologie Dietenbronn, Schwendi, Chairman of the DGLN

4.7.3.3 Objective of the Neurology Working Group

Disorders of the nervous system usually require technically specialized diagnostics. The early and effective use of laboratory tests can accelerate the process of developing a diagnosis and selecting appropriate treatment, possibly also helping to avoid other time-consuming or non-indicated diagnostic and therapeutic procedures, and in this way not only providing benefit to the patient but also ultimately reducing costs.

Despite all the advances in imaging techniques, a CSF examination is still frequently necessary to diagnose a CNS disorder, and in most cases of inflammatory processes even the first step. In contrast to the studies of blood or urine, CSF diagnostics require a number of peculiarities with an immediate impact on the diagnostic pathways.

Harald Renz und Dorte Brodje

4.8 Autoimmune disorders

4.8.1 Rheumatoid Arthritis Diagnostics

Rheumatoid arthritis (RA) is a chronic inflammatory disease with an etiology that is largely unknown. With a worldwide prevalence of approximately 0.5 to 1 %, it is the most common inflammatory joint disease, and affects women three times as often as men. The clinical picture of RA is often not very characteristic in the early stages. Since severe joint destruction can develop after an illness of rather short duration, an early diagnosis of RA is of crucial importance. Getting an early start with a suitable therapy can prevent or delay the progressive course of this disease.

4.8.1.1 Diagnostic Scheme

The clinical starting point for RA diagnostics is arthritis, in particular of the wrist, finger (MCP, PIP), and ankle joints. An early suspicion of RA is also raised when initially only one joint or several joints are affected, or the joint involvement does not occur symmetrically.

Specific attention is drawn to evidence of joint inflammation (synovitis) with soft swelling, pain on pressure, and limitation of movement (morning stiffness ≥ 60 minutes) over a period of at least six weeks (Guidelines of the German Society for Rheumatology (DGRh), ACR/EULAR 2010 Rheumatoid Arthritis Classification Criteria).

A new set of criteria for classifying RA was developed in 2010 by the ACR (American College of Rheumatology) and EULAR (European League Against Rheumatism) (Table ▶ 4.36). In this system, the number of affected joints (synovitis), serology, inflammatory markers, and the duration of symptoms are evaluated and assigned points. A diagnosis of RA requires at least 6 out of 10 points, provided that confirmed synovitis is present in at least one joint, absent other clear origins for the condition.

Table 4.36 ACR/EULAR Diagnostic criteria (2010).

A. Joint involvement (synovitis)	Point score
1 large joint	0
2–10 medium to large joints	1
1–3 small joints	2
4–10 small joints	3
> 10 joints (at least one small joint)	5
B. Serology	
Negative for RF and ACPA	0
Low positive for RF or ACPA	2
High positive for RF or ACPA	3
C. Duration of symptoms	
< 6 weeks	0
≥ 6 weeks	1
D.Inflammation markers	
CRP and BSG normal	0
CRP or BSG elevated	1

Laboratory Diagnostics

Laboratory diagnostics can offer an early diagnosis of RA through the detection of inflammation markers and autoantibodies typical for RA.

The assessment of inflammatory activity involves determination of the erythrocyte sedimentation rate (ESR) and/or C-reactive protein (CRP). A negative result significantly reduces the likelihood of an RA diagnosis, but does not rule it out. Hypochromic anemia is also often observed in the context of persistent inflammatory activity. Drug-induced gastrointestinal blood loss should be ruled out in this case.

The RA antibody diagnostics involve determining the IgM rheumatoid factor (RF) and antibodies to cyclic citrullinated peptides (ACPA). RF is rarely at detectable onset, and occurs with a frequency of 65–80 % in patients with RA. It is not specific for RA, but also occurs in other autoimmune diseases, in chronic inflammatory disease, and also in healthy individuals. The specificity of ACPA for RA is significantly higher (about 95 %) than that of RF at comparable sensitivity.

The rheumatoid factors and ACPA are determined once. Values 3 times greater than the standard value are referred to as highly positive. A negative result for both parameters makes rheumatoid arthritis unlikely, but does not rule it out completely. A positive result for both parameters increases the probability that RA is present to about 90–100 %. Discrepancies between the RF and ACPA results lead to ambiguity, but also increase the *a priori* probability of rheumatoid arthritis. The diagnostics process for RA is shown in the Figure ▶ 4.52.

4.8.1.2 Additional Reflections on Differential Diagnosis

To rule out the diseases of adulthood that are important from the differential diagnosis perspective, depending on the additional clinical indications, it is recommended to investigate the antinuclear antibodies (ANA; indication of collagenoses, also weakly positive with RA or even in healthy persons), antineutrophil cytoplasmic antibodies (ANCA; indication of vasculitides), HLA-B27 as an indication of spondyloarthritides, and uric acid and the infectious serology to rule out polyarticular gout (rare!) or infectious arthritides.

Literature

Mierau R, Genth E. Diagnostik und Prognostik der frühen rheumatoiden Arthritis unter besonderer Berucksichtigung der Labor-Analytik. J Lab Med 2005; 29(4): 251–256

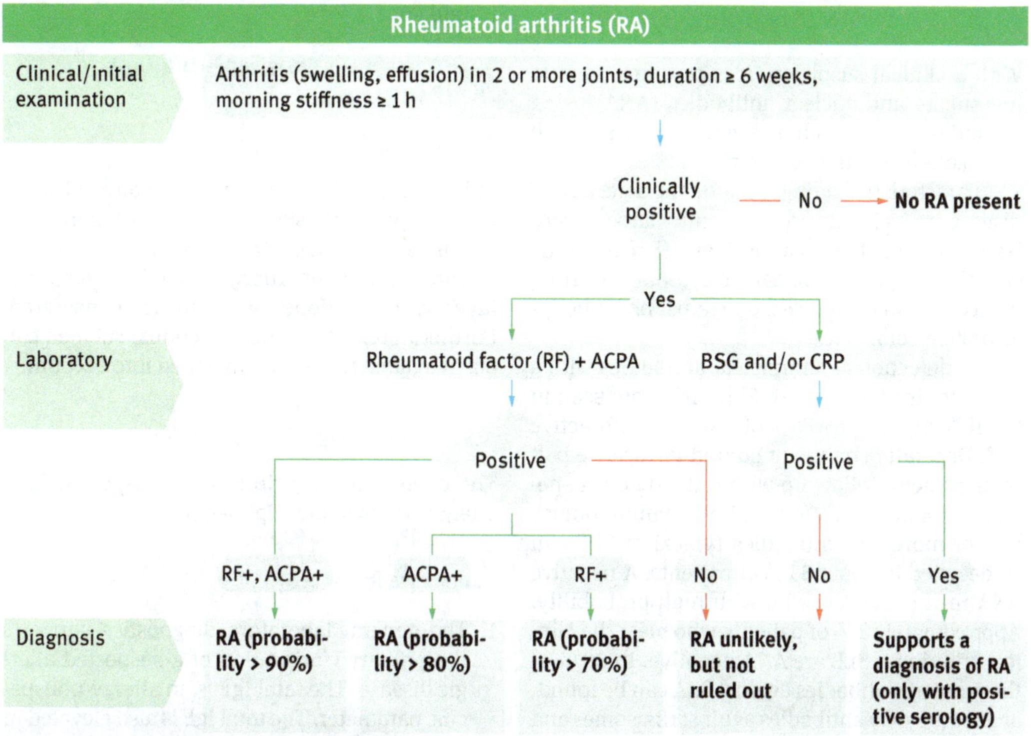

Rheumatoid arthritis (RA)

Clinical/initial examination

Arthritis (swelling, effusion) in 2 or more joints, duration ≥ 6 weeks, morning stiffness ≥ 1 h

Clinically positive — No → **No RA present**

Yes

Laboratory

Rheumatoid factor (RF) + ACPA — BSG and/or CRP

Positive — Positive

RF+, ACPA+ | ACPA+ | RF+ | No | No | Yes

Diagnosis

RF+, ACPA+	ACPA+	RF+	No	No	Yes
RA (probability > 90%)	**RA (probability > 80%)**	**RA (probability > 70%)**	**RA unlikely, but not ruled out**		**Supports a diagnosis of RA (only with positive serology)**

Figure 4.52 Diagnostic pathway for rheumatoid arthritis.

Aletaha D, Neogi T, Silman AJ, Funovits J, Felson DT et al. 2010 Rheumatoid Arthritis Classification Criteria. DGKL e.V., Arbeitsgruppe Autoimmundiagnostik. Rheumatoide Arthritis, www.dgkl.de

Schneider M, Lelgemann M, Abholz HH, Blumenroth M, Flugge C et al. Interdisziplinare Leitlinie. Management der frühen rheumatoiden Arthritis, 3. Auflage, Springer Verlag, 2011

Nishimura K, Sugiyama D, Kogata Y, Tsuji G et al. Meta-analysis: diagnostic accuracy of anti-cyclic citrullinated peptide antibody and rheumatoid factor for rheumatoid arthritis. Ann Intern Med 2007; 146(11): 797–808

4.8.2 Systemic Lupus Erythematosus

Systemic lupus erythematosus (SLE) is an autoimmune disease with a chronic course that potentially affects the entire body. SLE has an intermittent course involving many organ systems, such as the skin, joints, serous membranes, kidneys, blood cells, and the CNS. The 1982 classification criteria of the American Rheumatism Association (now ACR) are recognized worldwide, and were last modified in 1997.

Four out of a total eleven criteria must be fulfilled, not necessarily occurring simultaneously, which complicates establishment of the diagnosis.

The ACR criteria are:

1. Malar erythema
2. Discoid skin lesions
3. Photosensitivity
4. Oral ulcers
5. Arthritis
6. Serositis: pleuritis, pericarditis, also anamnestic
7. Renal symptoms: proteinuria >0.5 g/d, cell casts
8. Neurological symptoms: psychoses, epilepsy
9. Hematological symptoms: hemolysis, leukocytopenia, lymphocytopenia, thrombocytopenia
10. Positive ANA titer
11. Positive anti-DNA, anti-Sm, or cardiolipin antibody titer

Early clinical symptoms frequently include joint and skin involvement, and systemic symptoms such as fatigue, lassitude, or fever.

4.8.2.1 Laboratory Diagnostics

With a clinical suspicion, it is recommended to investigate anti-nuclear antibodies (ANA) using the indirect immunofluorescence test (IIFT) with Hep2 cells as the test substrate.

Characteristic findings include the detection of disease-typical, non-organ-specific autoantibodies against nucleosomal antigens (DNA-histone complex), against nuclear or cytoplasmic ribonucleoprotein complexes, or against phospholipid-protein complexes.

The detection of antinuclear antibodies with a high titer is indicative for SLE. ANAs are seen in the IIFT in almost 100 % of patients with active SLE. Depending on the immunofluorescence patterns present, follow up with tests to detect specific autoantibodies (e.g., ELISA, immunoblot). One or more autoantibodies typical of SLE can be detected in about 85 % of patients. A negative ANA result rules out SLE with high probability. Approximately 2 % of patients who meet the clinical criteria for SLE are ANA negative. In 80 % of these cases, antibodies against SSA can be found, and more rarely antibodies against ribosomes and phospholipid-protein complexes.

The diagnostics process for SLE is shown in the Figure ▶ 4.53.

4.8.2.2 Reflections on Differential Diagnosis

Differential diagnosis should be performed to differentiate from other systemic autoimmune diseases (suspected RA, systemic sclerosis, polymyositis, and mixed connective tissue disease) as well as systemic vasculitides and primary antiphospholipid syndrome.

Literature

DGKL e V., Arbeitsgruppe Autoimmundiagnostik-Systemischer Lupus erythematodes. (www.dgkl.de)

Gaubitz M, Schotte H. Frühdiagnose des des systemischen Lupus erythematodes (SLE). Z Rheumatol 2005; 64: 547–552

Sack U, Conrad K, Csernok E, Frank I, Hiepe F et al. Autoantikörpernachweis mittels indirekter Immunfluoreszenz an HEp-2-Zellen. Dtsch Med Wochenschr 2009; 134: 1278–1282

Hochberg MC. Updating the American College of Rheumatology revised criteria fort he classifikation of systemic lupus erythematodes. Arthritis Rheum 1997; 40: 1725

Harald Renz

4.9 Allergy Diagnostics – Diagnostic Pathways

Preliminary Remarks

This chapter addresses the importance of *in vitro* allergy diagnostics for the most important IgE-mediated immediate-type allergies.

Other forms of allergic reaction (e.g., delayed-type reactions, etc.) are not considered. Furthermore, intolerance reactions, such as can occur against foods, are not taken into account.

4.9.1 Food Allergy Diagnostics

The diagnostics algorithm for a suspected food allergy is shown in ▶ Figure 4.54.

Comments for Figure 4.54

1. The general laboratory diagnostics supports the primary clarification of a suspected allergic disease. The total IgE is an allergy-nonspecific parameter. The total IgE is also elevated in other diseases (smoking, nematode infection, certain immune deficiencies, infectious diseases such as HIV in the late stage, etc.), where the eosinophilic granulocytes are likewise elevated. Tryptase is released in the course of mast cell degranulation, and has a half-life of 24–48 hours, so that (especially intense) allergic reactions that are delayed by one or several days are also associated with increased tryptase values.

2. The measurement of specific IgE antibodies should be carried out quantitatively. Specific IgE levels do not necessarily correlate with the clinical response severity, so that an already severe clinical reaction can be present together with a relatively weaker increase in the specific IgE. When the individual allergen measurements are performed with native allergen material, one must consider that not all components are present in the respective allergen extract in sufficient quantity so that false negative results can be obtained in the course of the corresponding sensitization. A major cause of false positive results is the patient's IgE reactivity to cross-reactive carbohydrate determinants (CCD antigens). Any IgE produced in response to such carbohydrate side chains

will generally have no clinical relevance. A suspected CCD reactivity should always be investigated further if the patient exhibits polysensitization against a larger number of allergens. Tests to measure such CCD reactivity are available.

3. IgE-mediated food allergies are especially common in childhood. The foods listed in the primary screening here represent about 90 % of the relevant childhood foods. If semi-quantitative and qualitative tests are employed in the allergy screening procedure, it is necessary to break down a positive test result using single allergen determinations; the same is true with screening procedure that employs a "mixed allergen". The selection of the test allergens will be informed by the patient's medical history.

4. A new dimension has been achieved with the component-resolved *in vitro* allergy diagnostics that are now widely available. Allergens consist of mixtures of protein, and the most important components for many of the relevant allergens in our latitudes have now been molecularly characterized. Their sequences are known, so that they can be produced using recombinant techniques. The clinical evaluation of such component-resolved diagnostics is presently in a state of flux. At present, the component-resolved approach has a clinically relevant role in the diagnostics for individual allergies and allergens. Many of the proteins that occur in pollens and foods are related, so that the allergologically important protein families can be characterized and assembled. The detection of sensitization to members of individual families already plays a clinically relevant role, as can be show in the following examples:

a) A sensitization to storage proteins (e.g., Gly m 5/6 from soy, or Ara h 1, 2, 3, 6, and 7 from peanut) is frequently associated with severe clinical reactions.

b) A sensitization to PR10 proteins (pathogenesis-related protein family 10) is frequently associated with the development of oral allergy syndrome (OAS).

c) A sensitization to profilins is a quite common basis for multiple sensitization, but is only rarely associated with clinical symptoms.

d) A sensitization to members of the tropomyosin family is the origin of cross-reactions between shellfish and crustaceans, mites, cockroaches, and nematodes.

Significant examples are summarized in ▶ Tables 4.37 to 4.41.

Table 4.37 Protein family: storage proteins.

Storage proteins	Properties
• Peanut (Ara h 1, 2, 3, 6, and 7) • Soy (Gly m 5/6) • Hazelnut (Cor a 9) • Wheat (Tri a 19 gliadin)	• STable • Heat resistant • Also reaction after being cooked • Frequently associated with severe systemic reactions

Table 4.38 Protein family: Pathogenesis-related protein family 10 (PR-10)

Pathogenesis-related protein family 10 (PR-10)	Properties
• Birch (Bet v 1) • Peanut (Ara h 8) • Soy (Gly m 4) • Hazelnut (Cor a 1) • Apple (Mal d 1) • Kiwi (Act d 8) • Peach (Pru p 3) • Carrot (Dau c 1)	• Heat sensitive • Tolerates cooking • Most are linked to oral allergy syndrome (OAS) • Frequently associated with allergic reactions to fruit and vegeTables in Northern Europe

Table 4.39 Protein family: Non-specific lipid transfer proteins.

Non-specific lipid transfer proteins	Properties
• Peanut (Ara h 9) • Hazelnut (Cor a 8) • Peach (Pru p 3) • Wild herbs and weeds, e.g., *Artemisia* (Art v 3) • *Parietaria* (Par j 2)	• Stable to heat and enzymes • Reaction after being cooked • Frequently associated with severe systemic reactions

Table 4.40 Protein family: profilins.

Profilins	Properties
• Birch (Bet v 2) • Latex (Hev b 8) • Grasses (Phl p 12) • Peach (Pru p 4) • and many more	• Actin-binding proteins of wide distribution • Minor allergens • Rarely associated with symptoms • Frequently the origin of multiple sensitizations

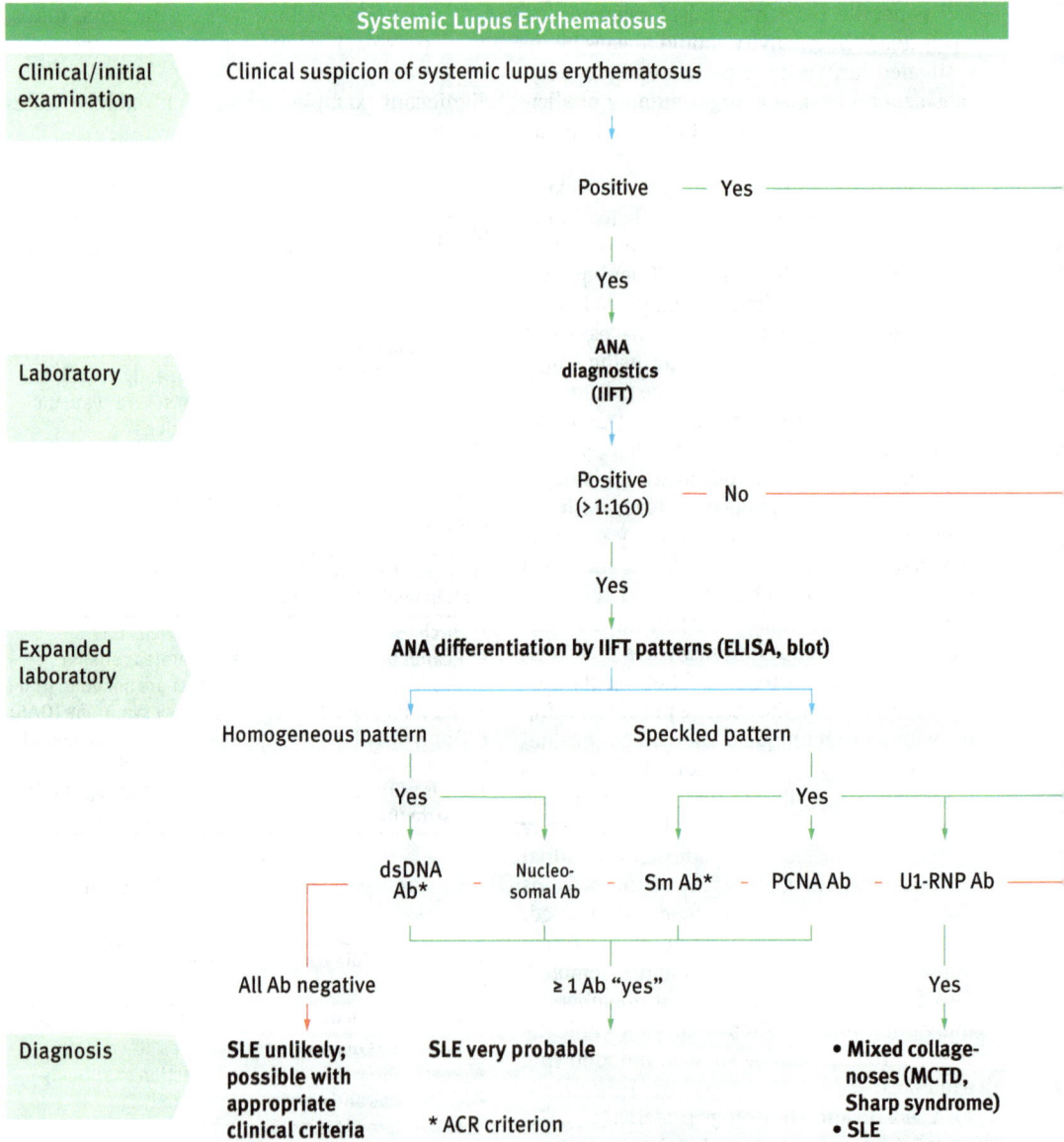

Figure 4.53 Diagnostic Pathway: Systemic Lupus Erythematosus.

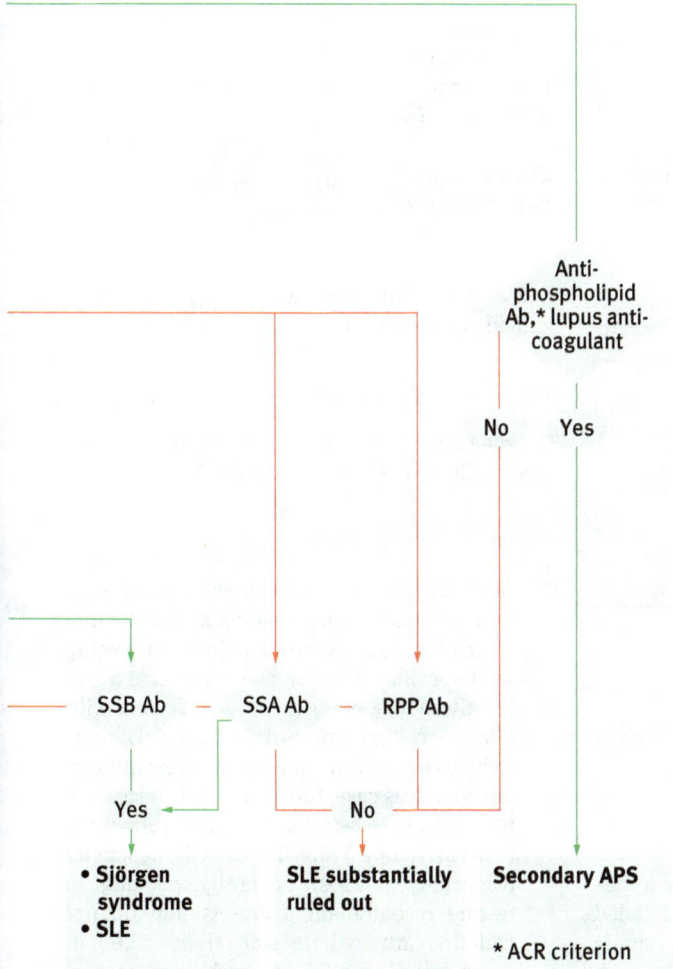

Anti-phospholipid Ab,* lupus anti-coagulant

No   Yes

SSB Ab — SSA Ab — RPP Ab

Yes   No

- Sjörgen syndrome
- SLE

SLE substantially ruled out

Secondary APS

* ACR criterion

Food allergy			
General diagnostics ①	**Screening** ③ • Eggs • Cow's milk • Cod • Wheat • Peanuts • Soy	Individual allergens ②	
Clinical and medical history			Component diagnostics with recombinant allergens ④
Total IgE, eosinophilic granulocytes Tryptase	⊕ ⊖ Provocation, elimination	⊕ Provocation, elimination	Cross-allergies, clinical relevance

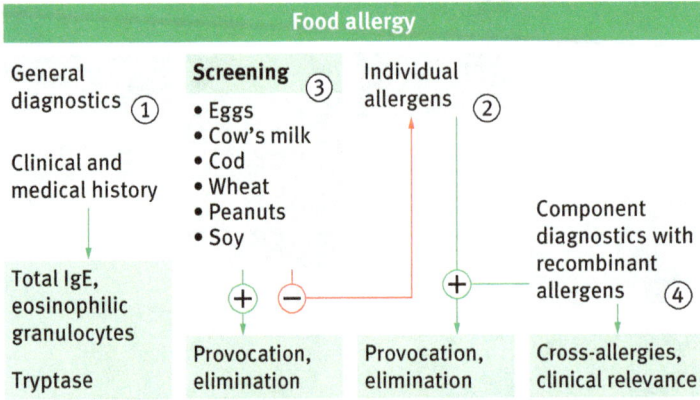

Figure 4.54 Diagnostic algorithm for suspected food allergy.

Table 4.41 Protein family: tropomyosin.

Tropomyosin	Properties
Mites (Der p 10), (Ani s 3), (Pen a 1)	Actin-binding proteins in the muscle cells as a marker for possible cross-reactions with: • Shellfish and crustaceans • Mites • Cockroaches • Nematodes

4.9.2 Inhalation Allergy Diagnostics

The diagnostic algorithm for a suspected inhalation allergy is shown in ▶ Figure 4.55.

Comments for Figure 4.55

5. The selection of the test allergens for a suspected indoor allergy is based on a detailed medical history. The same precautions apply to this screening as for a suspected food allergy (see comment 3).
6. The main trigger for outdoor air allergies is pollen. Attention should be paid to the respective local pollen calendar.
7. The main early blooming species are birch, hazel, and alder. These sources are broadly related so that the allergy diagnostics relating to birch cover the entire spectrum of early blooming species.
8. The same applies to the summer blooming grasses. Here again, there are broad affinities between the various grass families.

9. For year-round symptomatology, the exact medical history will contain combinations.

4.9.3 Insect Venom Allergy Diagnostics

The diagnostic algorithm for a suspected insect venom allergy is shown in ▶ Figure 4.56.

Comments for Figure 4.56

10. According to the Guidelines, testing with native bee and wasp venoms is still the first stage of *in vitro* diagnostics. However, testing with specified allergen components is a viable alternative at the first stage. Testing with allergen components is then essential if reactivity to bee and wasp is detected simultaneously. In this case, further study is necessary to differentiate between true cross-sensitivity (extremely rare!) and non-specific reactivity (especially to CCDs). Generally speaking, in testing recombinant allergens that do not contain carbohydrate side chains, i.e., in cases of IgE reactivity to carbohydrate side chains, the test result with recombinant allergen will be negative.

4.9.4 Drug Allergy Diagnostics

The diagnostic algorithm for a suspected drug allergy is shown in ▶ Figure 4.57.

Comments for Figure 4.57

11. The measurement of specific IgE antibodies plays a central role in the diagnosis of aller-

Inhalation allergy

Interior spaces
⑤

Outdoor air
⑥

Screening
- Mites (Der p 1; Der f 1)
- Cat
- Dog
- *Alternaria*

Invidual allergens

Spring — Birch (hazel-nut, alder) ⑦

Summer — Grasses, rye, herbs ⑧

Year-round — Combination interior and outdoor air ⑨

(+)

(−)

Diagnosis/ therapy

Diagnosis/ therapy

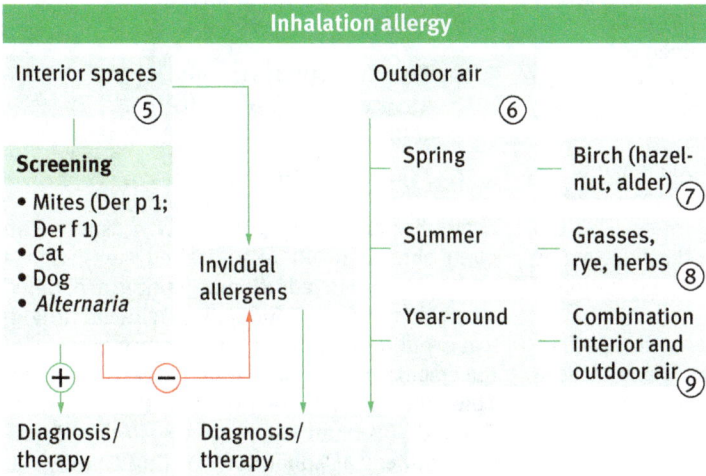

Figure 4.55 Diagnostic algorithm for suspected inhalation allergy.

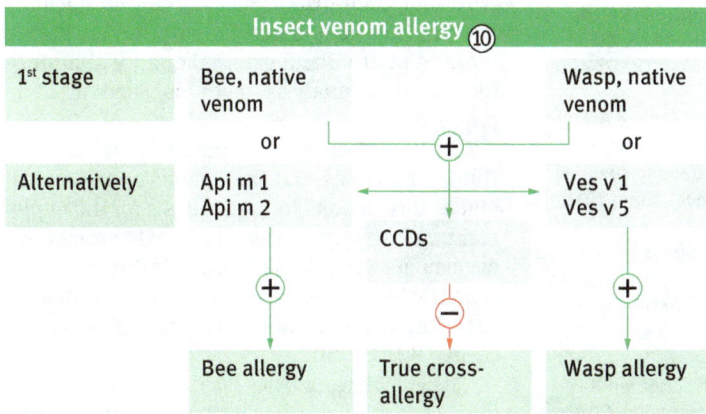

Insect venom allergy ⑩

1st stage

Bee, native venom

or

Wasp, native venom

or

Alternatively

Api m 1
Api m 2

Ves v 1
Ves v 5

(+)

CCDs

(+)

(−)

(+)

Bee allergy

True cross-allergy

Wasp allergy

Figure 4.56 Diagnostic algorithm for a suspected insect venom allergy.

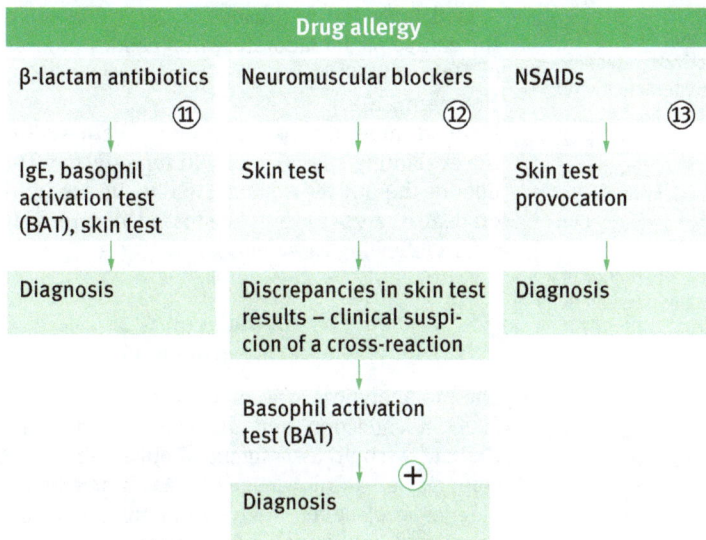

Drug allergy

β-lactam antibiotics
⑪

Neuromuscular blockers
⑫

NSAIDs
⑬

IgE, basophil activation test (BAT), skin test

Skin test

Skin test provocation

Diagnosis

Discrepancies in skin test results – clinical suspicion of a cross-reaction

Diagnosis

Basophil activation test (BAT)

(+)

Diagnosis

Figure 4.57 Diagnostic algorithm for a suspected drug allergy.

gies to β-lactam antibiotics. The most data show that the results obtained using the newer generation basophil activation test (BAT) are equally good in terms of sensitivity and specificity.

12. The BAT appears in the second stage of the diagnostic algorithm for the diagnosis of allergies to neuromuscular blockers. This test is especially valuable when the skin test results are negative, and there is a question of possible cross-reactivity.

13. IgE reactivity generally plays no role in diagnosing an allergy to NSAIDs (aspirin, acetaminophen, ibuprofen).

Literature

Renz et al, LaboratoriumsMedizin. Band 34, Heft 4, Seiten 177–195, ISSN (Online) 1439–0477, ISSN (Print) 0342–3026, DOI: 10.1515/JLM.2010.034, July 2010

Ito K, Sjolander S, Sato S, Moverare R, Tanaka A, Soderstrom L et al. IgE to Gly m5 and Gly m6 is associated with severe allergic reactions to soybean in Japanese children. J Allergy Clin Immunol 2011; 128: 673–5.

Nicolaou N, Poorafshar M, Murray C, Simpson A, Winell H, Kerry G et al. Allergy or tolerance in children sensitized to peanut: prevalence and differentiation using component-resolved diagnostics. J Allergy Clin Immunol 2010; 125: 191–7.

Eberlein B, Leon S, I, Darsow U, Rueff F, Behrendt H, Ring J. A new basophil activation test using CD63 and CCR3 in allergy to antibiotics. Clin Exp Allergy 2010; 40: 411–8.

Leysen J, Sabato V, Verweij MM, De Knop KJ, Bridts CH, De Clerck LS et al. The basophil activation test in the diagnosis of immediate drug hypersensitivity. Expert Rev Clin Immunol 2011; 7: 349–55.

Abuaf N, Rajoely B, Ghazouani E, Levy DA, Pecquet C, Chabane H et al. Validation of a flow cytometric assay detecting in vitro basophil activation for the diagnosis of muscle relaxant allergy. J Allergy Clin Immunol 1999; 104: 411–8.

Romano A, Torres MJ, Castells M, Sanz ML, Blanca M. Diagnosis and management of drug hypersensitivity reactions. J Allergy Clin Immunol 2011; 127: S67–S73.

Bilo BM, Rueff F, Mosbech H, Bonifazi F, Oude-Elberink JN. Diagnosis of Hymenoptera venom allergy. Allergy 2005; 60: 1339–49.

Mittermann I, Zidarn M, Silar M, Markovic-Housley Z, Aberer W, Korosec P et al. Recombinant allergen-based IgE testing to distinguish bee and wasp allergy. J Allergy Clin Immunol 2010; 125: 1300–7.

Eray Yagmur

4.10 Ejaculate Analysis and Quality Assurance in Male Fertility Laboratories

4.10.1 Introduction

A number of male fertility disorder aspects can contribute to result in undesired sterility in a male patient. In addition to taking a detailed sexual history and conducting a clinical urological examination, medical laboratory analysis of the ejaculate is a crucial qualitative component. Thus, the specific directive "Part B4 – Ejaculate Testing" (German Medical Association Directive on Medical Laboratory Testing Quality Assurance, RiLiBÄK, 2008), adopted at the end of 2010 and compulsory for all users of ejaculate analysis methods since January 2013, ensures uniform internal and external quality assurance for ejaculate analysis methods used in daily practice.

The WHO "Guide to Laboratory Examination of Human Ejaculate and the Spermatozoa-Cervical Mucus Interaction" forms the basis for the implementation, interpretation, and quality assurance of ejaculate analysis methods. This Directive is accepted as a basic reference by the German Medical Association and the German Society of Andrology (DGA) (WHO, 2010).

The ejaculate analysis results are documented in what is referred to as a spermiogram (▶ Table 4.42), and various origins of the clinically presumed male fertility disorder are evaluated in the course of the laboratory diagnostics process (▶ Figures 4.58 and 4.59) (Cooper, et al., 2010; Hoffmann, 2010)

In addition, the spermiogram is the basis for the evaluating sperm quality in reproductive endocrine therapy for women. Finally, the spermiogram also serves to verify the intended sterility in a man following vasectomy.

4.10.2 Pre-analytics and Macroscopic Physical Examination of Ejaculate

The pre-analytical aspects of ejaculate sampling (sample collection and abstinence), and also the macroscopic assessment of appearance and color as well as knowledge of the volume, are all diagnostic ejaculate analysis variables that are equally as important as the physical properties

Ejaculate analysis terminology

Oligoasthenozoo-spermia	Oligoteratozoo-spermia	Oligoasthenoterato-spermia	Asthenoterato-spermia
↓	↓	↓	↓
Sperm concentration or total sperm count ↓	Sperm concentration or total sperm count ↓	Sperm concentration or total sperm count ↓	Progressive motile sperm ↓
Progressive motile sperm ↓	Sperm morphology ↓	Progressive motile sperm ↓	Sperm morphology ↓
		Sperm morphology ↓	

Azoospermia	Cryptozoospermia	Necrozoospermia
↓	↓	↓
No sperms detected	Sperms detected after centrifugation	Immotility and reduced vitality

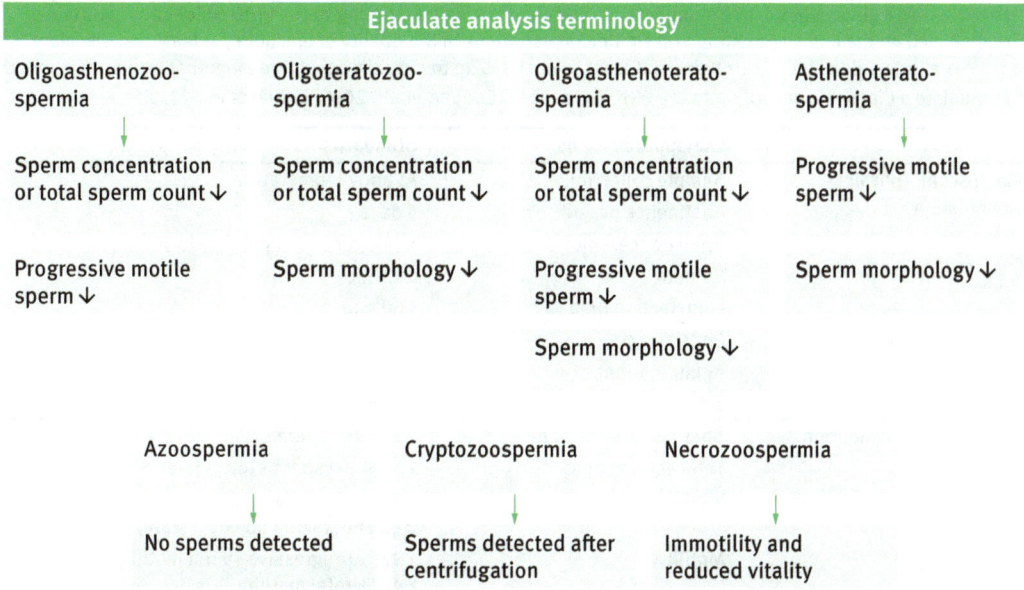

Figure 4.58 Ejaculate analysis terminology.

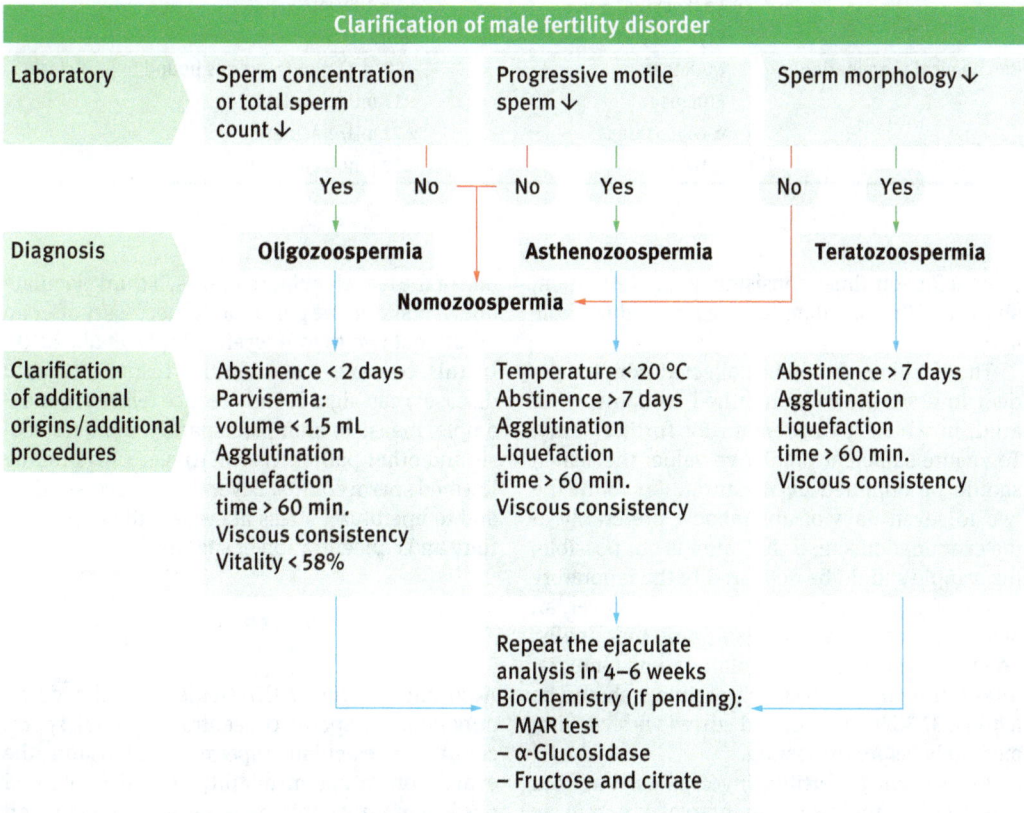

Clarification of male fertility disorder

Laboratory

Sperm concentration or total sperm count ↓   Progressive motile sperm ↓   Sperm morphology ↓

Yes — No ┬ No — Yes   No — Yes

Diagnosis

Oligozoospermia   **Asthenozoospermia**   **Teratozoospermia**

Nomozoospermia ←

Clarification of additional origins/additional procedures

Abstinence < 2 days Parvisemia: volume < 1.5 mL Agglutination Liquefaction time > 60 min. Viscous consistency Vitality < 58%	Temperature < 20 °C Abstinence > 7 days Agglutination Liquefaction time > 60 min. Viscous consistency	Abstinence > 7 days Agglutination Liquefaction time > 60 min. Viscous consistency

Repeat the ejaculate analysis in 4–6 weeks
Biochemistry (if pending):
– MAR test
– α-Glucosidase
– Fructose and citrate

Figure 4.59 Clarification of male fertility disorder.

Table 4.42 At a glance: Indicative standards for ejaculate analysis according to the WHO Guidelines (spermiogram). Based on the known potential and significant variations in the quality of ejaculate, at least two ejaculate analyses at intervals of four to six weeks (at least seven days up to a maximum of three months) are recommended to formulate a diagnosis according to the WHO Guidelines (Cooper, et al., 2010; Dohle, et al., 2010).

	Examination items	Standards
Macroscopic/physical examination	Sample collection	At body temperature
	Abstinence period	5 days
	Appearance/color	Homogeneous opal gray to yellow
	Volume	≥ 1.5 mL
	Liquefaction time	< 60 min
	Consistency	Forms droplets (after liquefaction)
	Agglutination	None
	pH	7.2 to 8.0
Microscopic examination	Sperm concentration	$\geq 15 \times 10^6$ sperms/mL
	Total sperm count	$\geq 39 \times 10^6$ sperms/ejaculate
	Vitality	$\geq 58\,\%$ of the sperms (cells not taking up eosin stain)
	Motility	$\geq 32\,\%$ progressive sperm motility $\geq 40\,\%$ total motility
	Morphology	$\geq 4\,\%$ normally formed sperms according to the "strict criteria"
	Leukocytes	$< 1 \times 10^6$/mL
	Erythrocytes	None
Biochemical examination	MAR test	$< 50\,\%$ of motile sperms bound to particles
	Fructose	≥ 13 mU/ejaculate
	α-Glucosidase	≥ 21 mU/ejaculate
	Citrate	≥ 52 μmol/ejaculate

of liquefaction time, consistency, agglutination, and pH of the ejaculate to be examined (▶ Table 4.43).

The ejaculate should be collected from the patient in a sterile, wide-mouthed container with a lid, in which it can remain for further study. To ensure sufficient predictive value, the semen should be obtained by masturbation following two to seven days of abstinence, preferably at the examination site; if this latter is not possible, the sample should be delivered to the laboratory within 60 minutes and kept > 20 °C. Moreover, an abstinence improves the result only marginally. To avoid exposing the ejaculate to low temperatures during the analysis, if possible it should be left in a 37 °C incubator, and stirred with care immediately before the testing.

Assessment of fertility involves carrying out two ejaculate analyses at an interval of four to six weeks. If pathological changes are observed in

one of the two ejaculate samples, a third ejaculate analysis should be performed if necessary after an additional two to four weeks (Dohle, et al., 2010). In this context, comorbidities (especially viral diseases) can significantly reduce fertility. For example, measles, mumps, hepatitis, mononucleosis and other pathogens can trigger substantially lowered sperm counts. Beyond the aspects of time and temperature, stress likewise reduces the motility and concentration of sperms.

4.10.3 Microscopic Examination of Ejaculate

According to the WHO Guidelines, the determinations of sperm concentration, total sperm count per ejaculate, sperm vitality, and the evaluation of sperm motility should be carried out solely on sample material after liquefaction using a phase-contrast microscope at a magni-

Table 4.43 The pre-analytical and macroscopic physical evaluation of the ejaculate. Documentation of the characteristics marked with an asterisk (*), i.e., appearance/color, volume, consistency, agglutination, and pH is done exclusively after liquefaction of the test material, which usually occurs after about 20 to 45 (max. 60) minutes.

Aspect	Description	Notes
Sample collection	At body temperature	• Avoid temperatures < 20 °C and > 40 °C • Cold leads to immobilization, therefore carry out the analysis promptly • No coitus interruptus (acidic vaginal secretions) • No use of condoms or lubricants (spermicide)
Abstinence period	5 days	• < 2 days: decreased sperm concentration and ejaculate volume • > 7 days: Impairment of sperm motility, morphology, increased sperm concentration • Due to the pronounced intra-individual variability in ejaculate properties, the number of days of abstinence should be maintained at a constant number for repeated analyses
Appearance/color	Homogeneous opal gray to yellow	• Brown: blood admixture • Watery and translucent decreased sperm concentration • Noticeably yellow: jaundice, vitamin preparations • The shorter the abstinence period, the more translucent: lower sperm concentration • The longer the abstinence period, the yellower: higher sperm concentration
Volume	≥ 1.5 mL (normosemia)	• No ejaculate: asemia • < 1.5 mL: parvisemia, DD partial retrograde ejaculation, central occlusion of the ejaculatory ducts, lack of stimulation of seminal vesicles, prostate disease, gonadotropin deficiency (testosterone determination), brief sexual abstinence, congenital malformation/absence (vas deferens, prostate, seminal vesicles) • > 6 ml: multisemia/hypersemia, DD long abstinence, inflammation; Note: pseudo-oligozoospermia
Liquefaction time	< 60 min	• Frequently within 20–40 min • > 60 min: viscosipathy
Consistency	Forms droplets after liquefaction	• Native and fresh ejaculate: gelatinous to viscous • Ropiness > 2 cm: viscosipathy • Determination of sperm concentration and motility can be faulty, therefore perform chymotrypsin liquefaction
Agglutination	None	• Agglutination present: sperm-agglutinating antibodies, diseases of the prostate or seminal vesicles • Agglutination indicates an immunological origin of the fertility disorder
pH value	7.2 to 8.0	• < 7.2: DD azoospermia, obstruction of the seminal tract, inflammation (chronic prostatitis, chronic vesiculitis, chronic epididymitis) • > 8.0: lubricants, signs of inflammation (acute prostatitis, acute vesiculitis, acute epididymitis) • With increasing time after ejaculation the pH shifts into the stronger alkaline range

fication of 400× (10× ocular lens, 40× objective lens). For the characteristics of concentration per mL and total sperm count per total volume, a calibrated Neubauer counting chamber can be used. The sperm vitality is assessed using eosin staining. Documentation of the characteristics of sperm morphology and cells is carried out using a bright field microscope after staining (e.g., Hemacolor) at a magnification of 400× (10× ocular lens, 40× objective lens), or 1,000× (100× objec-

Table 4.44 Interpretation of microscopic ejaculate analysis after liquefaction. In addition to sperm cells, the ejaculate contains other cells that are collectively referred to as "round cells". Thus, the ejaculate contains epithelial cells from the urogenital tract, spermatogenic cells (1st and 2nd order spermatocytes, early or late spermatids) and isolated leukocytes and erythrocytes. The lower limits (5th percentile) of ejaculate parameters for couples with a "time-to-pregnancy" of ≤ 12 months (Cooper, et al., 2010).

Appearance	Description	Notes
Sperm concentration	≥ 15 × 10^6/mL ejaculate (normozoospermia) Total count: ≥ 39 × 10^6/mL ejaculate	• No sperms: azoospermia • < 1 × 10^6/mL ejaculate or only after centrifugation: cryptozoospermia • < 15 × 10^6/mL ejaculate: oligozoospermia, DD inherent (undescended testicles), testicular inflammation, semen transport disturbances, stress, medications • > 50 to100 × 10^6/mL ejaculate: hyperzoospermia
Vitality	≥ 58 % unstained sperms	• Absence of eosin staining in sperms indicates vital cells • < 58 %: increasing oligozoospermia
Motility	≥ 32 % progressive motility; ≥ 40 % total motility (progressive and nonprogressive)	• None: immotility, necrozoospermia • Normal after a vasectomy, azoospermia for the first weeks to months • < 40 %: Asthenozoospermia • Orientation: • progressive: earlier WHO A and B; • nonprogressive: earlier WHO C; • immotile: earlier WHO D.
Morphology	≥ 4 % normal forms	• Normal forms: • Head: soft-oval configuration (length: 5–6 μm: width: 2.5–3.5 μm) • Acrosome (middle part): acrosomal region 40–70 % of the head area as the middle part (length: 6–7 μm; width: 1 μm), cytoplasmic droplets max. 30 % of the head area • Flagellum: uniform, slightly thinner middle part, not curled or bent (length: about 50 μm) • < 4 % normal forms: teratozoospermia, low fertility rate with defective spermatogenesis
Leukocytes Erythrocytes	< 1 × 10^6/mL None	• ≥ 1 × 10^6/mL: DD pyospermia, appearance dirty-yellowish, reduced motility, existing or recent infection, inflammatory process • Detectable: DD hematospermia spuria or vera, rarely tumor disorders

tive lens, oil immersion, 10× ocular lens). This key aspect of male fertility diagnostics has high prognostic value. The sperm morphology is assessed according to the WHO "strict criteria". The normal forms that conform to the strict criteria should represent ≥ 4 % of the sperms examined (▶ Table 4.44).

In healthy and fertile men, the sperm density fluctuates between 35–79 × 10^6/mL. Especially with increased sexual frequency, the sperm count decreases. By contrast, there are no significant fluctuations in sperm motility. However, the mo-

tility tends to deteriorate from the age of 40 years on. A very low sperm volume (< 1 mL) leads to reduced motility.

A higher percentage of highly mobile sperm correlates very well with a high conception rate. This means that even with extreme oligozoospermia, the existing sperms with very good progressive motility can induce pregnancy. At the same time, cases of pregnancy are known with the highest-grade motility disturbance and cryptozoospermia. When the motility is abnormal, usually the morphology is likewise abnormal.

Table 4.45 Further biochemical studies to estimate the accessory functions of the seminal vesicles, prostate gland, and epididymis.

Parameter	Description	Interpretation
MAR test	Negative	• Positive: ≥ 50 % of motile sperm bound to latex particles or erythrocytes; autoantibodies against sperms, detection of detection of immunological infertility
Fructose	≥ 13 mU/ejaculate	• <13 mU/ejaculate: DD seminal vesicle insufficiency, decreased testosterone levels • Decrease on prolonged standing of the ejaculate
α-Glucosidase	≥ 21 mU/ejaculate	• < 21 mU/ejaculate: epididymal insufficiency
Citrate	≥ 52 µmol/ejaculate	• Increased: strong prostate function activity, restriction of seminal vesicle function • < 52 µmol/ejaculate: inflammation-related functional prostate impairment

4.10.4 Further Biochemical Testing of Ejaculate

The biochemical features of ejaculate should only be analyzed using test material that has undergone liquefaction (▶ Table 4.45). In about 10 % of couples who have been unable to conceive, the man has spermatozoa-specific autoantibodies that lead to agglutination or immobilization. Immunoglobulins on the sperm surface membrane can be detected with the mixed antiglobulin reaction (MAR) test. The MAR test result is a good prognostic indicator for fertility. This test is based on the binding of polyacrylamide or latex beads to spermatozoa with the corresponding antibodies, which is detectable by phase contrast microscopy. A positive test result (≥ 50 % sperm binding to the particles) should be checked by studying the interaction between the sperms and the cervical mucus. Condition for implementing the test are good sperm mobility and a sperm concentration higher than 5×10^6/mL.

Fructose is unnecessary for fertilization, and is used in semen/seminal vesicle diagnostics. The fructose concentration provides an indication of secretory function of the seminal vesicles and the continuity of the ejaculatory duct. Nevertheless, though nonessential, fructose is a power source for the sperm motility. 90 % of the fructose is produced in the seminal vesicles, and 10 % in the ampulla of the vas deferens. The production of seminal plasma fructose is governed by testosterone.

α-Glucosidase is used in epididymis diagnostics. It is secreted in body and tail of the epididymis, and can be determined photometrically in the seminal plasma. Values below 21 mU/ejaculate indicate occlusion in the area of the efferent ducts. Obstructions in the area of rete testis do not affect the values in seminal plasma.

4.10.5 Quality Assurance in Ejaculate Analysis

The analysis of the sperm concentration, motility and morphology is highly subjective, and requires regular practice in assessing these diagnostic properties. The German Medical Association Directive on medical laboratory quality assurance testing has been a statutory requirement for internal and external quality assurance in ejaculate analytics since January 2013 (RiliBÄK, 2008).

All facilities that conduct ejaculate analysis must comply with the special section B4 of RiliBÄK in its entirety as a minimum requirement for quality assurance. In principle, this minimum requirement is the implementation of existing WHO and DGA specifications (WHO, 2010; Nieschlag and Behre, 2009). Thus, the spermatology workplace, the testing, and the methodology (counting chamber, staining) must all be documented. If multiple workplaces are present, respective workplace-specific quality assurance must be maintained.

Investigations of sperms to determine their concentration must be carried out in duplicate. In the duplicate determination, at least 2×200 sperms must be evaluated. If the sperm count after enrichment is less than 200/visual field, the requirement is dropped, i.e., a smaller number will be evaluated. The testing of sperm motility

Table 4.46 Internal quality assurance; calculation formulas for the contemporary evaluation of sperm concentration, motility ,and morphology, as well as for the retrospective evaluation of ejaculate tests.

Contemporary evaluation of sperm concentration	• Absolute value of the difference: $d = \lvert N_1 - N_2 \rvert$ • Arithmetic mean: $MW = \dfrac{(N_1 + N_2)}{2}$ • Check sum: $1{,}96 \times \sqrt{2 \times MW}$ • Check rule: $d \leq 1{,}96 \times \sqrt{2 \times MW}$
Contemporary evaluation of sperm motility and morphology	• Absolute value of the difference: $d = \lvert P_1 = P_2 \rvert$ • Arithmetic mean: $MW = \dfrac{(P_1 + P_2)}{2}$ • Check sum: $1{,}96 \times \sqrt{\dfrac{2 \times MW \times (100 - MW)}{n}}$ • Check rule: $d \leq 1{,}96 \times \sqrt{\dfrac{2 \times MW \times (100 - MW)}{n}}$

Retrospective evaluation of ejaculate testing	• Average of the differences: Sum $(d)/n$
	   – n, number of contemporary evaluations
	   – d, difference in the value pairs
	
	 • Standard deviation of the difference: $\sqrt{\left(1 / (n-1) \times Sum\left([d - MWd]^2\right)\right)}$
	
	 • Check rule: $MWd \leq 1{,}96 \times \sqrt{n}$

requires assessing the motility of spermatozoa in three stages: (i) progressive motile, (ii) locally motile, and (iii) immotile, each in duplicate. The designation of the percentual sperm morphological characteristics is also carried out in duplicate. The results must be fed into a contemporary (= current) evaluation and a retrospective (= long-term rating, at least 50 duplicate measurements required) evaluation.

The contemporary internal quality assurance looks at the difference between the duplicate determinations and their arithmetic mean, while the retrospective internal quality assurance considers the average of the difference in the respective duplicate determinations and the number of contemporary evaluations (▶ Table 4.46).

The external quality assurance is carried out semiannually with responsibility for the content. The DGA reviews the evaluations for the determinations of sperm concentration (count), motility, and morphology (the German Society of Andrology Quality Control (QuaDeGa); reference institution for RiLiBÄK).

Literature

Cooper TG, Noonon E, Eckarstein S, et al. World Health Organization reference values for human characteristics. Human Reproduction Update, Vol. 16, No. 3 pp. 231–245, 2010.

Dohle GR, Diemer T, Giwercman A, Jungwirth A, Kopa Z, Krausz C. European Guidelines on Male Infertility. European Association Urology 2010. http://www.uroweb.org/professional-guidelines/Hoffmann H. Andrologie. In: Jung G, Moll I (eds). Dermatologie. Thieme, Stuttgart, S. 467–470.

Nieschlag E, Behre HM (Hrsg) (2009) Andrologie – Grundlagen und Klinik der reproduktiven Gesundheit des Mannes, 3. Aufl . Springer, Berlin Heidelberg NewYork, S. 132.

Richtlinie der Bundesarztekammer zur Qualitatssicherung laboratoriumsmedizinischer Untersuchungen. Deutsches Arzteblatt 105, Heft 7: 15.2008 A341–A355.

World Health Organization. WHO Laboratory Manual for the Examination of Human Semen and Sperm-Cervical Mucus Interaction. 5th edn. Cambridge: Cambridge University Press, 010. http://www.who.int/reproductivehealth/publications/infertility/9789241547789/en/index.html.

Index

4-hydroxybutyric acid (GHB) 38
20210 polymorphism 179
Dexamethasone
– inhibition test 73
α_1-Microglobulin 130

A

Abdominal symptomatology, acute 99
Acanthocytes 131, 139, 144
Acetylcholinesterase 41
ACR criteria 203
ACTH 70
– syndrome, ectopic 70
– test 78
Acute care hospital 11
Acute demyelinating encephalomyelitis (ADEM) 196
Acute kidney injury 132
Acute lymphatic leukemia 161
Addison's disease 63, 79
ADEM 196
– distinguished from MS 196
Admissions Screening 27
Adrenal glands 61, 67
Adrenocortical insufficiency
– primary (Addison's disease) 75
Adrenocortical tumors 71
Adrenocorticotropic hormone (ACTH) 70
Aggregometry 171
Agreed objectives 18
AIT 61, 62
Albumin 137
Algorithm 5
Allergy 204
– diagnostics 204
ALT 95
Amanitin 44
Amyloidosis 55
– renal 137
Analgesic nephropathy 139
Analysis, toxicological
– exposure evaluations 38
ANCA 198
Anemia 150
Antibody diagnostics 202
Anti-glutamate decarboxylases 86
Anti-HAV IgM 114
Anti-HBc 114
Anti-HBs 114
Antineutrophil cytoplasmic antibodies (ANCA) 202
Anti-nuclear antibodies (ANA) 204
Antiphospholipid antibodies 179
Antiphospholipid syndrome 179
Antithrombin 182

aPTT Prolongation 168
Arterial hypertension 129, 137
Arthritis, rheumatoid 201
Ascites 56
AST 115
Autoimmune thyroiditis 61
AWMF 4

B

Bacteria 141
Bacteriuria, significant 143
Bands, oligoclonal 186
Basic diagnostic approach 77
Basic symptom 27
Bence-Jones proteinuria 135
Bilateral macronodular hyperplasia (AIMAH) 69, 71
Bilirubin 110
Biomarker 139
Bleeding diathesis 168
Blood 131
B lymphocytes 158
Bone marrow 186
– insufficiency 161
Budd-Chiari syndrome 56
Budget 19

C

CA19-9 126
Capillary electrophoresis 139
Cardinal symptom 27
Cardiovascular risk 93, 95
Cast 132
Cerebrospinal fluid (CSF) 52
– artificial 190
– Autoimmune-mediated 199
– Bleeding sources 192
– bloody 190, 192
– Changes 199
– Diagnostics 186
– Differential diagnosis 199
– Fistula 52
– inflammatory 192, 194, 199
– Pathogen-induced 199
– Syndrome 199
Ceruloplasmin 110, 200
Change management 18
Child-Pugh score 111, 118
Cholangitis 110
Choledocholithiasis 115, 118
Cholestasis 114
Cholinesterase 41
Chromatography 51
Chronic eosinophilic leukemia (CEL) 151

Chronic kidney disease (CKD) 133
– grade 5 128
Chyle 55
– Pseudochyle 55
Circadian Rhythm and Night Sleep 73
Classification 7
Classifier 7
Clinical chemistry 5
Clinical treatment pathway 3
CMV 111, 190
CNS diseases
– Chronic Inflammatory 194
– Multiple sclerosis 194
– Syndrome, clinically isolated 194
CNS infections
– Aspergillosis 189
– Focal encephalitis, septic 189
– Neurotuberculosis 189
– Opportunistic 189
– Toxoplasmosis 189
– Viruses 190
Cocaine 39, 44
Cockcroft-Gault formula 132
Cockroache 205, 208
Codeine 39
Complement consumption 198
Conductivity 131
Confirmatory analysis 51
Congenital erythropoietic porphyria 105
Control, glycemic
– Diabetes Control and Complications Trial (DCCT) 90
– United Kingdom Prospective Diabetes Study
  (UKPDS) 90
Coproporphyrinogen oxidase 103
Corticotropin-releasing hormone (CRH) 69
Cortisol 72
– Free in 24-hour urine 73
Course assessment 39
Cr51-EDTA clearance 132
Creatinine 39
– clearance 132
Creutzfeldt-Jakob disease 200
CRH syndrome, ectopic 69
CRH Test 75
Crigler-Najjar syndrome 110
CRP, sensitive 95
Crustaceans 205
Crystals 131
CT 123
Cut-off value 39
Cyclic citrullinated peptides (ACPA) 202
Cystatin C 6, 96

D
DCCT 90
D-dimer 31, 172
decision trees 3, 9, 11, 187
Dementia syndrome 186
Demyelinating disease 195
Density 131
De Ritis ratio 110, 118

Dexamethasone 70
Diabetes Mellitus
– American Diabetes Association (ADA) 84
– Antibodies 86
– German Diabetes Association (DDG) 85
– World Health Organization (WHO) 83
Diazepam 40
Diphenhydramine 41
Disease management 21
D-penicillamine glomerulonephritis 137
Drainage dialysate 52
DRESS syndrome 150
Drug allergy 208, 209
Drug intoxication 39
D-SCORE 96
dsDNA 198
Dubin-Johnson syndrome 118
Dyslipidemia 92, 97
Dysplasia, bilateral micronodular 69, 71

E
EBV 111
ECG 122
E. coli 141, 189
Effusion 10, 52
Elastase concentration 127
Encephalitis 187
Eosinophilia 150
EPH gestosis 137
Epstein-Barr virus 111
Erythrocyte casts 139, 144
Erythrocyte protoporphyrin 105
Erythropoiesis 85, 148
Erythropoietic protoporphyria 105
Erythropoietin 150, 164
Extravascular fluid 52
Exudate 52, 56

F
Factor V disorder 179
Factor XII deficiency 168
Fanconi syndrome 139
Fasting plasma glucose 83
Flow diagram 86, 91
Folic acid deficiency 150, 151
Food allergy 204
free T3 63
free T4 63
fT4 62
fT4 level 62
Fungi 142, 189

G
Gallstones 107
Gammopathy, monoclonal 135
Gas chromatography/mass spectrometry 39
General unknown screening 41, 44, 51
Gestational hyperthyroidism 61
Gilbert's syndrome 110
GLDH 110
Glomerular filtration rate (GFR) 132

Glomerulonephritis 137
Glucocorticoids 62, 100
Glucose-6-phosphate dehydrogenase
    deficiency 141
Glucose tolerance test 11, 127
Gold nephropathy 137
Graves' disease 61
Guillain-Barré syndrome (GBS) 190

H

Haemophilus influenzae 189
Hair analysis 40
Hansel staining 142
HbA1c 11
HBsAg 111
HDL cholesterol 88, 92
Health insurer 15
HELLP syndrome 111, 115
Hematuria 129, 132
hematuria, paroxysmal nocturnal 141
Hemochromatosis 9, 110
Hemoglobinuria 135
Hemolysis 72, 118
Heparin 150, 173
Hepatitis A 114
Hepatitis, acute viral 111
Hepatitis viruses 114
Hereditary coproporphyria 99
Heroin 39
Herpes simplex virus (HSV) 111
HIT 173
HIV 71
HLA-B27 202
Homocysteine 181, 182
Hospital information system 144
HPLC 50
HSV 1 190
HSV 2 190
Hurst syndrome 196
Hydroxymethylbilane synthase 103
Hyperbilirubinemia 115, 118
Hypercholesterolemia 99, 101
Hypercortisolism 67, 70, 71
Hypereosinophilic syndrome 151
Hyperlipidemia 99, 100
Hyperlipoproteinemia 101
Hypersplenism 163
Hyperthyroidism 61
Hypertriglyceridemia 92, 93
Hypnotic toxidrome 44
Hypocortisolism 75
Hypolipidemia 100
Hypothyroidism 62

I

IAS 98
ICD codes 17
IFCC 84
IgA nephritis 137
IgA nephropathy 138, 141
IgG 63, 114, 137

IgG/albumin ratio 140
IgG band, oligoclonal 195
Immune hemolysis 151
Immunoassay 39, 47
Immunofixation 135, 137
Immunophenotyping 161, 186
Impaired fasting glucose 84
Inefficient erythropoiesis (MDS) 150
Inhalation allergy 208, 209
Insect venom allergy 208
International Association of Diabetes and Pregnancy
    Study Groups (IADPSG) 88
International Atherosclerosis Society (PROCAM score
    and algorithm) 96
Iohexol clearance 132
Iron deficiency 85, 150
Islet cell antibodies 90
IT implementation 22

J

JAK2 mutation 164
Jaundice 107, 115
Joint European Guidelines 96, 98

K

Kidney disease 128
Kidney injury molecule-1 (KIM-1) 135
Kidney transplant rejection, acute 137

L

Laboratory profile 11, 27
LDH 118, 122
LDL cholesterol 90
Legal Rulings 5
Length of stay 19
Leukocytes 199, 212
Leukocytosis 158
Leukocyturia 141
Leukopoiesis 149
Lewy body dementia 199
Liability lawsuits 5
Lipase 122
Lipid metabolism 93
Lipid metabolism disorder 97
Liquorrhea 52, 53
Listeria 189
Liver and Pancreatic Disorders 107
Liver cirrhosis 55, 56, 57
Lp(a) 95, 96
LSD 39, 44, 51
Lupus nephritis 137, 141
Lymphoma 143, 151, 158
Lymphopoiesis 149

M

Malar erythema 203
MALDI-TOF 139
MDRD formula 132
Medical Association 4, 130
Meningeal carcinomatosis 192
MGUS 158

Microalbuminuria 90
Minimal-change glomerulopathy 137
MRZ reaction 198
Myelodysplastic syndrome (MDS) 163
Myoglobinuria 135

N
NAFLD 111
NGSP 84
NMDAR (N-Methyl-D-Aspartat receptor) 198
Normoblasts 148

O
OCB 198
OGTT 84
Opioid toxidrome 44
Optic neuritis 194, 196
Order Entry system 144
Order ticket 27
Oxazepam 40

P
Palmar erythema 115
Pericardial effusion 58
Peritoneal dialysate 52
Peritoneal dialysis (PD) 52
Peritonitis 52, 53
Petrosal Sinus Catheter 75
Photodermatoses 104
Plasma cell 158, 195
Plasma fluorescence scan 99
Pleural effusion 57
Pneumococci 189
Poison control center 38
Poisoning 41
Polycythemia 69, 158, 163
Polycythemia vera 164
Porphobilinogen 99
Porphyria 99
Porphyria variegata 105
Post-genomic era 16
PR3 cANCA 198
Pre-diabetes mellitus 85
Pregnancy Outcome (HAPO) study 89
Prevalence 12
Prion disease 199
Proerythroblasts 148
Profile testing 10, 11
Protein 14-3-3 200
Protein C deficiency 179
Protein/creatinine ratio 130, 137
Protein S deficiency 179
Proteinuria
– glomerular 90, 135
– prerenal 135
– tubular 135
Proteome analysis 139
Prothrombin 179
Prothrombin 20210 polymorphism 182
Protoporphyrinogen oxidase 103
Protozoa 142, 189

Pruritus 107, 111
Pseudocholinesterase (PCHE) 114
Pseudochyle 55
Pseudo-Cushing syndrome 69, 71
Psilocybin 44
Pyelonephritis 139
– acute 143
– chronic 142, 143

Q
Quality standard 21
Quantification 38
Quick time reduction 170, 171

R
Radicular syndrome 187
Radiculitis 190
Remuneration system 19
Reticulocytes 148
Rheumatoid factor (RF) 202
RiliBÄK 4, 215
Ristocetin cofactor 172
Rivaroxaban 181
Rotor syndrome 118

S
SAH 187, 190
Secretin-pancreozymin test 127
Sedatives 38
Sensitivity 12
SGB V 21
Shellfish 205
Spider naevi 115, 123
SSA 204
Staphylococci 189
Steatorrhea 123
Stepwise diagnostics 10
Subarachnoid hemorrhage 9, 190
Sympathomimetic toxidrome 44, 47
Systemic lupus erythematosus (SLE) 196, 203

T
Tau protein 200
Test strips 11, 54, 110, 131
Thrombocytopenia, heparin-induced 173
Thromboembolism, acute venous 172
Thrombophilia 29, 173
– screening 173
Thrombopoietin 148
Thrombosis 168, 172, 173
Thymus 149
Thyroglobulin antibodies (Tg Ab) 63
Thyroid gland 61
Thyroid hormone resistance 62
Thyroid peroxidase antibodies (TPO Ab) 63
Thyroxine (T4) 61
Total protein 135, 137
total T3 63
total T4 63
Toxidrome 41
TPO antibody determination 65

Transudate 52, 56
TRH deficiency 62
Triglycerides 88, 90
Triiodothyronine (T3) 61
Tropomyosin 205, 208
TSH 61
Tuberculosis, renal 142
Turnaround time 173

U
Ultrasound 107
Urinary sediment 142
Urine biomarker 139
Urine Leakage 56
Urine protein differentiation 134, 137

V
Varicella virus 111
Vasculitides 137, 195
Viruses 111
Vitamin B12 118, 150, 151
von Willebrand disease 168, 171

W
Wegener's granulomatosis 77, 137, 198
Wells score 173
Wilson ATP7B gene 201
Wilson's disease 110, 186, 187
Withdrawal syndrome 44

X
Xanthochromia 190

www.ingramcontent.com/pod-product-compliance
Lightning Source LLC
Chambersburg PA
CBHW081515190326
41458CB00015B/5373